Introduction to
Computers *for*
Healthcare
Professionals

Fourth Edition

Irene Joos, PhD, MSIS, RN
La Roche College

Nancy I. Whitman, PhD, RN
Lynchburg College

Marjorie J. Smith, PhD, CNM, RN
Winona State University

Ramona Nelson, PhD, RN, BC, FAAN
Slippery Rock University

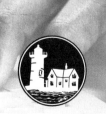

JONES AND BARTLETT PUBLISHERS
Sudbury, Massachusetts
BOSTON   TORONTO   LONDON   SINGAPORE

World Headquarters
Jones and Bartlett Publishers
40 Tall Pine Drive
Sudbury, MA 01776
978-443-5000
info@jbpub.com
www.jbpub.com

Jones and Bartlett Publishers International
Barb House, Barb Mews
London W6 7PA
UK

Jones and Bartlett Publishers Canada
2406 Nikanna Road
Mississauga, ON L5C 2W6
CANADA

Jones and Bartlett's books and products are available through most bookstores and online booksellers. To contact Jones and Bartlett Publishers directly, call 800-832-0034, fax 978-443-8000, or visit our website www.jbpub.com. Substantial discounts on bulk quantities of Jones and Bartlett's publications are available to corporations, professional associations, and other qualified organizations. For details and specific discount information, contact the special sales department at Jones and Bartlett via the above contact information or send an email to specialsales@jbpub.com.

Cover image © Photos.com

Library of Congress Cataloging-in-Publication Data
Introduction to computers for healthcare professionals / Irene Joos
... [et al.]. — 4th ed.
     p. ; cm.
  Rev. ed. of: Computers in small bytes. 3rd ed. c2000.
  Includes bibliographical references and index.
  ISBN 0-7637-2883-7 (alk. paper)
  1. Medicine—Data processing. 2. Nursing—Data processing.
3. Medical informatics. 4. Nursing informatics. 5. Computer
literacy. 6. Computers.   I. Joos, Irene Makar. II. Computers in
small bytes.
  [DNLM: 1. Computers. 2. Computer Literacy. 3. Computer User
Training—methods. 4. Medical Informatics. 5. Software.
W 26.55.C7 I613 2005]
R858.I58 2005
610'.285—dc22
                            2004030325

Acquisitions Editor: Kevin Sullivan
Production Director: Amy Rose
Production Assistant: Alison Meier
Associate Editor: Amy Sibley
Marketing Manager: Emily Ekle
Manufacturing Buyer: Amy Bacus
Cover Design: Kristin E. Ohlin
Printing and Binding: Malloy Inc.
Cover Printing: Malloy Inc.

Printed in the United States of America
09 08 07 06 05   10 9 8 7 6 5 4 3 2 1

Preface

The fourth edition of *Introduction to Computers for Healthcare Professionals* (formerly *Computers in Small Bytes*) reflects the ever-changing world of computers and the "real" world of today. It features updated lesson content and exercises, which incorporate more Internet information and activities as well as the latest version of Microsoft Office.

This book aims to assist the novice computer user in developing computer skills useful in both the school and work settings and a basic understanding of health care informatics. Each chapter highlights basic terminology and concepts necessary for understanding its topic. Exercises develop the user's skills in each area progressively, and assignments help assess the user's level of understanding and skill. Each chapter is designed to stand alone, so that the user can order them in the sequence that meets his or her needs. Where appropriate, the user is referred to other chapters in the book that provide information related to the current chapter.

Each chapter emphasizes basic concepts and terms that reflect changes in the computer world and provide a foundation for understanding and using computers. The first chapter incorporates more information about information literacy and its importance in the work world. Chapter 2, "Computer Systems: Hardware, Software, and Connectivity," which presents basic information necessary to understand current technology, has been expanded to reflect changing technology. Chapter 3, "The Computer and Its Operating System Environment," now includes more Desktop and Windows management concepts and exercises, while still providing basic material on managing files and folders. The next chapter, "Software Applications: Common Tasks," provides information and activities common to Windows software programs. These include using online help; creating, opening, saving, deleting, and copying files; and so forth. The software chapters were updated to reflect the basic skill set needed to use the Office suite effectively. The Internet and communications chapters were updated to reflect the evolving world of the Internet and related communication activities. The chapter "Information: Access, Evaluation, and Use" includes concepts and exercises about searching and search strategies and the subsequent evaluation and use of the retrieved information. A redesigned privacy and security chapter replaces the legal and ethics chapter and addresses threats to and procedures for protecting privacy, confidentiality, and security of data and of the computer. The book concludes with a chapter called "Health Care Informatics and Information Systems," which provides the learner with an introduction to information systems concepts and theories related to heath care.

It is our sincere hope that this book will serve as a sound foundation for developing basic computer skills for health care professionals. Once basic skills and knowledge exist, it is amazing how quickly intermediate and advanced knowledge and skills develop.

About the Authors

Irene Joos

Irene Joos is currently the director of online learning at La Roche College as well as a faculty member in the IS Department. Prior to this position, she was the director of library and instructional technologies at La Roche College. Dr. Joos received her baccalaureate degree in nursing from Pennsylvania State University. She holds a master's degree in both medical-surgical nursing and information science, as well as a doctorate in education from the University of Pittsburgh.

Dr. Joos has taught medical-surgical nursing, foundations, basic nursing concepts and theories, professional nursing role, and nursing informatics courses at diploma, baccalaureate, and master's programs. With a FULD grant, she was instrumental in the installation of interactive video units in the skills laboratory and also managed both the microcomputer and skills laboratories at the University of Pittsburgh School of Nursing, Learning Resources Center. She teaches office automation, management of information systems, cyberspace, computer based training, introduction to databases, and introduction to information system courses to undergraduate students in both on campus and online formats. She serves as the faculty advisor for the website of the student's literary journal, *Nuances*.

Dr. Joos's area of interest is the use of technology to help do work in an efficient and effective manner. This includes using technology in whatever arena you might find yourself—education, research, and practice. This has been the focus of her publications and presentations.

Nancy Whitman

Nancy I. Whitman is currently associate dean of the College at Lynchburg College in Virginia. Prior to this she was dean of the School of Health Sciences and Human Performance and professor of nursing there. Dr. Whitman received her baccalaureate degree in nursing from Alfred University, her master's degree in pediatric nursing from University of Virginia, and a doctorate in nursing from University of Texas, Austin. She is a member of Sigma Theta Tau, Omicron Delta Kappa, and Phi Kappa Phi.

Dr. Whitman has taught health education, pediatric nursing, patient education, nursing research, introduction to nursing, and professional issues courses. She developed and taught an elective in computers in nursing for both master's and undergraduate students. She has been active in a variety of nursing assessment and college program assessment activities.

Dr. Whitman has made presentations to nursing faculty, practicing nurses, and other health care educators on a variety of topics including those related to computers and computer-assisted instruction. She developed an interactive video program that teaches concepts and correlated basic nursing skills for infection control and designed a number of Web-based course materials. Dr. Whitman received the New Investigator Award from the NLN Society for Research in Nursing Education Forum (1989). In 1989 she was one of the first HBOC scholars. She has co-authored three editions of the book *Health Teaching in Nursing Practice: A Professional Model*, currently published by Appleton & Lange.

Marjorie Smith

Marjorie J. Smith, PhD, RN, CNM, is an emeritus professor of nursing at Winona State University, Winona and Rochester, MN, where she was formerly the director of the master's program in nursing. Dr. Smith received her baccalaureate degree in nursing from the University of Wisconsin, Madison. Her master's degree in childbearing family nursing and doctorate in adult education are from the University of Minnesota. She is a certified nurse midwife and was a member of Sigma Theta Tau and the American College of Nurse Midwives.

Dr. Smith has taught medical-surgical nursing, pediatric nursing, and obstetrical nursing at the undergraduate level in diploma, associate degree, and baccalaureate programs. She has also taught advanced courses in nursing theory, research, women's health care, instruction and evaluation, nursing informatics, and health care technology and computers. She was chief editor of the textbook *Child and Family: Concepts of Nursing Practice*, published in 1982 and 1987 by McGraw-Hill. She has also written a computer assisted learning program, *The Client Using the Birth Control Pill*, published in 1991 by Medi-Sim. In 2000 she received the Outstanding Nurse Educator award from the Minnesota Association of Colleges of Nursing. In retirement Dr. Smith has continued her work related to CenteringPregnancy®, a model of group prenatal care. She also continues her work with computers and enjoys an active travel and family life.

Ramona Nelson

Ramona Nelson is a professor of nursing at Slippery Rock University where she teaches Web-based distance education courses on health care informatics as well as community health. In addition, she co-directs the SRU health care informatics program. Dr. Nelson holds a doctorate in higher education from the University of Pittsburgh. She holds both a master's degree in nursing and a master's degree in information science from the University of Pittsburgh. Her BSN is from Duquesne University.

In 1988 Dr. Nelson was accepted in the first nursing informatics post-doc program at the University of Utah and in 1989 as one of the first HBOC Scholars. Through her numerous publications and presentations, she has provided national leadership for articulating the scope of nursing informatics. Because of her leadership role, she has been selected as a fellow in the American Academy of Nursing, asked to serve on the ANA taskforce defining the current scope and standards of practice for nursing informatics, and has reviewed grants for Department of Health and Human Services. Her current research is focused on consumer informatics and distance education.

Contents

On the Way to Computer and Information Literacy

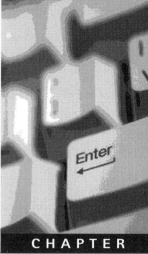

Health care professionals increasingly rely on information systems to assist them in providing quality care. They realize that a large percentage of their practice is the management of information. Computers help them to perform functions such as sorting and addressing patient materials; documenting care; organizing, calculating, and managing patient financial data; providing remote patient care through telemedicine facilities; and organizing and accessing health care literature. To take advantage of evolving computer technologies, health care professionals must be computer and information literate.

This book is designed to help students develop computer and information literacy. Its focus is the introduction of basic concepts that cross specific application programs and the development of practical computer skills. The exercises provide practice in applying the concepts and skills, with examples from the health care arena.

► 1.1 LITERACY

Health care providers learn to use a stethoscope as a tool to assess patients. This involves understanding the function and purpose of the stethoscope as well as developing skill in using it. Just as health care providers learn to use the stethoscope, they also must learn the function and purpose of computers in health care as well as developing skill in its use. In other words, health care providers must become "computer and information literate."

Literacy	Literacy means the ability to locate and use printed and written information to function in society, both personally and professionally.
Computer Literacy	Add computer to the term literacy and it refers to the ability to use the computer to do practical tasks. A variety of different beliefs exist about what actual skills computer literacy entails, but there is agreement that it involves the skill of using computer applications to accomplish work in any discipline.
Information Literacy	This is used to describe a set of skills that enables a person to identify an information need, locate and access the needed information, evaluate the information found, and communicate and use that information effectively. With the information explosion and the growth of information as well as misinformation, information literacy has become a major topic in all educational settings. Given information literacy's growing importance, Chapter 11 further expands the information literacy topic.

People who are computer and information literate

- Use the computer and associated software as tools to complete their work in a more effective and efficient manner.
- Recognize the need for accurate and complete information as the basis for intelligent decision making.
- Find appropriate sources of information using successful search strategies.
- Evaluate and manage information to facilitate their work.

- Communicate information in its various formats.
- Integrate technology and information strategies into their daily professional lives.

Many professional organizations and accrediting agencies now include information and computer literacy requirements as part of their criteria. For example, the Association of College and Research Libraries produced a document defining and outlining specific criteria and standards for demonstrating information literacy (Association of College and Research Libraries, 2000).

▶ 1.2 ORGANIZATION OF THE BOOK

This book consists of 13 chapters and an index that features highlighted computer terms. With the exception of this chapter, each is organized in the same way, beginning with a lesson that introduces the content, describes key concepts and terms, and in application chapters, provides descriptions of common application functions and keystrokes. Each chapter also includes one or more exercises for use in the classroom or computer laboratory to practice application of lesson concepts and one or more assignments intended for users to demonstrate knowledge and skill with the chapter topic.

The first chapter provides material that is useful to understanding and using this book. Chapters 2, 3, and 4 contain content about hardware, operating systems, and software. Computer hardware and software terms are introduced in Chapter 2. Chapter 3 focuses on managing the computer environment. Chapter 4 covers tasks that are common to most application programs. This means that many applications in a graphic environment have common looks and functions.

The next four chapters include lessons and practice exercises for word processing, presentation graphics, spreadsheets, and databases. Microsoft Office 2003 is used to illustrate the basic concepts of each of these chapters.

Basic Internet concepts for connecting and browsing, and related software such as Netscape and Internet Explorer are then introduced. Chapters 10 and 11 discuss use of the Internet for communicating and accessing informational resources. Every attempt was made to select Internet sites that would exist while this book is used and that demonstrate the concepts presented; however, Internet sites do change. The remaining two chapters outline privacy and security issues in using computers in health care and introduce the concept of informatics in health care.

► 1.3 BEFORE BEGINNING: SOME HELPFUL INFORMATION

Every computer system and every computer laboratory have subtle differences that can cause problems for the beginner; therefore, learning something about the computer environment used is essential. Teachers or computer laboratory personnel can help to answer the following questions:

Accounts: Is an account needed to use the computer laboratory? If so, what is the process for getting one? Many places have at least a 24-hour wait time before the laboratories can be used. On the other hand, some schools automatically create an account when a student registers or provide facilities and directions to create an instant account.

Computer Laboratories: Where are the computer laboratories located, and who has access to them? Is an identification card needed to use the equipment and software? Are some laboratories reserved for specific student populations, that is, health professional students or engineering students, or are all the laboratories general purpose and available to all students, staff, and faculty?

Cost: Is there a user charge for accessing and using the computer equipment and software? Do the rates vary (less at night or during off peak times)? Is a computer fee included in tuition charges? What does the fee cover?

Documentation: Does the computer laboratory have user documentation? Where is the documentation? Are there handouts available in the computer laboratory, or are the documents available online to read and/or print? What documentation is needed to start? Most computer laboratories have user documentation that provides help starting and learning specific software programs. For example, the laboratory might have a document called "Getting Started with Outlook" or "Accessing the Network from Home."

Equipment/Storage:

What type of hardware will be used? What types of diskettes are needed, and where can they be purchased? How is the equipment turned on? Where can students store data files?

Laboratory Hours:

What are the laboratory hours? Do they change during the term? Are they open over the week-end? Some laboratories expand their hours of operation toward the end of the term when many papers and projects are due. Does a laboratory assistant need to be present for the laboratory to be open, or is the laboratory left unattended?

Lease or Buy:

Does the university have a program whereby students lease or buy a laptop computer for use at home, in the dormitory, or in the classroom? If so, how long does it take to get a computer? How does the university support this program in terms of repair, software, etc.? Is an option available to buy the computer at the end of the lease?

Logging In:

Is there a log-in procedure (a series of steps to access the computer software)? If so, how does one log into the system? Is there a help sheet to follow?

Policies:

What are the policies that govern use of the computer laboratory? Policies can include anything from how often to change a password to how many pages can be printed each term to respecting the rights of others. What are the penalties for not adhering to the policies? Penalties can be anything from a warning for a minor offense to dismissal for a major offense. Most computer laboratories and organizations or businesses provide the policies to each account holder or give directions for viewing them online. If this is not a student account but an employee account, certain policies related to confidentiality of data and protection of a password need to be acknowledged and followed.

Printing:	What printing capabilities are available in the laboratory? Is there access to color printing? Is there a charge for printing? Some schools use a prepaid print card, keep an electronic record of printing that allows individual billing, or use a software program such as PaperCut to keep track of printing costs. When the printing credits go to 0, the student must add more print credits to continue printing. Other schools permit unlimited printing.
Rules:	What are the rules that govern use of the laboratory? Many laboratories prohibit eating and drinking, chatting, and game playing. Laboratories can be restricted to academic use only. Some laboratories also check all diskettes that are brought into the laboratory for viruses.
Support/Help:	What support is available when help is needed? Many laboratories provide helpers to assist patrons who have questions or are having problems. Others provide online help services and quick reference guides for their users. Are there orientation classes for the laboratories and/or training classes on specific software? What is the telephone number for the help desk? What is its e-mail address?

► 1.4 GETTING STARTED WITH THE WORKBOOK

It is wise to review the material in this section before beginning work on a computer.

Enter	Used throughout this workbook, enter refers to the *enter* or *return* key. When the word enter appears, do not type it. Press the enter or return key; it is usually marked with a left pointed arrow.
Bold	Instructions in bold indicate what to click on, what keys to press, or what to type. Computers are very exacting. A misspelled word or failure to

	place a blank where a blank is needed results in error messages. Make sure what is typed is exactly what is bolded.
Ctrl + X	When a Ctrl, Alt, or Shift appears followed by a plus sign (+) and function key number or letter, press the first key, and then while holding it down, press the correct function or letter key. Release both keys together.
Version	The specific sequence and location of commands vary with different versions of software. Microsoft Office 2003 is used for the word processing, presentation graphics, spreadsheet, and database content, and Internet Explorer and Netscape Navigator 7.0 are used for the two browsers. If the computer is a Mac with Office 2004 or Safari (browser), some of the specific commands will be different.
MacOS/Windows	Although the exercises written for Word, Excel, Access, PowerPoint, Internet Explorer, and Netscape Navigator were done using a Windows operating system, Mac-based programs can just as easily be used for these exercises. Most of the keystrokes are exactly the same. A few menu items and a few keys on the keyboard are different.

Some additional tips described here are helpful as computer and information literacy is developed through use of this book.

1. Do not try to complete all of the book exercises at once. Sometimes it is helpful to come back later, especially when the exercises are not going well or when fatigue sets in.
2. Pay attention to messages on the screen. They are the computer's way of trying to provide help.
3. Use the software sequences found at the end of each lesson on an application program to complete the exercises or assignments for that software program. It is not necessary to memorize the commands, mouse clicks, or sequences of events. Use the screen clues, prompts, and online help for guidance through the sequence.

4. Try additional functions by referring to other reference sources such as online help, manuals, or reference books. The functions given in this book were chosen to help the user complete the exercises and learn some basics of how the programs work. Many more functions can be done with each of the software programs presented.

5. Always back up files. This is especially important for the beginner so that hours of work are not lost.

6. Practice doing assignments from all courses using the computer. It takes practice to develop computer literacy. The more the computer is used, the easier and faster tasks will become.

7. Be patient. Learning a new vocabulary and developing new skills take time and energy.

► 1.5 FOR THE PROFESSOR

Using the Workbook

- It is easy to use the entire book or parts of it within a computer course. Reorganize the lessons as necessary to fit the course outline. Those who teach about computers have found, however, that the general information about computers and operating systems is important before learning about specific software applications. In addition, Chapters 4 and 5 are best introduced before the other lessons about specific software programs. Commonalities among the various Office programs help get the students ready for the individual application chapters. Word processing is one of the most readily useful applications for students and thus one of great interest. Learning to use the keyboard and mouse for word processing provides the basis on which to build other computer skills. In addition, the student can convey knowledge of other computer concepts using word processing, thus providing further opportunity to practice and expand word-processing skills as they progress through the book.

- Use selected chapters of the workbook within individual courses to prepare students to use the computer as a tool in health care settings. For example, introducing the database and information literacy chapters in an introductory nursing course guides students on the use of computerized literature databases and helps students begin to organize nursing care plans. The spreadsheet chapter fits ideally into an administration or leadership course, and the presentation graphics chapter enhances courses about patient teaching.

- Use the book as a stand-alone for students lacking the required computer and information literacy competencies. The student then could demonstrate the required competencies by completion of selected assignments.
- If the book is used in an informatics course, it is helpful for students to contract for projects and a final grade. This allows students to set their own objectives dependent on their experience, skill level, and learning needs.

Organization of Chapters

Lessons

Lessons provide a foundation for classroom presentations. The lessons were developed to introduce concepts related to the topic as well as to provide direction for some of the exercises that follow. Supplemental readings in current textbooks, journals, and on the Internet expand the content and provide examples of applications for health care settings. Appropriate concepts and terms are introduced in each chapter lesson. Sometimes the concept or term is repeated in other chapters as necessary to aid understanding of the new material.

Exercises

Exercises for each lesson are designed for use in the classroom or computer laboratory setting. All or part of them can be used. The step-by-step exercises designed to introduce a computer skill were developed to require minimal assistance. However, because novice users can find the most imaginative problems, it is helpful if the teacher or a laboratory assistant is available to help students handle problems and decrease initial frustration. Some of the exercises work well as a foundation for class discussions for either the entire class or for small groups.

Assignments

The assignments included with each lesson provide a means for independent evaluation of individual students or small groups. Use all or part of them. Requiring assignments within 1 or 2 weeks after the class presentation encourages students to practice the concepts immediately and helps them identify misconceptions or problems in applying the material. Grading criteria for assignments requiring use of software programs can include competence, accuracy, and pleasing visual presentation. Teachers may distribute grade points to these assignments in any way they wish.

Orienting Students

Throughout the workbook, wherever possible, content that is generic to any computer is used. Supplementing the workbook with some specific information that students need to be successful with the computer exercises and assignments may be needed. Because computer laboratories are set up in a variety of ways, students need an orientation to the computers that they will be using. Even starting the computer can be a challenging and fear-provoking experience for the novice computer user. Step-by-step instructions on starting the computer and accessing each software program are essential.

Information about where the computer stores data is also important. Some computer programs are configured to save data automatically on a floppy disk (diskette); others have space set aside on subdirectories of the hard drive or file server. Even on the same computer, various programs may be configured differently. Students may have difficulty initially understanding data storage concepts and often think files are lost when they are saved on the hard drive or file server data space. Explanations and written guidelines about the data storage configurations for each program the students will be using can save the student many hours of frustration.

SUMMARY

This chapter provides an orientation to the terms computer and information literacy. It describes how this book is organized and the conventions used to denote user actions. Some helpful information about getting started using the school or laboratory facilities is also presented.

References

Association of College and Research Libraries. (2000). *Information literacy competency standards for higher education*. Chicago: Author. Retrieved August 31, 2004, from http://www.ala.org/ala/acrl/acrlstandards/standards.pdf

Exercise 1: Developing Literacy
Objectives
1. Develop a personal definition of information literacy.
2. Recognize the appropriate format for electronic references using American Psychological Association (APA) style.

3. Compare information literacy tutorials in terms of ease of use.

4. Describe the relationship between information literacy and e-portfolios.

Activity

1. Go to the directory of online resources for information literacy at **http://bulldogs.tlu.edu/mdibble/doril/**.

   a. Click on **Definitions**. Review them. What is the definition of computer literacy?

   b. Click the **Back** button to return to the first web page.

      Click on **The Information Literacy Process**.

      Scroll to the number **4. Using and communicating information, Citation section, American Psychological Association section,** and select **APA: Electronic Reference Formats Recommended by APA**.

      What does APA recommend for electronic reference formats?

   c. Use the **Back** button to return the original site. Click **Information Literacy Standards**.

      Review the **Information Literacy Competency Standards for Higher Education**.

      What did you learn about the information literacy standards for higher education?

   d. Use the **Back** button to return to the original site. Click on **Tutorials**.

      Compare the following 4 tutorials in terms of ease of use, ability to move around them, content, and their value to you.

      Information Literacy Tutorial. University of Wisconsin-Parkside Library

      Information Literacy and You. Penn State University Libraries

      Information Literacy Tutorial. Minneapolis Community & Technical College

      Information Literacy Tutorial. Five Colleges of Ohio

2. **Go to http://portfolio.psu.edu/**. Click the **About** link.

   What is an e-Portfolio?

   How does it relate to information literacy?

Assignment 1: Learning About Your School's Computer Policies
Directions

Use the school's intranet site to find the answers to the following questions:

1. Find your school's website.

2. Is there a technical support center? Is it known by another name?

3. What are the policies and procedures of the academic computing center?

4. Can you download these policies?

5. How does a student set up network and e-mail accounts?

6. What operating systems/software does the center support?

7. Is there a laptop lease/buy program at your school?

8. Does your school have an e-portfolio system for students?

9. Is there an e-learning center? If so, what classes are available?

10. What are the hours for technical support?

11. What was the most valuable thing you learned from this assignment?

Turn in a summary of what you learned answering these questions.

Computer Systems: Hardware, Software, and Connectivity

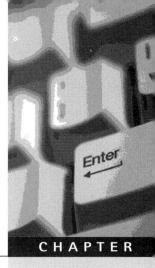

OBJECTIVES

1. Define information systems.
2. Describe the major components of computer systems and their related functions.
3. Define basic terminology related to hardware, software, and connectivity.
4. Describe the main classes of computer software.
5. Appreciate the language of information systems.

People live in an information age and use information systems to help them deal with the wealth of information that is available. A system is a set of interrelated parts; an information system is a system that produces information using the input/process/output cycle. The basic information system consists of four elements: people, procedures, communication (connectivity), and data, whereas a computer information system adds the elements of computers and software. Types of information systems include transaction systems such as payroll and order/entry systems, management information systems that facilitate the running of organizations, decision support systems that facilitate decision making, and expert systems that provide advice or make recommendations regarding diagnosis or treatments.

The purpose of an information system is to provide information to the users that will facilitate the work of the organization. Chapters 11 and 13 provide more information about health care systems. People are the most important part of the system; they and ultimately their organizations benefit from the information provided by these systems. Two basic types of users are end users and technical professionals. End users are the people who use the computers but do not have much technical knowledge about them. Technical professionals are the information technology users who develop, maintain, and evaluate the systems.

Procedures are the step-by-step directions for how the system works and how things are done to accomplish the end results. Most systems have manuals or documentation that include the directions and/or instructions, rules or policies, and special guidelines for using the system. Many of these are now online.

Communication (connectivity) refers to the electronic transfer of data from one place to another. This is an area of rapid developments that changes how work is done. Chapters 9, 10, and 11 review some of the basic concepts regarding communication.

Data and information are described in detail in Chapter 13.

Hardware, an introduction to software, and connectivity are the focus of this chapter. Later chapters contain more information about specific software programs.

▶ 2.1 INTRODUCTION TO COMPUTER SYSTEMS: HARDWARE

The hardware for a computer system consists of input devices, the system unit (processing unit, memory, boards, and power supply), output devices, and secondary storage devices. The following definitions are important to understanding the upcoming sections on hardware. Refer to the definitions as these terms are encountered throughout this chapter.

Common Computer Terms

A computer is an electronic device that converts data into information. As an electronic device, it does not understand spoken words. The computer uses a series of *0*s and *1*s to describe data and to represent information. A **bit** is the smallest unit of data, the lowest level, and is an abbreviation for binary digit. A bit represents one of two states for the computer, 0 or 1, off or on like a light switch. Everything the computer understands uses combinations of *0*s and *1*s. A **byte** is a string of bits used to represent a character, digit, or symbol. It usually contains 8 bits.

Computers come in various sizes and configurations. Listed here are the common types of computers:

Mainframe	A large computer that accommodates hundreds of users simultaneously is a mainframe. It has a large data storage capacity, a large amount of memory, multiple input/output (I/O) devices, and speedy processor(s). Many universities and hospitals run their computer systems on mainframe computers.
Minicomputer	A minicomputer is a term that describes medium-sized computers that are faster and store more data than personal computers (PCs) and are cheaper than mainframes. In terms of size, they are between mainframes and personal computers. Many departments in larger companies use minicomputers to house specific software related to the department's function. For example, a pharmacy or laboratory department might have a minicomputer running pharmacy or laboratory department software.
Workstation	A workstation is a computer with capabilities beyond a normal PC. It looks like a PC but generally uses a different central processing unit (CPU) design known as RISC (reduced instruction set computing). Most of these use the UNIX operating

system (OS). They are used in some departments for higher level processing than can be handled with a PC or on research projects requiring higher level processing than a PC can deliver.

When used in a network context, workstation means a computer node on a network.

Microcomputer

A small, one-user computer system with its own CPU, memory, and storage devices is a microcomputer. Microcomputers are growing in processing power, speed, and storage. They are also referred to as PCs and desktops.

Portable PC

Two classes of portable computers exist: notebook and laptop. Notebooks are usually $8\frac{1}{2}" \times 11"$ and fit into a briefcase. Laptops are slightly larger than notebooks and usually have full-size keyboards. The configuration of portable PCs is similar to that of microcomputers. These computers provide mobility for the end user.

PDA

PDAs, the acronym for personal digital assistants, are increasing in popularity in all walks of life. They are the smallest portable computers and are currently less powerful than PCs. There are two basic types: handhelds, which are larger and heavier and usually come with their own miniature keyboard and small touch screen, and palm sized, which are smaller and lighter than handhelds and use a stylus touch screen and handwriting for data input. PDAs are designed to complement desktop computers.

PDAs consist of the same functional components as PCs but have no hard drives. A PDA has a processor, OS, memory, power source (batteries), display (liquid crystal display [LCD]), input device, I/O ports, and software. PDAs are used to store contact information, check and send e-mail, play games, listen to music, and download information from the Internet. Their ability to store information such as drug references, laboratory tests, and other diagnostic reference material makes them increasingly popular in the health care field.

Some people like to think of cellular phones as computers, but currently, they are really I/O devices with some storage capacity. They permit accessing e-mail, websites, instant messaging and sending/receiving pictures in addition to voice communications.

Before describing the four basic computer components, three more terms need to be defined.

Boot	Boot is a term that means to start the computer so that it can execute the necessary startup routines.
Default	Default is a term used to explain the setting the computer uses unless told otherwise. This is an important term because users will have difficulty retrieving or finding files if they do not know where the computer is storing them. Most college laboratories require their users to store data on a removable storage device or folder on the file server. Most will not let students store their data in the Microsoft Office My Documents folder.
Toggle	To toggle means to switch from one mode of operation to another. For example, pressing the insert key toggles between insert mode and typeover mode.
Upgrade	Upgrade is a term that is used to describe enhancing a piece of equipment or buying the newest release of a software program. Many computers are "upgradeable," meaning that the user may add more memory, additional storage devices, and so forth.

Input Devices

Input devices are hardware components that convert data from an external source into electronic signals understood by the computer. The user interacts with the computer through an interface and an input device. In this interaction, a frequently used term to describe the "visible indicator" on the screen that marks the current location and the point at which the work begins is the **cursor**, which is also referred to as a **pointer**. The cursor can appear as a pointer (generally an arrow), a vertical or horizontal line, a rectangle, or an I-beam that looks like a capital letter *I*. The cursor also changes to reflect processes and functions. For example, in Windows, it changes to an hourglass when the program is processing a command. In Netscape, an Internet browser, it changes to a hand when placed over linked text or objects (text or objects that provide more information either at this site or at another site).

Two major input devices are the keyboard and the mouse.

Keyboard

The keyboard is an input device that looks like a typewriter but has more keys. The most common layout includes the typical typewriter keys (alphanumeric keys) with the function keys at the top and the cursor movement keys and the numeric keypad (calculator layout) on the right. However, laptop computers have a slightly different layout because of size limitations. Newer keyboards may also add keys for Internet and media functions. Most keyboards are attached to the system unit through the keyboard port. Cordless keyboards use radio waves or infrared light waves to communicate to the system unit via an IrDA or Bluetooth port (both defined under ports) attached to the system unit. Laptop keyboards are built into the top of the system unit. Newer keyboards are designed to reduce the chance of wrist and hand injuries and are therefore referred to as "ergonomic" keyboards.

Described next are some of the common special keys for many keyboards.

Alphanumeric keys resemble the typewriter keyboard layout and are used for data entry.

The **Caps Lock** key is a toggle key used to switch between uppercase and lowercase letters. Use it when the need is for large amounts of text to be in all caps.

The **Backspace** key is used to delete characters to the left of the cursor.

The **Delete** key is used to delete text to the right of the cursor. It is sometimes labeled Del and is located above the arrow keys on most keyboards.

The **Enter** key is pressed after entering commands or at the end of paragraphs. Also use it to accept the outlined button in a Windows dialog box. Some texts use symbols (<CR>) to represent the enter key. This text uses Enter to mean "press the enter key."

The **Insert** key is above the arrow keys on most keyboards. The default is to insert characters at the location of the cursor, moving all other characters to the right. In many programs, Insert serves as a toggle switch to

move between typeover and insert modes. If characters are being replaced, press the Insert key to toggle it back to insert mode.

The **Shift** key functions like a typewriter shift key. It produces uppercase
letters when used in combination with the letter keys. On many keyboards, an up arrow (↑) represents the shift key.

The **Tab** functions like a typewriter Tab. It moves the cursor along the
screen at defined intervals or to the next field in a dialog box. For example, pressing the tab key moves the cursor five spaces at a time in many
application programs.

▶ Function/special keys

The **Alt**, **Ctrl**, and **Shift** keys extend the number of functions possible
with the F1–F12 keys to 48. These keys, in combination with other keys,
initiate commands or complete tasks. These keys also provide keyboard
shortcuts to some commands. For example, Ctrl + S represents the Save
command in many applications.

The **Esc** key generally backs out of a program or menu one screen or menu
at a time.

The **Fn** key is short for function. It is used in conjunction with other keys
to produce special actions that vary with applications. It is most commonly found on portable computers without full-size keyboards.

The **Function** keys are special keys that are used by application programs to
complete tasks. They are most frequently located at the top of the keyboard.
Their specific function varies for each software program. They are typically
labeled F1, F2, and so on, usually up to F12. With the advent of the windows
environment, the use of these keys has diminished in favor of mouse clicks
and shortcut keystrokes such as Ctrl + P for print and Ctrl + O for open.

The **Print Screen** key is used alone or in combination with the Alt key to
place the screen or active window onto the clipboard. Once on the clipboard, the image can be pasted into an application program.

▶ Cursor keys (control)

The **Arrow keys** are generally clustered together in a group of four and have
directional arrows on them. On most keyboards, they are on the lower
right. Pressing an arrow key moves the cursor around on the screen in the
direction of that key's arrow. Some people refer to these keys as cursor keys.

The **Page Up/Down**, **Home**, and **End** keys are used to move quickly from
one place in the document or on the screen to another. These keys are
above the arrow keys on most keyboards.

▶ Numeric keypad

The **Numeric** keys are used to enter numbers and function like a numeric keypad. Some keyboards require the Num Lock indicator light to be on when using the numeric keypad numbers because they function as cursor movement keys when the Num Lock light is off.

▶ Special Windows keys

The **Application** key is located under the right shift key between the Ctrl and Windows logo keys. It displays the shortcut menu for the selected item. For example, it will display the shortcut menu for this text if pressed while the cursor is in this paragraph. This is a new key introduced on the new natural keyboards.

The **Windows logo** key displays or hides the Start menu. It is also used in combination with other keys to execute commands. For example, pressing the Windows logo key and *F* opens the search for a file or folder dialog window. This key was introduced with the Windows 95 and natural keyboards and is located on the bottom left between the Ctrl and Alt keys and the bottom right between the Alt and application key of the keyboard.

Mouse

Currently, most computers come with another input device, a mouse. The traditional mechanical mouse has a ball on the underside of it. To use it, the user slides it over the mouse pad or desktop. Newer "optical" mice do not have a ball on the underside but sense changes in light reflection to detect mouse movement. A mechanical mouse has a ball on its underside, whereas an optical mouse has no moving mechanical parts.

Some laptops have a trackball, pointing stick, or touch pad that serves as the mouse or pointing device. A trackball is a stationary mouse with the ball on the top part of it. The user moves the ball instead of the mouse. A pointing stick looks like a pencil eraser and uses pressure to detect mouse movement. A touch pad is another stationary pointing device in which the user moves the finger around on the pad to move the cursor. These were designed for mobile computers because there may not be a desktop space to move the mouse along.

The mouse connects to the computer via a cord plugged into the mouse port. A growing number of them are now cordless and use radio waves and infrared light waves to communicate to the system unit.

The mouse is used to access menus or functions, open application programs, and create graphic elements without using the function or cursor keys. A button is a place on the mouse that is pressed to invoke a command or activity. It clicks when pressed. Most mice today have two buttons. Many newer ones also contain a wheel on the top.

Described here are common mouse operations:

Point means to move the mouse so the cursor is on or over a particular command or icon on the screen.

Click (press) means to press and hold the mouse button down, as on a menu item to see the commands, or to scroll through a window until the command is selected. Often this means to single click.

Single click means to press and release the left mouse button once to activate a command or select an icon or menu option. Use a single click to insert the I-beam (cursor in the shape of a capital *I*) at the point in the document where typing is to occur.

Double click means, with the cursor on an icon or option, press and release the left mouse button twice in quick succession. Use the double-click operation to start an application program, open a file or folder, or select a word for editing.

Right click activates the shortcut menu. To right click, press and release the right mouse button once. Make sure to right click the appropriate place. Different menus appear for different areas of the desktop or a window. Use it when instructed to right click; otherwise, use the left mouse button.

Triple click means to press and release the left mouse button three times. In word processing programs, this is used to select a paragraph.

Drag means to left click an icon, menu option, or window border; then, without lifting the finger off the mouse, roll the mouse to move the object to another place on the screen. This can change a window's size, copy a file or document, select text, or take something to the trash.

Right drag means to hold down the right mouse button, move the mouse to a different location, and then release the mouse button. This generally results in the appearance of a shortcut menu from which to select a command. The commands vary depending on the object right clicked.

Rotate wheel means to move the wheel forward and backward. This action is used to scroll up and down in a document or at a website.

Press wheel button means click the wheel once and move the mouse on the desktop. This action causes the mouse pointer to scroll along the document automatically until pressed again.

Other Input Devices

Described here are additional input devices used as an interface to the system unit.

A **digital camera** is used to take pictures and then upload them to the computer or to a special picture printer, thus bypassing the need to store the image on film and then have the film developed.

A **light pen** is a light-sensitive, pen-like device. Some require a special monitor to enter data. Some hospital clinical information systems use this input device. Light pens and electronic pens are not the same; electronic pens permit electronic signatures and require the user to hold the pen and write on a special pad. Light pens enable the user to enter data only with special screens.

A **microphone** (voice input device) permits the user to speak into the computer to enter data or give instructions. These are sometimes used with paraplegics to give commands to computer-controlled robots that help the person complete activities of daily living or do work. Many people who do not type well also prefer speaking to the computer.

A **PC video camera** is an input device that is used to capture video. It is used to send video images as e-mail attachments, to make video telephone calls (video conferencing), and to post live, real-time images to a web server. When used to capture and display images on a web server, the input device is called a **web cam**.

A **scanner** is an input device that converts character or graphic patterns to digital data (discrete coded units of data). It can take a picture, scan it, and put it on the screen. Software programs then import this converted data. Two main types of scanners are image (for text and graphics) and barcode (for database work) readers. Growing in popularity are data collection devices that collect the data at remote places and then upload the data to the main computer. In high-security areas, some scanners now collect biometric data such as a fingerprint, voiceprint, or retinal scan to verify the user. Many hospitals use bar code scanners to input data such as supplies used by patients and medications administered.

A **touch screen** is a special screen that allows the entering of commands or actions by pressing specific places on the screen with the finger. Most PDAs and interactive video programs use touch screens as the main input device.

A **stylus** or **digital pen** is used with tablets to create an image on the tablet surface. These tablets then convert the marks or images to digital data that the computer can use. A special stylus, used to select options from a screen, is the main input device for many PDAs.

Cradles or **docking stations** are input devices primarily used by PDAs, laptops, iPods, and cameras to input data from the mobile device to the desktop computer. They are connected to the computer to ease the movement of data from one device to the other. The user places the device in the cradle or on the docking station and many times presses a button. The data then move from the mobile device to the desktop computer.

System Unit

The system unit contains the control center or "brains" of the computer; it is not visible to the eye on most computers unless the cover of the computer is removed. The system unit is contained in a case, which varies in size and shape.

Processing Unit	This consists of several semiconductor chips mounted on a single circuit board (called by many the motherboard or system board), often referred to as the CPU and memory.
Chip	A chip is a tiny piece of semiconducting material, usually silicon, that packs many millions of electronic elements onto an area the size of a fingernail. Computers contain many chips that are placed on circuit boards. A specialized chip, CPU, contains an entire processing unit, whereas memory chips contain only memory.
CPU	The CPU is the computer circuitry that interprets and executes program instructions. It is sometimes referred to as the processor, microprocessor, or central processor. It has two parts: the control unit and the arithmetic/logic unit. The control unit coordinates the computer's activities. It receives, interprets, and implements instructions. The arithmetic unit performs math functions such as addition, subtraction, multiplication, and

division. The logic unit compares two values of data to determine whether they are equal or whether one is greater than or less than the other. The arithmetic/logic unit temporarily uses registers and memory locations to hold data being processed. Microprocessors (CPUs) are of two types: CISC (complex instruction set computing, commonly found in small computers) and RISC (reduced instruction set computing), commonly found in Macs and workstations.

Microprocessors are referred to by specific names and manufacturers, such as Intel Pentium series, Intel Xeon MP, and AMD64. This is the heart of the computer. It controls and coordinates many functions. Large computers found in hospitals have many chips plugged into circuit boards that communicate with each other. Intel no longer uses the processor speed in its name but refers to the processor by a series. For example, Intel Pentium M 7xx.

Memory

Memory storage (primary) is fast but has low density (amount of data stored per square inch) and costs more per amount of data stored than secondary storage. Read-only memory (ROM) is memory burned on the chip at the factory; the computer can read instructions from it but cannot alter them. This memory is permanent. Computer startup instructions reside in ROM; these are instructions that tell the computer what to do when turned on (see Chapter 3 for more on startup). There are other variations of ROM, such as PROM (programmable read only memory), which permits programming instructions once, and EPROM (erasable programmable read only memory), which permits a user to program the instructions many times.

Random access memory (RAM) is memory that stores data the computer needs to use temporarily. It is volatile and gets erased when the power is turned off. The common unit of measurement for RAM is the byte, which is the amount of storage it takes to hold a character. The more RAM a computer has, the more it can do. When a software program is started, the files that are needed to run the program are stored in RAM as well as in the user's data file. As additional functions are requested, the computer loads additional software files. If the memory is not large enough, software files are swapped, slowing down the work.

A newer type of memory is called Flash memory. It is a type of nonvolatile memory that can be erased and rewritten, making it easier to update its contents. Some computers hold their startup instructions in this type of memory so that it can be upgraded. **Cache** is a form of fast memory that is discussed later in the chapter.

Motherboard

This is the main circuit board of the computer to which all other internal components connect.

Ports

Ports, carrying information, are the highways that lead into, out of, and around the computer. Many of them are the interfaces between the computer and peripheral devices. These are plugs, sockets, or hot spots located on the back and front of most system units. Ports allow the computer to communicate with peripheral devices. For example, many computers have built-in game, mouse, keyboard, and monitor ports. This allows the computer to talk with these devices. The ports described here are also considered external data buses (a bus is a series of connections or pathway over which data travels). Most computers have at least one serial port, one parallel port, and at least two USB (universal serial bus) ports. Newer computers can be configured with FireWire, IrDA, and/or Bluetooth ports that connect to some of the newer peripheral technologies such as digital cameras, PDAs, and MP3 players.

Serial

A serial port, called by most people a "com" port, arranges data in serial form one bit at a time. This allows data to move from the internal, parallel form in the computer to external devices. Because it allows two-way communication, the reverse data flow occurs from external devices back to the computer. Most modems connect to serial ports.

Parallel

A parallel port is a unidirectional port set up to send parallel data. Parallel data are data moving abreast in groups of eight bits or a byte of information. Parallel ports commonly connect the computer to a printer (one-way communication). A version of this port is the enhanced parallel port (EPP), which permits bidirectional communication.

SCSI

A small computer system interface, or "scuzzy," is a parallel port that supports faster data transfers than traditional parallel ports. Scuzzy ports permit attachment of up to seven peripheral devices in a linked chain fashion. This interface also contains a set of command protocols or instructions for data transfer. There are many varieties of SCSI ports from SCSI-2 to Fast SCSI to SCSI-3; they vary in terms of the pin connectors and data transfer rates.

USB

A universal serial bus is a port standard that supports faster data transfer rates (12 million bits per second). USB supports up to 127 peripheral devices as well as plug and play technologies.

FireWire

A firewire port is a special purpose port. It is similar to a USB port in that multiple devices can be attached to it. It is used to connect devices (cameras, camcorders, etc.) that require faster data transmission than normal ports. A FireWire port supports up to 63 devices.

IrDA	An infrared light beam port is used to connect wireless devices using light waves to the computer. The wireless device must line up with the port on the computer just like the remote control on a television for it to work. These are used for wireless keyboards, mice, and PDAs.
Bluetooth	A Bluetooth port competes with the IrDA ports using radio waves to communicate between the devices instead of infrared light waves. The advantage to this type of port is that there is no line-of-sight requirement. Although some current devices such as PDAs, cell phones, baby monitors, garage doors, and other electronic devices are Bluetooth enabled, Bluetooth is not the current default standard for wireless technology.
MIDI	A MIDI port permits the connection of musical instruments to the computer.
Expansion Slots	Expansion slots are places on the system board where cards, adapters, or other computer boards can be added. Cards or adapters provide the option to run additional devices such as internal modems, sound cards (containing synthesizers for playing sound files), network cards, and hard drives (secondary storage devices). On laptops, these personal computer memory card international association (PMCIA) slots permit adding devices such as modems, memory cards, sound cards, and hard drives via credit card-like expansion modules.
Power Supply	A power supply box provides the conversion from the power available at the wall socket (120-volt 60-MHz, AC current) to the power necessary to run the computer (+5 and +12 volt, DC current). The power supply must ensure a good, steady supply of both 5- and 12-volt DC power for the computer to operate effectively.

In addition to the processor of the computer, other factors in the system unit affect how fast the computer works. These are the registers, the RAM, the clock speed, the internal data bus, and cache.

Registers

Registers are temporary storage spaces used by the CPU when processing data. Registers are part of the processing unit, not the memory. The size of the registers affects processing speed. The larger the register, the faster the computer processes data. For example, a 32-bit register is slower than a 64-bit register.

RAM

The amount of RAM increases the speed of processing. A program runs faster when more of it fits into RAM simultaneously. Keeping the program in RAM means the computer does not have to access files it needs from the hard drive, which is much slower than accessing the files from memory.

Clock Speed

The clock speed is determined by the quartz crystal circuit that controls the timing of computer work. The faster the internal clock (used to time process operations) runs, the faster the computer works. Measurement of clock speed is gigahertz (GHz or 1 billion cycles per second). Older machines worked at the megahertz (MHz or one million cycles per second) level. Theoretically, the higher the number, the faster the computer works.

Bus

Internal data buses move data around in the computer on a data bus, which is a collection of wires. A data bus is a path between computer parts such as the CPU, memory, and other devices. The wider the bus (number of wires or pins), the faster it can move data. All buses consist of two parts: an address bus (where the data is going) and a data bus (the actual data). What is critical about the bus is its width (16, 32, and 64 bits) and speed. The width determines how much data it can move at a time, and the speed determines how fast it moves the data.

ISA The industry standard architecture (ISA) bus is the most common in PCs and is also the slowest. It generally provides connections for the mouse, modem, and sound cards.

PCI The peripheral component interconnect (PCI) bus is the current standard for connecting higher speed devices such as the local hard drive, network cards, sound cards, and video cards.

AGP The accelerated graphics port (AGP) bus is the default internal bus between the graphics controller and the main memory. It is dedicated and designed specifically for a video system.

Cache Cache is a memory space similar to RAM but extremely fast. The amount of cache a computer has also affects how fast the computer works. It is time consuming to move data back and forth between the CPU registers and memory. Data stored in a cache are accessible faster than other data.

Output Devices

Output devices take the processed data, called information, and present it to the user in display, print, or sound form. Described here are some common output devices.

Monitor

Display screen, CRT (cathode ray tube), and LCD (liquid crystal display) are terms used to describe the monitor. *Monitor*, however, generally refers to the entire box, whereas *display screen* refers to just the screen. CRTs are used with desktop systems, and flat panels are used with laptop and increasingly with desktop computers. Flat panels have grown in popularity because of their smaller footprint, smaller power requirement, and no-flicker effect, but they are more expensive than CRTs. Most mobile computers use LCD technology for the display device. Large businesses sometimes use gas plasma monitors that permit displaying images on a larger scale, such as 50 inches. Monitors vary in size, color, resolution, refresh rate, and dot pitch.

Size

Size refers to the diagonal measurement from corner to corner of the monitor for CRTs. Active viewing area refers to the actual measurement from left to right and top to bottom and is used to describe LCDs. The size needed depends on what is being done. Common sizes are 15, 17, and 19 inches; larger sizes are used for desktop and Internet publishing.

Color

Color refers to whether the monitor is monochrome (one color, usually green or amber, on a black background) or color. The number of colors displayed varies from 256 and to much higher numbers. Most monitors sold today for general purpose use are colored. Monochrome monitors may be seen in such places as retail sales systems or hospital information systems. Display mode refers to the numbers of colors and the maximum resolution of a monitor. For example, UEGA (ultra extended graphics array) displays 16.8 million colors at a 1600 × 1200 resolution.

Resolution

This term describes how densely packed the pixels are. The monitors display images via pixels (tiny dots) and vary in number of pixels per screen (resolution). The more pixels on the screen, the sharper the image. A common resolution is 1024 × 768 pixels, but many monitors are capable of 1600 × 1280 pixels and higher.

The capabilities of the video card influence the quality of the images a monitor displays more than the monitor itself. The video card or controller is an interface between the CPU and the monitor. It contains the memory and other circuitry necessary to display information on the screen.

Resolution can be altered. For example, a 1280 × 1024 can be set to 800 × 600 without losing any sharpness while gaining the ability to display larger sized objects. This is not true for LCD displays. If a user completes the previously mentioned change, the image will no longer be sharp. Using the highest resolution available to the display is not always the best choice, as many menu items and toolbars will appear very small.

Refresh Rate   Refresh rate is the number of times a monitor scans the screen vertically each second. This applies to CRTs and not LCDs. Hertz (Hz) is the measurement unit used for refresh rates. The higher the refresh rate, the less flickering happens on the monitor. To avoid flickering, the refresh rate should be at least 72 Hz. Another important term related to the refresh rate is **noninterlaced**. Noninterlaced monitors scan every line with each refresh; interlaced monitors scan every other line with each refresh.

Dot Pitch   Dot pitch is the measure of the distance between the red, green, and blue phosphors that make up the colors of the monitor. The closer together they are, the sharper and denser the screen colors are. Here, the smaller the number, the better the colors. Dot pitch measurement is in millimeters.

The last point about a monitor relates to its conformance to standards. First, a monitor needs to be energy efficient and conform to the Energy Star guidelines. This requires a monitor to idle down to 30 watts or less when not in use. The second guideline relates to emissions. This refers to the amount of electromagnetic emissions produced by a monitor. The monitor should comply with the MPR-III or the more rigorous TCO92, TCO95, TC098, or TC099 standards.

Printers

Printers produce either black and white or color output. Use black and white printers for papers, correspondence, handouts, and reports. Use color printers for overheads, poster presentations, and documents in which color enhances the message.

Nonimpact

A nonimpact printer is one in which the mechanisms do not touch the surface of the paper. Some examples are laser, thermal, and ink jet printers. Laser printers are the most expensive of the printers. They produce high-quality print, are fast, and produce little noise. Ink jet printers are less expensive than laser printers. They produce a better quality output than dot matrix and serve as an excellent middle ground between laser and dot matrix printers. Many ink jet color printers are very reasonably priced. Growing in popularity are the photo printers that use ink jet technology to produce color pictures in varying sizes. Some plotters also use ink jet technology to produce large banners and architectural drawings.

Impact

An impact printer is one whose mechanisms touch the surface when printing. Some common examples are dot matrix and line printers or plotters. Dot matrix printers are the least expensive but are noisy and produce lower quality print. Use dot matrix printers for carbon forms such as invoices and statements. Plotters are used for graphic design work such as design plans.

Other Output Devices

As end users become more adept at using technology, the demand for other output devices increases.

**Speakers and
Headsets**

Stereo speakers and headphones come with most computers today. These are for reproducing and displaying high-quality sound on the computer. These speakers can be mounted on the monitor or stand separately on the desktop. Some high-level multimedia computers also come with a subwoofer to deal with the bass sounds. Most computer laboratories now require users to wear headphones when using the computers so that the sounds do not dis-

	turb other users. If no headphones are used, then the sound must be turned off.
Data Projectors	A data projector is used to display graphic presentations to an audience. This is a device that takes the image on the computer screen and projects it onto a larger screen. Data projectors can be portable or ceiling mounted. As with all electronic devices, the price and quality range from the low end to the high end.
Multifunction Devices	These devices are all-in-one I/O devices. They contain a printer, scanner, copier, and fax machine. Some advantages of these over separate devices are that they are cheaper than purchasing each device separately and they take up less space. Two disadvantages are that when the device is broken all devices are down and that in order to gain increased functionality the user sacrifices some advanced features.

Secondary Storage

A place or space for holding data and application programs is referred to as storage. The computer has both primary (memory) and secondary (floppy diskettes, hard drives, optical drives, and tape drives) storage spaces. Primary storage was discussed under memory.

Secondary storage is media that holds the application programs and user data when not in use. Secondary storage takes longer to access data, has a higher density or amount of data per square inch, and is less expensive than primary storage. Two main types in use today are magnetic and optical. Floppy disks, hard disks, and tapes are examples of magnetic media. CDs, laser, and DVD drive discs are examples of optical media. Data storage uses the same units to measure size as memory does—bytes. Kilobytes, megabytes, gigabytes, and terrabytes are size terms that describe the amount of data a medium holds. A kilobyte is 1024 bytes or characters. A megabyte (MB) is 1 million+. A gigabyte (GB) is 1 billion+, and a terrabyte is 1 trillion+ bytes or characters. The trend for data storage is to use smaller physical sizes that hold larger amounts of data.

Floppy Drives	Floppy drives read floppy diskettes. Floppy diskettes store programs or data files. Most disk drives are high density and read high-density

(HD) and double-density (DD) diskettes. A floppy diskette holds 1,444,000 characters and comes in 3.5″ size. Many computers no longer come with floppy drives; they must be purchased separately.

Zip Drives

Zip drives, although considered floppy disk drives, use disks that are slightly larger in size and approximately twice as thick. They hold at least 100 MB and up to 750 MB of data and are commonly used to store graphic files and larger program files and sometimes to back up data on hard drives. Most computers do not come with zip drives; they must be purchased separately and can be installed internally or externally.

Flash Drives

Flash drives (memory sticks, USB drives, thumb drives, memory keys) are replacing floppy drives as a convenient method for transferring data between systems. They do not require installing— just plug them into a USB port. Many computers now have USB ports on the front side of the computer for easy access. These drives come in sizes varying from 14 to 512 MB, with some even larger (in the GB range). Most of them are the size of a cigarette lighter and can attach to a key chain.

Hard Drives

A hard drive is a data storage device fixed in a sealed case that reads data stored on platters in the drive. It stores more data (in the gigabyte range) and permits faster retrieval than floppy drives. Hard drives are either external to the system unit or contained within the system unit (fixed). They are also available as hard cards inserted in an expansion slot or as portable drives inserted in a bay or connected to a USB port. Some interface standards for moving the data between this storage device and the processor are EIDE (enhanced integrated drive electronics) and SCSI as well as FireWire and USB ports. When purchasing a computer or hard drive, these terms are used to describe the hard drive.

Tape Drives

Tape drives are secondary storage devices that allow the backup or duplication of data stored on a hard disk. They store data sequentially (one right after the other) in magnetic form, much like an audiotape. They are declining in popularity except for larger computer systems and are being replaced by optical backup devices.

Optical Drives—CDs

Optical drives are the main alternative to magnetic storage. They hold large amounts of data, usually written (pressed) once and accessed many times. The most common example is the CD-ROM (compact disc—read-only memory). This storage device typically holds 650 MB of data, although some can go as high as 1 GB.

CD-Rs (compact disc-recordable) permit writing to once, whereas CD-RWs (compact disc-rewritable) permit writing and erasing many times. No erasing can be done with CD-Rs. This storage device can store digital audio, full-motion video, graphics, and animation in addition to text data.

**Optical Drives
DVDs**

The latest addition to the CD-ROM storage technology is the DVD technology. Earlier DVDs were designed to accommodate video and thus were named digital video discs. As their use as a data storage medium increased, the name changed to digital versatile disc. These discs hold more data such as a full-length movie than CDs.

There are five versions of DVDs: DVD-R, DVD-RW, DVD+R, DVD+RW, and DVD-RAM. DVD drives are needed to read these discs. New on the scene are hi definition DVDs.

Labeling disk drives

Disk drives are referred to with letters. Letters and icons with letters help users direct the computer to the drive from which they want to access stored information or to the one they want to assign as the default drive. The letters *C* and *D* usually refer to the hard disk. CD-ROM and zip drives usually use the letters *D*, *E*, *F*, or *G*. The computer reserves the letters *A* and/or *B* for floppy drives. In the Windows environment, words appear next to the letters describing the na-

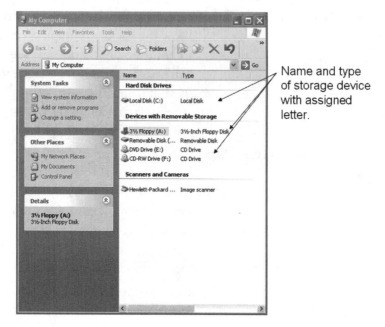

Name and type
of storage device
with assigned
letter.

Figure 2.1

Example of Storage
Device Names and
Letters

ture of that storage device as well as the letter assigned to it. For example, 3.5"
floppy appears next to the letter A (see Figure 2.1 for an example of drive names
and letters). Because there are many variations for drive labeling, consult the
laboratory assistant or instructor for the conventions used in your laboratory.

Other Peripherals

Two other peripheral devices should be considered when looking at hardware: the surge protector and the uninterruptible power supply (UPS).

Surge Protector   A surge protector is a device that is located between the electrical outlet and the computer sup-
ply source. This device protects the computer from
low-voltage surges in electrical power by directing
the extra power to the outlet's grounding wire. Although it offers protection from normal surges in
voltage, it cannot protect the computer from
lightning strikes. The other names for a surge protector are power strips and surge suppressors.

UPS   An uninterruptible power supply device is a
power supply that takes over in the event of a
power outage. It runs on a battery and keeps the

computer going for several minutes after the outage. This valuable time permits the user to save data and shut down the computer. There are two types: standby and online. Standby monitors the power line and switches to battery power when a problem is detected. The online type constantly provides power even when the power line is functioning properly, thereby avoiding the momentary lack of power when the UPS switches from power to battery. These are more expensive units. Think of these as standby generators much like hospitals use in case of a power outage, but on a much smaller scale.

Generally, printers, speakers, and scanners are plugged into surge protectors, whereas the computer, monitor, and storage devices are plugged into the UPS. Printers cause a large drain on the battery of a UPS.

► 2.2 CONNECTIVITY

Most people now assume that a computer has the ability to communicate with other computers. Communication refers to the process of moving data and information from one computer device to another. That means that users expect to be able to communicate from a PC to a laptop to a hand held to a web server.

The basic communication process includes a sender and receiver, a channel, and a communication device. Chapter 9, "Using the World Wide Web," and Chapter 10, "Computer-Assisted Communication," discuss some of the services people use when connected as well as what it takes to get connected to the Internet. Described here are relevant terms for understanding basic computer communications or connectivity.

Communication Devices

A communication device is any type of hardware capable of transmitting data and information from one computer to another. Examples of communication devices are dial-up modems, cable modems, digital subscriber line (DSL) modems, and network interface cards.

Dial-up Modem

This is a device that prepares the data to be transmitted over a telephone line. This means converting digital data into analog (wave) form and then reversing the process at the other end. Many people still use this means of connecting to the Internet as other choices are either not available or too expensive.

DSL Modem

This is a modem used when one is connecting to the network over a DSL connection. These are usually obtained through the telecommunications company that provides the connection service.

Cable Modem

This is a modem used when connecting to the network using the television cable services.

Wireless USB

Adapters are now available to bring wireless USB 2.0 data rates to wireless connections between computers and peripheral devices for the purpose of transferring music, photos, and data. It was being designed to compete with Bluetooth wireless technology but will bring data rates of 480 MB over a distance of two meters. It uses UWB (ultra-wideband) radio technology at the 3.1- to 10.6-GHz spectrum, whereas Bluetooth uses the 2.4-GHz portion (Kolic, 2004).

Ethernet Cards

An Ethernet card is inserted into the computer to provide connectivity to a network. It is generally used in schools, offices, and businesses to connect all the computers and peripherals to the school's or company's network.

Communications Channel

This is the transmission media that the data takes to arrive at the other end.

Dial-up

Dial-up is also referred to as plain old telephone service (POTS). It is still the most common way to connect to the Internet as it is widely available, but it is much slower than other media. Upper speed here is 56 Kbps.

DSL A DSL connection uses a faster connection, usually through the phone system. The limitation here is that it is not available to a wide array of users, as there are severe distance limitations. The user must be within 18,000 feet of a phone switching station, and the further away from the switching station, the slower the data rate. It reaches speeds of 128 Kbps to 9 Mbps.

Cable The cable lines coming into most homes provide another option for a communications channel. This channel is faster than the previous two but degrades in speed as more people access the cable.

T1 and T3 These are communications media that are used for large businesses. Services are generally provided by a telecommunications company.

Wireless This channel employs radio (broadcast, microwave, and satellite) and light waves (infrared) to transmit the data.

Networks are connections between various devices for the purpose of sharing resources, communicating, and accessing information. Chapter 10, "Computer-Assisted Communication," and Chapter 12, "Security and Privacy," address additional terminology related to networks and connectivity. Most businesses use a combination of wired and wireless network connectivity. Growing in popularity are WLANs (wireless local area network) and home networks. WLANs connect devices to the network over short distances using Wi-FI (wireless fidelity) standards. Wi-FI is now a generic term used to describe 802.11b, 802.11a, or 802.11g standards for wireless technologies.

▶ 2.3 INTRODUCTION TO COMPUTER SYSTEMS: SOFTWARE

Computers are multipurpose machines. They are, however, unable to complete any task without directions from software programs. Software programs consist of step-by-step instructions that direct the computer hardware to perform specific tasks such as multiply, divide, fetch, or deliver data. They provide instructions for the computer. All computers require software to function. When the computer is using a specific program, users say they are running or executing the program.

The following are three major categories of software.

Operating System (OS)

The OS is the most important program that runs on a computer. The OS tells the computer how to use its own components or hardware. No general-purpose computer can work without an OS.

Operating systems perform some functions necessary to all users of the computer system. Some of the basic tasks that they perform include keeping track of files and folders, communicating to peripheral devices such as printers, receiving and interpreting input from the mouse or keyboard, displaying output on a screen, and managing how data moves around inside the computer. In other words, operating systems coordinate the computer hardware components and supervise all basic operations.

The most common operating system for PCs is the Windows family (Windows 98, 2000, XP, and NT) and for Apple computers the Macintosh operating system (OS 10). Some computers also use variations of UNIX called Linux and Xenix. Portable computers may use Windows CE. Larger computer systems and workstations may use VMS and Unix or a Unix variation such as Solaris. The important point to remember here is that all computers need an operating system to work and that they will change to reflect changes in technology and user needs. Chapters 3 and 4 provide more detail about working in the Windows environment.

Languages

Language software presents a simplified means, called a language, to execute a series of instructions. It consists of a vocabulary and an accompanying set of rules that tell the computer how to work. Languages permit the user to develop programs that do specific tasks. Some common languages are C, C++, COBOL (Common Business Oriented Language), JAVA, and Visual Basic. Users do not need to be programmers to use the computer; however, programming skills are helpful when trying to do more advanced things on the computer.

There are four levels of programming languages. Machine-level languages are the lowest level and consist of numbers only. Assembly languages are the next level, and they give the programmer the ability to use names instead of numbers. High-level languages are what users normally think of when they say programming language. They include the previously mentioned languages such as Visual Basic, C, and JAVA. They consist of a set of keywords or commands and related syntax for organizing the program. The last level of programming languages is called fourth-generation languages or 4GL. This level of programming language is the closest to human language. These are usually used in artificial intelligence type programs. LISP (List Processor) is one example.

Although many people include HTML (HyperText Markup Language) and SGML (Standard Generalized Markup Language) as programming languages, in reality they are not. They are considered organizing and tagging languages designed to manage the layout and formatting of documents between different computer systems.

Applications

Application programs meet specific task needs of the user and are considered the core of any computer system. Applications use language software to write the application program. Major types of applications or programs include the following:

- General-purpose software such as word processors, spreadsheets, database managers, presentation graphics, and communications programs
- Educational programs
- Utility programs such as virus scanners, hard disk managers, and menu systems
- Personal programs such as calculators, calendars, and money managers
- Entertainment programs such as games and simulations

This book covers some common general-purpose application software.

General Purpose Software

Communications software permits one computer to "talk" to another by using standard communication protocols (rules and procedures that govern the communication).

Database software helps organize, store, retrieve, and manipulate data for the purpose of later retrieval and report generation.

Desktop publishing software permits the user to create high-quality specialty publications such as newspapers, bulletins, and brochures. It handles page layouts better than word processors and permits the importing of a variety of text and graphic files from other application programs.

Graphics software facilitates the creation of a variety of graphics. Three types of graphics programs exist. **Presentation** graphics permit the user to create or alter symbols, present a variety of chart styles, make transparencies and slides, and produce slide shows. **Paint programs** permit users to create symbols or images from scratch. **Computer-aided drafting** programs meet the schematic drawing needs of architects and engineers.

Integrated software includes in one program some capabilities of word processing, database, spreadsheet, graphics, and communication programs.

Spreadsheet software permits the manipulation of numbers in a format of rows and columns. Spreadsheet programs contain special functions for adding and computing statistical and financial formulas. Use them for financial functions and number crunching.

Statistics software permits statistical analysis of numeric data.

Suites are value packages that include a word processor, a spreadsheet, a database, a presentation graphics program, and sometimes a personal information manager. The main advantage of these suites is the cost (lower than each program individually) and the ability to share data easily between each program.

Word processing software permits the creating, editing, formatting, storing, and printing of text. Most have spell and grammar checkers built into them.

Education

Computer-assisted instruction software is a set of programs that help users learn concepts or specific content related to their discipline or area of study. In some circles, these programs are also referred to as training software.

CD-ROMs and DVDs hold educational programs that provide integrated sound and motion to provide a lesson.

Utilities

Utilities are a group of software programs that help with the management or maintenance of the computer. Some examples are hard disk managers, virus detectors, compression/decompression programs, and viewers. There is a new brand of utilities that deal with blocking spam, blocking or finding keyboard logger programs or spyware, and protecting users from unwanted intrusions.

Personal

Personal software programs help people manage their personal lives. Some examples are appointment calendars, checkbook balancing applications, money management applications, and calculators.

Entertainment

A class of software programs that is designed for fun is called entertainment software. Many games exist to provide diversion, including golf and football; others challenge problem-solving abilities. Still others are more video arcade-type programs.

When discussing software developments, the trend is for easier-to-use, graphic, or icon-driven programs that are available in suites.

SUMMARY

This chapter presents sufficient terminology and concepts necessary to become an intelligent computer user. To that end, the term *information system* was defined, and the major components of computers were described. Software basics were presented, including the three major classes. Although some of the specifics of the computer system will change as technology develops, the basic concepts will remain. Users will always need the input–process–output cycle and some form of software.

Reference

Kolic, R. (2004). *Wireless USB brings greater convenience and mobility to devices.* Retrieved August 2, 2004, from http://deviceforge.com/articles/ AT9015145687.html

Additional Resources

DVD Frequently Asked Questions (and Answers). (2004). Retrieved June 12, 2004 from http://www.dvddemystified.com/dvdfaq.html

Iomega. (2004). *Iomega: Frequently asked questions about Iomega super DVD writers.* Retrieved March 16, 2004, from http://www.iomega.com/dvd/dvd_faq.html

Minasi, M. (2004). *Complete PC upgrade and maintenance guide* (15th ed.). Alameda, CA: Sybex, Inc.

Mueller, S. (2003). *Upgrading and repairing PCs.* Indianapolis, IN: Que Publishing.

Rupley, S. (2004). *Wireless USB: The Next Video Data Channel?* PC Magazine. Retrieved June 20, 2004, from http://www.pcmag.com

White, R. (2003). *How computers work* (7th ed.). Indianapolis, IN: Que Publishing.

Online Resources

How Stuff Works (http://www.howstuffworks.com) is an excellent site for learning about computer hardware and connectivity.

Online Computer Directory for Computer and Internet Terms and Definitions (http://pcwebopedia.com/) is a great site for definitions and understanding basic concepts. It has a great interface and is simple and easy to use. Another site of this type is Tech Target at http://whatis.techtarget.com/.

PC Magazine (http://www.pcmag.com) is an excellent site for reviews and the latest happenings regarding hardware and connectivity.

PC Tech Guide (http://www.pctechguide.com) covers a lot more detail and technical issues regarding technology.

Exercise 1: Identify Computer Components
Objectives

1. Identify the specific computer hardware being used.

2. Use the proper terminology to describe the computer and related components.

Activity

1. Computer.

   What type of computer is being used?

   Make: Model:

(Make refers to the company that manufactures the computer. Some examples are HP, Gateway, Compaq, Dell, and Apple. Model refers to the specific computer manufactured by the company.)

Why is this important to know?

How is this computer turned on?

2. Monitor.

Is the monitor part of the system unit or separate from the system unit?

What type of monitor is it (CRT or LCD)?

What size is it?

Does it need to be turned on separately from the system unit?

If so, how is it turned on?

3. Storage.

What storage devices are available on this computer? (Describe them here.)

Is there access to a network file server?

Where are users permitted to store data?

What type of removable disks can be used?

Why is this important to know?

Draw and label the disk drive setup.

4. I/O devices.

What types of input devices are available with this computer?

What types of output devices are available with this computer?

Does the computer share a printer?

5. Connectivity.

Are there places to plug in a mouse, modem, printer, or other peripheral devices?

Is the computer connected to another computer that serves as a file server (a file server is a computer that contains software and data shared by those using the system)? Is the computer networked?

Turn on the equipment. Are user identification and password needed to access the system?

6. Software.

List the software available for use on this computer.

Exercise 2: Computer Configuration
Objectives

1. Identify questions to ask and information needed when buying a computer.
2. Relate information from a newspaper computer advertisement to the material presented about hardware.

Activity

Using the following advertisement information, fill in the blanks below:

Dell OptiPlex SX280, 256 MB RAM, Pentium 4 520 with HT technology (2.8 GHz) processor, 60 GB SATA hard drive, 40X Max Variable CD-R, Iomega Zip 100 MB, modem, integrated 10/100/1000 NIC, Dell mouse, Dell 19″ monitor, Microsoft Windows XP Professional, Microsoft Office 2003.

Microprocessor _____   Memory _____

Computer Speed _____

Storage Devices _____

Monitor Type and Size _____

Keyboard _____ Yes   Mouse _____ Yes

Connectivity _____

Sound System _____

Operating System _____

Questions:

What type of removable storage disks (discs) can be used? _____

What software is provided? _____

Can a flash memory or key storage device be used? _____

List additional questions that should be asked before buying this computer.

Exercise 3: Computer Specifications
Objectives

1. Specify minimum hardware requirements for different scenarios.
2. Identify software needs.
3. Justify the recommendations for the requirements for both hardware and software.

Activity A

You are in charge of a local health clinic. The budget requests are due to the clinic board, and you are submitting a request for a microcomputer, related peripheral devices, and software. You want to use the computer to help with the clinic management duties. Itemize and justify your request.

Activity B

You are the systems analyst in the center for research in your institution. The director decides to purchase computers for the center. You must now specify the hardware and software to meet the computing needs for the center. The center staff consists of a director (PhD), two associate directors (PhDs), three research associates (master's degree prepared), one statistician, and three members of the clerical staff.

Activity C

You want your parents to purchase a computer, a printer, and related software as a present for you. They need some help from you to determine what type of computer and software you need and whether the cost is reasonable. Itemize what you want and justify it to them.

Use hardware and software advertisements from newspapers, computer magazines, computer retailers, and the Internet to obtain hardware and software specifics.

Exercise 4: Accessing Application Software
Objectives

1. Start application programs using a variety of techniques.
2. Identify the software programs available on the computer.
3. Identify the operating system.
4. Shut down the computer.

Activity

1. Start an application using the double click method.

   Turn on the computer system. *Text appears on the screen as the computer goes through start up routines.*

   If necessary, press **Ctrl + Alt + Del** to obtain the log-in screen. That means to hold down the Ctrl key, hold down the Alt key, and then press Del. **Release** all three keys.

If necessary, type your log-in (**User ID**) and **Password** and press **Enter**. Use the **Tab** key to move between the User ID text field and the Password text field.

Double click the **Internet Explorer** 🖅 icon on the desktop. *The browser program opens.*

Click the **Close** ✕ button on the browser window to close the application.

2. Start an application using the Start button on the taskbar.

Click the **Start** button on the taskbar. *A menu appears.*

Select **All Programs**, **Accessories**, and **WordPad**. *WordPad, a word processing program that comes with Windows, now starts.*

Click the **Close** ✕ button on the WordPad window to close the application.

3. Start an application using My Computer (If it is on the desktop).

Double click the **My Computer** 🖳 icon.

Double click the **Local drive** icon (usually C:), the **Windows** folder, and then the **System32** folder. If files are hidden, click **Show the contents of this folder** to display the files. *You will need to scroll through the window to find the calculator icon.*

Double click the **Calc** 🖩 icon. *The calculator program opens.*

Click the **Close** ✕ button on the calculator window to close the application.

4. Identify application programs on the system.

Click the **Start** start button on the taskbar.

Select **All Programs**.

List the applications programs that are accessible on this computer.

5. Identify the operating system.

Click the **Start** start button, and select **Control Panel**. *The control panel window opens.*

Click the **Performance and Maintenance** option. *The performance and maintenance window opens.*

Double click the **System** 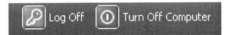 icon. *The system information window appears.*

If using a different version of Windows, look around the control panel for system information.

What version of Windows are you using? _____

What is the processor for this computer? _____

What is the speed and RAM for this computer? _____

Click the **Close** button on the top right of the System Properties window.

Close all remaining open windows.

6. Shut down the computer.

Click the **Start** button (see Figure 2.2).

Figure 2.2

Shutting Down

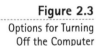

Click **Turn off the computer.** *The following screen appears* (Figure 2.3).

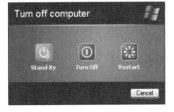

Figure 2.3

Options for Turning
Off the Computer

Click **Turn off** from the options.

At work and in some laboratories, users do NOT turn off the computer. In that case, select the option for logging off and follow the directions given. Some computers automatically turn themselves off when shutting down; others require the user to physically turn them off. The same applies to the monitor.

Assignment 1: Compare Two Computers, Surge Protectors, and UPS Devices

Directions

1. Obtain two advertisements for a microcomputer from the newspaper, from computer magazines, or from a store that sells computers.

2. Compare the two computers by filling in the following form.

3. Make a recommendation for one.

4. Turn in both the form and the computer advertisements.

5. Recommend a surge protector and UPS.

NAME: _____

Features/Specifications	Computer 1	Computer 2
System Unit:		
Make/model		
Microprocessor type		
Speed	GHz	GHz
RAM	MB	MB
Number of expansion slots		
Number and type of ports		
Secondary Storage:		
Hard drive	GB	GB
Floppy drives	Yes/No	Yes/No
Zip/Super drive	Yes/No	Yes/No
CD-ROM	Yes/No	Yes/No
If yes, speed		
Writable	Yes/No	Yes/No
DVD drive	Yes/No	Yes/No
Tape drive	Yes/No	Yes/No
Flash stick	Yes/No	Yes/No
I/O Devices:		
Keyboard included	Yes/No	Yes/No
Mouse included	Yes/No	Yes/No
Monitor included	Yes/No	Yes/No
Monitor type and size		
Printer included	Yes/No	Yes/No
If yes, make		
If yes, type		
Connectivity:		
Modem	Yes/No	Yes/No
Modem type		
Ethernet card	Yes/No	Yes/No
Wireless enabled		
Additional Information:		
Sound system	Yes/No	Yes/No
Operating system	Yes/No	Yes/No
If yes, specify		
Additional software		
If so, specify	Yes/No	Yes/No
Cost:		

Recommendation:

Rationale/Comments:

Surge Protector and UPS:

Because computers and their peripherals are an investment, users need to protect them. Evaluate two surge protectors and two UPS devices. Make a recommendation of which one a user should purchase and why.

Surge Protectors

Criteria	Surge #1	Surge #2
Response time (less than 10 nanoseconds)		
Joules (How much electricity can be absorbed—at least 600)		
Indicator Light (unit is working)		
Cost		

UPS

Calculate what size is needed (add the amps used by the monitor, CPU, and storage devices and anything else intended to be plugged into the UPS. Multiply that total by 110 volts). Find a site that evaluated UPS and support your decision with a review for the unit recommended.

Assignment 2: Compare PDAs and Select Software
Directions

1. Compare two PDAs using the following criteria.

   Use—What do you want to do with a PDA?

   Software—What software is available for this PDA?

   Size—How important is size?

   Input device—What is the data entry type that is available for this unit?

   Operating system—Is the operating system Palm OS or PocketPC (formerly MS CE)?

   Display—What type of display comes with this model?

   Memory—How much memory comes with it? Can more be added?

   Power supply—Does it come with alkaline (AAA) or rechargeable (lithium) batteries?

   Ports—How does the PDA interact with the computer?

   Cost—How much does it cost?

2. You just won a PDA (Palm M515) and were also awarded $100 for software. Develop a list of software and justify your need for each piece of software. Include both free software programs and those with a cost attached. If there is a cost, is it a one-time fee or a yearly fee?

   Here are some sites to start your search:

Medical PDA Software	http://www.medspda.com/
Collective Med.com	http://collectivemed.com/
Palm Gear	http://www.palmgear.com/

The Computer and Its Operating System Environment

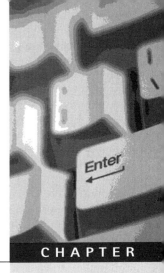

CHAPTER

3

OBJECTIVES

1. Describe the Windows operating system environment.
2. Describe the boot process.
3. Describe a graphical user interface and operating system trends.
4. Identify the process for managing the desktop and windows.
5. Identify basic concepts of file and disk management, including file-naming conventions.

E very desktop computer relies on an operating system to function. Computers without a functioning operating system are just pieces of hardware with the exception of simple, single-purpose computers such as those that control a microwave or oven. Although there are many operating systems for different types of computers, such as the OS for MAC and UNIX/Linux for workstation and larger computers, this chapter describes the operating system environment for the majority of personal computers (PCs): Windows.

Windows is based on a friendly interface between the user and the hardware. This is called a graphical user interface (GUI) and is designed to take advantage of the computer's graphic and mouse capabilities to make using the commands and applications easier. The user no longer needs to remember commands but uses the mouse in a point-and-click approach to issuing commands.

Critical to working in any operating system environment is the ability to manage files and folders. Files contain data and information, whereas folders are storage places for files. This chapter also includes information on managing files and folders using My Computer and Windows Explorer.

► 3.1 OPERATING SYSTEM ENVIRONMENT

Operating systems are responsible for many of the "housekeeping" tasks needed by the computer. The operating system "wakes" the computer through a set of commands and routines that lets the computer recognize the central processing unit, memory, keyboard, disk drives, and printers. The purpose of the operating system is to supervise the operation of the computer's hardware components and to coordinate the flow and control of data. Without the operating system, the user cannot run language or application software.

Today, most operating systems (platforms) come preinstalled on the hard drive of the computer. Several versions of the Windows operating system are in use: 98, 2000, ME, NT, XP, and others that are in the works. There are also versions of operating systems designed for mobile devices such as PDAs where the operating system resides on a read only memory (ROM) chip. The general trend in these versions is the integration of Internet capabilities, the ability to perform multiple tasks at the same time, the ability to work in network environments, and increased inclusion of security and multimedia capabilities.

To become proficient in using the computer, a basic understanding of how the system works and how to manage the desktop environment is needed. This means learning how to customize the desktop, manipulate the windows, switch between applications, and manage files and folders.

Starting the Computer: The Boot Process

The boot process refers to turning on the computer and initiating a series of actions. A cold boot is starting the computer when it has been powered off. It also includes using the restart button on the computer if it has one. A warm boot is the process of restarting a computer that is already on by pressing the **Ctrl + Alt + Del** keys together or selecting the **Start** button, the **Turn Off Computer** option, and clicking the **Restart** ❄ button. Use a warm boot when installing new software or when the computer stops responding.

POST TEST: When the computer is turned on, the power supply sends an electrical signal to the processor, causing it to reset itself and find the BIOS (basic input and output system) instructions on the ROM (read only memory) chip. The BIOS performs a POST, or Power On Self Test. This test analyzes the buses, clock, memory, drives, and ports to make sure that all of the hardware is working properly. The results of this test are compared with data stored in the CMOS (complementary metal-oxide semiconductor) chip.

SYSTEM FILES AND KERNEL: Once this is completed, the software loaded in ROM activates the computer's disk drives and looks for a bootable sector of a disk—the part of the disk containing a program that loads the system files into memory. Depending on the computer this could involve checking the floppy, CD, and/or hard drive. Once found, the system files are loaded into memory. This central module of the operating system is referred to as the kernel. It is the part of the operating system that loads first and remains in memory as long as the computer is turned on. The operating system in memory is now in control of monitoring system resources. This startup procedure runs very quickly on new computers, and if problems are found, the computer makes beeping sounds and then stops running. If all goes well, the user will be asked to log-in or on PCs to select their account, and the desktop will appear.

This information is not critical to using a computer. It does, however, increase the ability to problem solve when something goes wrong during the boot process. For example, when a message "non-system disk error" appears, this means that a nonbootable disk is in the *A* drive. The user left a data disk in the drive and the data disk does not have the necessary system files for the computer to proceed. If the data disk is removed and any key pressed, the computer will proceed with configuring the computer for use. If the on button is pressed and no activity is heard, the computer may have been unplugged. It cannot initiate the startup because it needs electricity to trigger the boot process, and thus, it does nothing.

► 3.2 GRAPHICAL USER INTERFACE (GUIs)

Both Windows and Macintosh OS use GUIs for the user to interact with the operating system. Figure 3.1 shows a typical Windows desktop with its graphical interface.

Although the focus of this chapter is the windows operating system, some features common to both Windows and Mac OS are listed here.

Desktop

The desktop is the area on the screen where the icons and taskbar are displayed. It is the primary workspace in the Windows environment that fills the screen. This is what displays when the computer is turned on or, if necessary, when the user logs in. The desktop may be customized to suit the user. That means the colors and the location of objects can be changed, images can be added to the background of the desktop, and screen savers can be installed. The default look of the desktop changed with Windows XP.

Dialog Box

The dialog box is a special window that requires the user to make selections to implement the commands. It contains options from which the

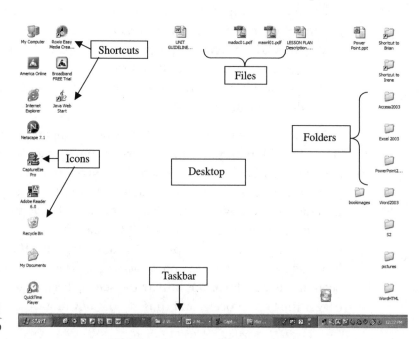

Figure 3.1

Windows XP Desktop

user selects. This may require typing information into a textbox (such as a file name), selecting from a list box (such as selecting fonts and sizes in a print dialog box), clicking a square or circle to make a selection (such as print all pages, current pages, or certain pages in the print dialog box), using a drop-down box, or clicking a button.

Menus

Menus are lists of commands that are available by selecting a command category from the menu bar.

Mouse

A device used to select objects and issue commands is a mouse. The idea is to make issuing commands faster, especially for the nontypist. GUIs depend on the mouse or other pointing devices to select objects or commands from menus and toolbars. Most of the commands accessed with the mouse also have their equivalent keyboard strokes. Refer to Chapter 2 for a description of mouse actions.

Objects

Small pictures or graphic representations of icons, files, folders, and shortcuts located on the desktop are referred to as objects. Placing the pointer on an object, and clicking selects it. Double clicking the object opens it. Right clicking an object opens a shortcut menu, sometimes called a content-sensitive menu.

Pointer

A pointer is the symbol used to represent the insertion point. Many application programs change the look of the pointer to reflect the process the system is expecting. For example, the pointer changes to a double-headed arrow ($\leftrightarrow$) to represent resizing the window. Use the pointer to select commands from menus and toolbars. Different pointer shapes will be presented as they occur in discussions about application programs.

Taskbar

The taskbar is generally at the bottom of the desktop. It is used to access applications and files. All open windows become items on the taskbar.

The default look of the taskbar changed in Windows XP; it is no longer gray but is blue with a green start button.

Windows A window is a place on the desktop where the contents of application programs, files, or folders are displayed. Each program or file has its own window. Each window contains a title bar, menu bar, one or more toolbars, and a status bar. If all of the contents of the window cannot be displayed because of the window size, the window will also contain scroll bars. Additional window controls include close, maximize, minimize, and restore.

The GUI provides the user with a consistent look and easy-to-use commands. The common features and looks enable the user to adjust quickly to other applications and to move between the applications easily.

► 3.3 MANAGING THE DESKTOP

This section discusses the layout of the desktop and how to manage the desktop. Most workers enjoy arranging their own desks in a specific order that makes them more comfortable and productive in their work environment. Personal items are added to their desk. The computer desktop is designed to mimic one's personal desktop.

Objects on the Desktop

The desktop displays several objects by default. Default means that, unless told otherwise, the computer uses a certain setting or configuration. Figure 3.1 shows some of these default objects: icons, folders, shortcuts, files, and the taskbar.

Icons Icons represent applications, such as Internet Explorer and MSN, and special programs, such as the Recycle Bin. The following list describes some of the common icons found on the desktop in a Windows environment. Windows XP places the Recycle bin icon on the desktop by default. All other programs are located through the Start button or Quick Launch area of the taskbar unless they are added to the desktop when a new program is installed on the computer or the default settings are changed. Every computer may not have all of the following icons; also, some may have additional icons not shown here.

My Computer

In earlier versions of Windows, My Computer was on the desktop. In Windows XP, it is located through the **Start** button, **My Computer** by default. A user can add it to the desktop by right clicking the entry on the start menu and selecting **Show on desktop**. Use this icon for viewing and accessing all storage drives and devices connected to the computer.

Recycle Bin

The recycle bin stores deleted files until emptied. Files from external storage devices (3.5" floppy drive and zip drives) are not temporarily stored here. They are deleted immediately. This icon is placed on the Windows XP desktop by default.

My Documents

The My Documents folder is used to store Microsoft Office documents by default. In Windows XP, it is located through the **Start** button, **My Documents** by default. A user can add it to the desktop by right clicking the entry on the start menu and selecting **Show on desktop**.

Internet
Explorer

This icon starts Internet Explorer. Use it to access the World Wide Web (WWW or Web). In earlier versions of Windows, it may be on the desktop; in Windows XP, it is on the Quick Launch area of the taskbar.

My Network
Places

If the computer is connected to a network, the user has access to the My Network Places icon. Use it for viewing and accessing network resources.

Other icons may be added to the desktop or quick launch area of the taskbar. For example, when a laptop is used regularly, there may be an icon called My Briefcase that is used to synchronize files between the desktop and the laptop.

Folders

Folders are holding places for files and may also be located on the desktop. Pictures of yellow file folders represent them (🗀). Folders provide a way to organize work by storing like programs and files in them. Folders may be embedded within other folders to create a hierarchical structure to the system. How to create folders is discussed later in this chapter.

Files

Files contain data and are created in applications such as Word, Excel, PowerPoint, etc. Files are where work is done. Icons representing the file take the look associated with the application. For example, a Word file is represented by a *W* symbol on the icon representing the file. Files are created when work is saved in an application or when the Create New File command is selected from the shortcut menu.

Shortcuts

These are pointers to an actual application, folder, or file. They contain the path to the executable file for the application, to the folder, or to the file. Deleting one only deletes the shortcut, not the application, folder, or file. Shortcuts are represented by a right curved arrow on the bottom left of the icon. In Figure 3.1, there are shortcuts to QuickTime, AOL demo, and a few other programs. Use shortcuts to provide quick access to commonly used applications, folders, or files. The process of creating them is presented later in this chapter.

Taskbar

The taskbar, by default, is located at the bottom of the screen and may be moved to any screen edge. The taskbar is actually four separate components, although it looks like one object. At the far left is the **Start Button**, which opens the **Start Menu** and provides access to programs, documents, the find feature, settings, help, and shutdown. To the right of the Start button is the **Quick Launch** area. Add frequently used applications to the Quick Launch area to keep the desktop uncluttered. To the far right is the **Notification area**. This contains the clock and often icons for programs that usually run in the background and need only occasional user input. Examples of these types of programs are Norton Anti-Virus AutoProtect and the volume control. The remainder is the body of the taskbar itself. Most programs place a button on the taskbar when they are opened. Similar applications are located together. Clicking one of these buttons allows the user to bring that application's window to the foreground and make it active. The taskbar helps the user to switch from one application to another.

The Start *start* button changed with Windows XP. It has expanded to replace many of the icons that were formerly on the desktop (Figure 3.2). What used to be called Programs is now called All Programs. The Start menu now contains the username at the top with an icon next to it that can be changed or customized. On the left

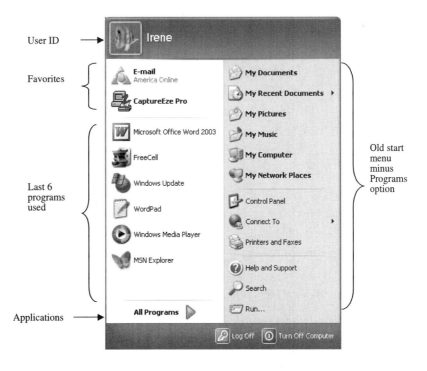

Figure 3.2
Start Menu

side are the most recently accessed programs and a list of favorite programs. This is Microsoft's attempt at cleaning the desktop. A practice exercise at the end of this chapter demonstrates how to customize the start menu.

Pointer Shapes

Before working in the windows environment and moving things around, it is important to discuss the varying pointer or cursor shapes. During different actions in the Windows world, the pointer changes shape. When it does that, the computer expects to complete certain operations and responds accordingly.

 This is the ready arrow. The program is waiting for commands. Use it to select objects, double click objects, right click objects, drag objects, or choose menu or icon commands.

 Use the I-beam to insert text. It appears when the user is over a text field along with the insertion point (blinking vertical bar). The user is expected to type text. The text is inserted at the location of the vertical bar or insertion point, not the I-beam location, which could be over any text field.

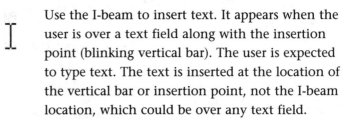 These are the window-sizing pointers. Use them to resize windows. Sizing pointers appear when the cursor is over a window border. There are four versions: left–right, up–down, left slanted, and right slanted. Left–right arrows widen the window. Up–down arrows lengthen the window, and slanted arrows widen and lengthen the window simultaneously.

The hourglass means that the computer is processing and cannot process any further commands until it finishes processing. Wait. Do not type or click the mouse button until the hourglass disappears. If the user clicks before the ready arrow appears, the computer may freeze, stop working, or crash.

The hand means that the mouse pointer is over a linked object or linked text. Clicking the text or object will bring more information from this site or another site. Use the hand to obtain additional information.

 When the mouse pointer looks like this, the action attempted is not available. This is the no-mouse pointer look.

Additional pointer shapes are discussed as they appear in specific applications.

Changing the Appearance of the Desktop

The default theme for the Windows XP desktop is Windows XP with a Bliss background and a blue color. In earlier versions of windows, the desktop was teal. Many users never change the default theme, background, or color scheme; others like change and stimulation in the workday world, and thus, they change it regularly. Windows provides for both types of users by letting the user choose the desktop theme and color scheme. If the default theme is changed, the new settings remain until changed again.

▶ **To change the default theme:**

Right click a blank area of the desktop.

From the short cut menu, select **Properties**.

Click the **Themes** tab.

Select a theme from the theme drop-down menu.

To see the theme before exiting the dialog box, click **Apply**.

When satisfied with a theme, click **OK**.

▶ **To change the desktop background and color:**

Right click a blank area of the desktop.

From the short cut menu, select **Properties**.

Click the **Desktop** tab.

Select the **Background** and **Color** desired.

Click **Apply** to see the changes.

Click **OK** when the correct changes are selected.

The desktop may also be changed from the control panel. To access the control panel, select the **Start Button** on the taskbar, the **Control Panel** option, and **Appearances & Themes**, or double click the **My Computer** icon, select **Control Panel** from the Task Pane on the right, and select **Appearances & Themes**.

Moving Objects on the Desktop

Any object on the desktop may be moved and placed anywhere on the desktop. Windows provides an option to change the location of any object. The taskbar can be located on any of the four edges of the screen. The default is to place the taskbar on the bottom of the screen.

► **To change the location of the taskbar:**

Place the mouse pointer on a **blank** area of the taskbar.

Drag the taskbar to the **left**, **right**, **bottom**, or **top** of the screen.

Release the mouse button.

When dragging the taskbar, it initially appears not to move. Keep dragging the mouse toward the edge of the screen; eventually the taskbar will move.

► **To change the location of an icon, folder, shortcut, or file:**

Select the object, and **Drag** it to the new location.

Right click a **blank area** of the desktop.

From the short cut menu, select **Arrange Icons By** and **Align to Grid** (Figure 3.3).

The objects (icons) will now be in the general area where they were moved but will be in a straight column or row. An invisible checkerboard is

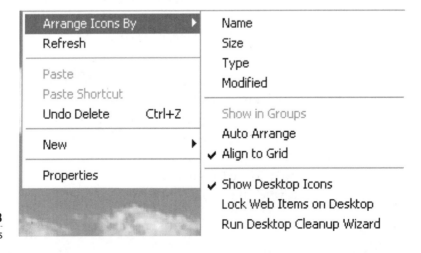

Figure 3.3

Arrange Icons

on the screen, and when issuing the command **Align to Grid**, the icons are snapped into the closest square to produce straight rows and columns. If the objects (icons) snap back into place when they should be moveable, right click a **blank area** of the desktop, select **Arrange Icons By** and **Auto Arrange** to remove the check mark for that selection (see Figure 3.3). The check mark causes the icons to snap back into place.

There are four choices under Arrange Icons By: name, size, type, and modified. The icons will then be arranged on the left side of the desktop in the order selected. The disadvantage to this option is that every time new objects are added, they will be in different spots on the desktop. Most people like their objects in a consistent place on the desktop so they do not need to spend time looking for them.

Choosing a Screen Saver

Screen savers are moving or static pictures displayed on the desktop when no activity takes place for a specified period of time. They were initially designed to protect the monitor from having images burnt onto it. Today, they are primarily used for decoration. Many screensavers come with the operating system, and others may be obtained free from the Internet or purchased at computer software stores.

▶ To set up a screen saver:

Right click a **Blank area** of the desktop.
Choose **Properties** from the shortcut menu.
Click the **Screen Saver** tab.
Click the screen saver **Down Arrow**, and select a **Screen Saver Image**.
Make any appropriate adjustments with the **Settings button**.
Click **Apply** and **OK**.

Shutting Down the System

When the user finishes working with the computer, it is important to shut down the system before turning off the computer. Shutting down the computer saves the current settings and prevents the corruption of files (see Figure 3.4).

▶ To shut down the system:

Click the **Start** button on the taskbar.
Select **Turn Off Computer**.
Select the appropriate option (in most cases, **Turn Off**) and click **OK**.

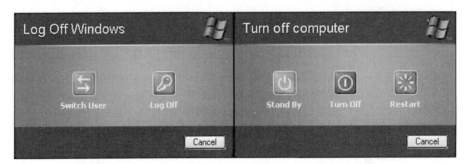

Figure 3.4
Log Off and Turn Off
the Computer

▶ **To log off and prepare the computer for another user:**

Click the **Start** button on the taskbar.

Select **Log Off**.

Select the appropriate option (in most cases, **Log Off**) and click **OK**.

Most of the time, the appropriate option will be either Log Off or Turn Off. In most computer laboratories, the user logs off and does not turn off the computer. The computer saves all of the current user settings, closes all programs, and then prepares to receive another user. The computer remains turned on, and a log in window appears with instructions (press **Ctrl**, **Alt**, **Del**) for how to log in. The log-in screen appears for the user to type a user ID and password. On a nonnetworked computer, a message appears on the screen to click your user name. Be careful with the Switch User option. This option lets another user log on while keeping the previous user's programs and files open.

At the end of the work day or as appropriate at home, the best choice is to select Turn Off. The computer will proceed with shutting down. Most computers today will turn off their system unit automatically, but the monitor may still need to be turned off. The Stand By option puts the computer in a low-power state but will let the user quickly resume working. The computer looks like it is turned off, but the yellow power lights remain on. To restart the computer, press the power button on the computer, or in some laboratories, press the spacebar key. Use the Restart option when updating or installing new programs. The computer will turn off and then restart itself.

▶ **3.4 MANAGING WINDOWS**

This section describes the layout of most application windows and the process of controlling the windows and changing the windows display options. All applications, files, and folders display in a window. Each window shares similar

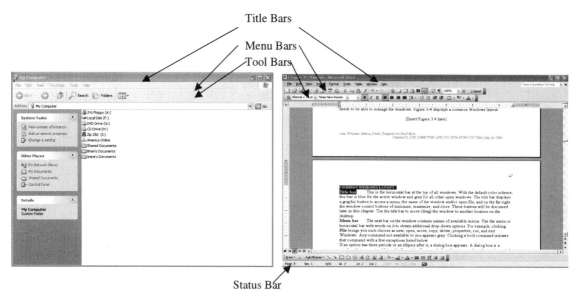

Figure 3.5

Typical Windows

attributes. To be able to work in the Windows world efficiently, the user needs to be able to manage the windows. Figure 3.5 displays a common window's layout on the left and an application window's layout on the right.

Common Windows Layout

Title Bar

This is the horizontal bar at the top of all windows. With the default color scheme, this bar is dark blue for the active window and light blue for all other open windows. The title bar displays a graphic button that can be used to access a menu or the name of the window and/or open file, and on the far right, there are the window control buttons that minimize, maximize, and close the window. These buttons are discussed later in this chapter. Use the title bar to move (drag) the window to another location on the desktop.

Menu Bar

The next bar on the window contains names of available commands. Use the menu or horizontal bar with words on it to obtain additional drop-down options. For example, clicking **File** brings up such choices as new, open, create shortcut, delete, rename, properties, and close, depending on the open program. Any command not available at this time appears dimmed. In Windows

XP, frequently used commands migrate to the top of the drop-down menu.

To display all of the commands for a specific group, click the menu command, and wait a few seconds. The full menu will appear. Another way to display all the commands for a specific group

is to click the double down arrows ( ) at the bottom of the drop-down menu.

To change the default to display the full set of options in the drop-down menu,

> Click **View**, **Toolbars**, **Options** tab, and place a **check** in the Always show full menu box. Click the **Close** button. Now the full list of options will display in the drop-down menu.

If an option has three periods or an ellipsis after it, a dialog box appears. A dialog box is a window that requests additional information from the user before the command can be implemented. For example, in Figure 3.6, the commands New, Open, Save as, and Print will all bring up a dialog box. Complete the information as appropriate in the dialog box and click OK for the command to be executed.

If an option has a right arrow, another menu appears. In Figure 3.6, the Permissions and Send To commands will bring other menus. This other menu is sometimes called a nested or submenu.

Toolbars

Most windows display one or more toolbars. The standard toolbar provides access to commonly used commands such as Create a new file, Open a file, Save a file, Print a file, and Cut/ Copy/Paste data or images (see Figure 3.7 Toolbars). These commands are discussed in detail in Chapter 4. Additional or different commands may appear in some applications because of the nature of particular programs. For example, the Web browsers

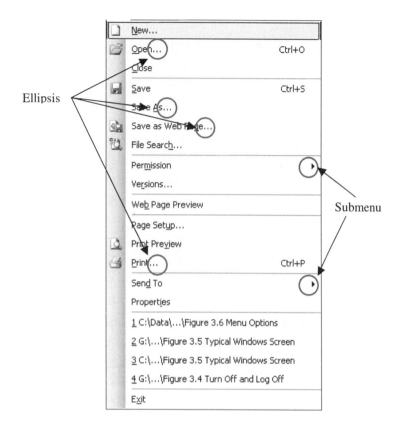

Figure 3.6

Menu Options

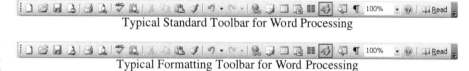

Typical Standard Toolbar for Word Processing

Figure 3.7

Toolbars

Typical Formatting Toolbar for Word Processing

(discussed in Chapter 9) require a different set of commands. The standard toolbar in this type of application contains access to commands such as Back, Forward, Stop, Refresh or Reload, Home, and Search.

If there is a second toolbar, it is generally a formatting toolbar. The toolbar provides for quick access to commonly used character, paragraph, and page formatting commands. The second toolbar under the top toolbar in Figure 3.7 is a formatting toolbar. By default, Windows XP has the standard and formatting toolbar sharing the same line. Frequently used toolbar commands migrate to the visible section of the toolbar.

To see commands not showing on the toolbar,

double click the vertical dotted line (⋮) to the left of each toolbar. To always display two toolbars, click the **Toolbar options** button to the far right of the toolbar, and select the **Show Buttons on Two Rows** option (Figure 3.8).

Windows gives the user the ability to display additional toolbars through the **View**, **Toolbars** command. Additional toolbars, such as the ruler bar and draw toolbar, are discussed in the appropriate application chapters.

Status Bar

Some applications use a horizontal bar at the bottom of the window to display such things as the number of objects in the window, a description of menu commands, the number of pages in a document, the location of the cursor, and special tog-

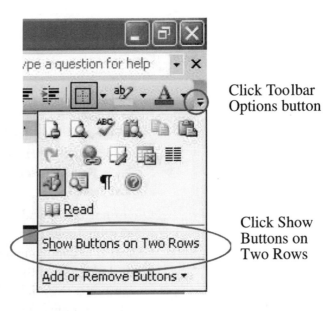

Click Toolbar
Options button

Click Show
Buttons on
Two Rows

Figure 3.8

Set Toolbars to Two
Rows

gle switches such as overwrite, num lock, and cap lock. Contents of the status bar depend on what is important in the application. For example, in Excel it displays whether the num lock and cap lock keys are on or off.

Scroll Bars

Located along the right and bottom of the window are the scroll bars. They appear when there are more data than can be displayed in the window. Figure 3.5 displays both a horizontal and vertical scroll bar. Use them to move through a document or to view data when the entire document is not visible. There are arrows at the top and bottom of the vertical scroll bar on the right and at the left and right for the horizontal scroll bar on the bottom with a box somewhere between them. Clicking the arrow buttons moves the user slowly through the window. The box or elevator in the scroll shaft indicates the current locations relative to the total document. Dragging the elevator in the scroll bar gives more control over viewing the contents of the window. The elevator shaft may also be clicked to go to an approximate location in the document.

Task Pane

A task pane appears on the left side of the My Computer window and on the right side of application windows. In the My Computer window, it lists common file and folder management tasks (to be discussed later) and other places the user might want to access while using that particular window. In application windows, it changes based on what is being done in the application.

Opening a Window

Several ways are available to open a window or program:

- Double click the icon representing the window to open it.
- Right click the icon representing the window to open it, and select **Open** from the menu.

- Select **Start** from the taskbar, and then select the **Window** to be opened. For example, to open a recently used file, select **Start**, **My Recent Documents**, and the **Name of the file**. To open the control panel folder, select **Start** and **Control Panel**.

Once the window is open, perform the appropriate tasks. Because more than one window may be opened at a time, the user will need to control the window display.

Controlling the Window

Several controls are available for working with windows. Use these controls to move a window to another location on the desktop, change the size of a window, or close a window. The resize features permit the user to control the actual size of the window; the maximize and minimize buttons use default standards to control the size of the window. Maximize expands the window to fill the screen. The minimize button places a button on the taskbar and removes the window from the desktop. The program remains open but is running in the background. The restore button returns the window to the size it was before it was maximized.

These buttons are used when running multiple programs, opening multiple windows, or opening several files. This permits the user to view or work on each while placing the others in the background.

In addition, windows may be arranged on the desktop in cascade, tile horizontally, or tile vertically. When many windows are open, the cascade option works well to see all the open windows. All open windows will be cascaded from the top of the screen down showing the title bar of each open window. Tiling horizontally and vertically is used to partition the screen into quadrants depending on the number of opened windows. Use this feature for dragging and dropping data from one window to another.

Function	Directions
Move a window	Click a blank area in the **Title Bar** of the window to move.
	Hold down the mouse button and drag the window to a new location and release the mouse button.
Resize a window	Select the window to resize by clicking the **Title Bar**.
	Point to a window **Border** or **Corner**.

	When the cursor becomes a double-headed arrow (↔ ↕), drag the **corner** or **border** until it is the desired size.
	Release the mouse button.
Enlarge a window	Select the window to enlarge by clicking the **Title Bar**.
	Click the **Maximize** ( ) button in the upper right corner of the Title Bar. This button is a toggle button and shares space with the restore button.
Reduce a window	Select the window to reduce by clicking the **Title Bar**.
	Click the **Minimize** ( ) button in the upper right corner of the Title Bar.
Restore a window	Select the Window to restore by clicking the **Title Bar**.
	Click the **Restore** ( ) button in the upper right corner of the Title Bar. This button is a toggle button and shares space with the maximize button.
Close a window	Select the Window to close by clicking the **Title Bar**.
	Click the **Close** ( ) button in the upper right corner of the Title Bar.
Arrange a window	Right click a blank area of the **Taskbar**.
	Select **Cascade** or **Tile windows horizontally** or **vertically**.

▶ 3.5 MANAGING FILES AND FOLDERS

This section deals with managing files and folders. The file system is the core for working efficiently and effectively with a computer. Knowing how to find, access, and manage files is important to managing the system. There are two main ways to access files—My Computer and Windows Explorer—and several different views to see those files once they have been accessed. Windows XP provides easy access to common file and folder management tasks through the left-side task pane in the open window. Once a file or folder is selected, the appropriate commands appear in the left task pane.

Some basic file and folder management concepts are introduced here. The specifics of creating, renaming, moving, copying, and deleting files and folders then follow.

Designating Default Disk Drives

A default drive is the drive the program uses to find and save files unless told otherwise. Remember from Chapter 2 that the drive letter designation for the hard drive is generally *C*, for a 3.5" drive *A*, and for a CD ROM or zip drive *B*, *D*, or *E*. Most programs use a default folder on the *C* drive to store new files created. For example, Microsoft Office uses the My Documents folder on the *C* drive to store all Microsoft Office files. All programs provide the ability to change the default storage drive and folder. To do this, find the preferences or options command, which generally is located in the tools or edit menus. One of the options in the dialog window is usually the ability to change the location of files.

When not permitted to alter settings in the computer laboratory or work environment, use the File, Save as command to change the location of files each time the program is accessed. In the Save as dialog window, click the down arrow button in the Save in textbox area and select the correct storage device.

Diskette Preparation Command (Format)

The **Format** command initializes a diskette by placing sectors and tracks on the diskette and creates the file allocation table, an index to where the files are stored physically on the diskette. This process magnetically maps the diskette. Diskettes cannot be used unless formatted. Many diskettes and most zip disks come preformatted, and there is no need to reformat them unless they are being recycled. Formatting erases all data on the diskette.

Sector	A sector is a pie-shaped segment of tracks on a disk.
Track	Tracks are concentric rings on a disk or diskette.

CDs also need to be prepared to receive data. CD drives generally come with software for preparing the disc for a variety of functions. One of these functions is to prepare the CD as a data CD or with Drag-to-Disc format (Drag-to-Disc option is part of Roxio's Easy Media Creator software that backs up data to a recordable CD or DVD). Files may be added to the disc by dragging them to the CD using My Computer or Windows Explorer. This feature functions like other magnetic storage media.

Function	Directions
Format—Floppy	Double click the **My Computer** icon.
	Right click the **A drive** icon.

	Select **Format...**
	Click **Start**.
	Click **Close** to finish format.
Format—Zip	Double click the **My Computer** icon.
	Right click the **Zip drive** icon.
	Select **i–Format...**
	The zip drive utility format command for preparing the disk must be used. In this example, the format is for the Iomega drive and appears as i-format.
	Follow the directions on the screen to reformat the disk.
Format—CD	First, there must be a writable CD drive on the computer.

Next, use the software that comes with the drive to prepare the disc to receive data. These directions use Roxio's Easy Media Creator software version 7.

To format a blank disc manually:

- With Drag-to-Disc running, insert a blank, rewritable disc into the recorder.
- From the Drag-to-Disc menu, choose **Format Disc** or right click the CD-R drive and select **Format**.
- Select the appropriate options in the Format Options dialog box.
- Click **OK**.

For most CD recorders, the Drag-to-Disc command automatically begins formatting when files are added to a blank rewritable disc. When preparing CDs, follow the directions that come with the software for the disc drive.

When reformatting a diskette, always check to make sure that it does not contain any important files because formatting the diskette will erase those files.

Creating Folders

Organize and manage files by creating folders and saving work in them. A folder is a storage place for files and other folders. How they are organized depends on what is being done. For example, a folder might contain all files that are related to a specific course, another for personal items, and yet another for articles or publications. Storing files in the appropriate folders allows for easy retrieval and backup of data. Associating files with projects or tasks allows for easier cleanup when projects or tasks are completed. Saving all files in **My Documents** or **My Files** folders makes retrieving and deleting more difficult and time consuming. An icon 📁 represents each folder.

▶ To create the folder:

Point to a **blank area** of the desktop or open storage device window.

Click the **right** mouse button. *A shortcut menu appears.*

Click the menu item marked **New**. *Another shortcut menu appears.*

Click the menu item labeled **Folder**. *A new folder appears on the desktop or in the storage device window. The folder name is highlighted.*

Type a **Name** for the folder and press **Enter**. *The folder now has the new name.*

When in many applications, a new folder can be created from the Save As dialog box by clicking the New Folder 📁 button located on the toolbar. When in a nonapplication window such as My Documents or My Computer, click the Make a New Folder on the left task pane.

Naming Files and Folders

All files and folders have names. There are three parts to naming a file: filename, delimiter, and file extension. A sample file is My Smiley Face.bmp. Folders have a name, but no delimiter or extension.

Filename

In the previous example file, the portion to the left of the period (My Smiley Face) is the filename. Filenames use letters, numbers, or some special characters up to 255 characters. Legal characters are letters of the alphabet (A–Z), digits (0–9), and all the special characters except * ? < > \ / " : and |. Blank spaces between the characters of the filename may be used to make the filename more readable and understandable; use them with caution, however, as some programs cannot handle file names with spaces or names larger than eight characters. Filenames are not case sensitive. They may be typed in all lowercase, a combination of uppercase and lowercase, or all uppercase. Use a unique filename for each file; there can be no duplicate filenames in the same folder.

Delimiter   The delimiter is the period that separates the file-name from the extension. This is optional; users do not need to use the delimiter unless typing an extension to the filename.

Extension   The portion to the right of the delimiter is the ex-tension. Extensions help to identify the nature of the file. For example, doc is the extension at-tached to Word documents. In most cases, the de-fault option in the Windows environment is to hide the extensions. This means that the user does not need to type the extension. It is assigned to the file by the application used to create the file. In this environment, the extension is then used to identify what application was used to cre-ate the file; when double clicked, the file opens in the appropriate application.

Before working with files, think about some standards to apply to naming files for personal work, for a clinical area, or for a department. There are many ways to do this depending on what work is being done, who does it, what is being shared, how it is shared (on network or diskettes), how it is accessed, and who retrieves it. The important point here is to use an understandable convention that enables the file to be recognized 6 to 12 months after it is created.

To name files and folders, follow the directions given here.

Function	Directions
Name File (Application)	Start an **Application** such as Word or Excel.
	Create the file.
	Select **File**, **Save** or click the **Diskette** button.
	Select a location from the **Save in** text box.
	Type the **File name** in the **File name** text box.
	Click **OK** or press **Enter**.
Name File (On Desktop)	Right click a **blank area** of the desktop or in a Window.
	Select **New**.
	Select the **Type** of file (Word, Excel, etc.).
	Type the **File name**.
	Click **OK** or press **Enter**.

Name Folder	Right click a **blank area** of the desktop or window.
	Select **New** folder.
	Type the **Folder** name.
	Click **OK** or press **Enter**.
	or
	Click the **Make a new folder** command in the task pane of an open nonapplication window.
	Type the **Folder** name and press **Enter**.

Viewing Files and Folders

Once the files and folders are created and named, most users will need to access them. Two choices are available for accessing files and folders: My Computer and Windows Explorer.

My Computer

Double clicking My Computer opens a window that displays the storage devices and folders stored on this computer (Figure 3.9). The screen divides into several areas and lists the appropriate content for each area. Double clicking a storage device or folder results in the current folder being replaced with the new folder. Repeat the double clicking until the file or folder is displayed.

The user may toggle between the command and structure task pane on the left side of the win-

Figure 3.9

My Computer and
Windows Explorer

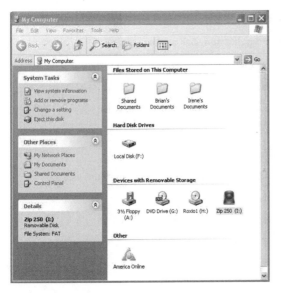

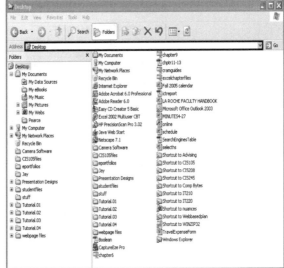

dow by clicking the folders ![Folders icon] Folders button on the toolbar.

Windows Explorer   Windows Explorer provides a different view of files and folders. The left side of the screen shows the organizational structure, whereas the right side shows the contents of the selected device or folder. In Figure 3.9, the top of the structure is the Desktop. All the icons on the desktop are displayed on the left side (My Documents, My Computer, My Network Places, Recycle Bin, etc.). Under My Computer are the storage devices (*A*, *F*, *H*, etc.) and selected folders and shortcuts located on the desktop. The right side of the screen shows the contents of the Desktop.

A plus sign next to an icon on the left side means that there are more objects below it that are not displayed. A minus sign means that level of the structure is fully expanded and visible. The look can be changed by collapsing and expanding each level of the structure on the left side by clicking the plus or minus signs. Clicking an object on the left side results in the contents of that object displaying on the right.

The display of the icons in the window depends on the view selected. There are five options for the display of the icons in the My Computer window and Windows Explorer: thumbnails, tiles, icons, list, and details. If using the Picture folder, there is also another option called filmstrips. Here is a description of each option.

Show in Groups   This option permits the user to group files by any aspect of the file like name, size, and type. Use this view when looking for like files, for instance all Word documents. The default is to group by type.

Thumbnails   This view displays the images a folder contains on a folder icon so the contents of the folder can be quickly identified. Use this view to see the contents of folders quickly.

Tiles	The tiles view displays files and folders as icons. This used to be called large icons. The icon name appears to the right of the icon.
Icons	This view displays files and folders as smaller icons than the tile view. The file name is displayed under the icon.
List	The list view displays files and folders as very small icons followed by the file or folder name. Use this view when there are many files and folders to see.
Details	This view provides the user with details about the file and folder in a list form. Use this view to see more details about the objects.
Filmstrip	This view is available in the pictures folder. A single row of thumbnail images appears.

To use My Computer and Windows Explorer, follow these directions.

Function	Directions
View—My Computer	Double click the **My Computer** icon on the desktop or click **Start**, **My Computer**.
	Double click the **Storage device** where the file is located.
	Double click the file wanted or
	Double click the folders until the correct file displays.
	Double click the file.
View—Windows Explorer	Click **Start**, **Programs**, **Accessories**, **Windows Explorer** or right click the **Start** button and select **Explore**.

To change how files and folders display in the window, follow these directions.

Function	Directions
Change View—Menu	Select **View** from the menu bar.
	Click **Thumbnails**, **Tile**, **Icons**, **List**, or **Detail**.

Change View—Toolbar	Click the **View** button down arrow on the toolbar.
	Click **Thumbnails, Tile, Icons, List**, or **Detail**.

To change how items are grouped, follow these directions.

Function	Directions
Change Grouping	Select **View** from the menu bar and **Arrange Icons by**.
	Click **Name, Size, Type**, or **Modified**.

Copying Files and Folders

The copy command copies one, several, or all of the files from one place to another. That means there will be two of the same files. There are several ways to copy files and folders: use menu systems, use drag and drop, or use the shortcut menu. The process for copying files and folders is the same. When using drag and drop from the *A* drive to another drive such as *C*, the default is to copy. When using drag and drop from the *A* drive to another folder in the *A* drive, the default is to move. The default option can be overridden by right dragging the file. When dropping it in its new location, select copy from the pop-up menu. These directions work for both My Computer and Windows Explorer, except for the task pane. Windows Explorer has no task pane option.

Function	Directions
Copy one file—menu bar	Click the **File** to be copied.
	Select **Edit, Copy** from the menu bar.
	Go to the **new location** and **Click**.
	Select **Edit, Paste**.
Copy one file—task pane	Click the **File** to be copied.
	Click **Copy this File** from task pane.
	Select the **storage** location from the dialog window.
	Click **Copy**.
Copy one file—drag and drop	*This works going only from one drive to a different one.*
	Both file and destination must be visible.
	Select the **File**.
	Drag it to its **new location**.
	Release the mouse button.

	If copying from A to A or C to C, etc.:
	Right drag the **File** to its additional location.
	Release the mouse button.
	Select **Copy here**.
Copy one file—shortcut menu	Select **File**.
	Right click **File**.
	Select **Copy**.
	Go to the **new** location.
	Right click in the **new location**.
	Select **Paste**.
Copy adjacent files	Click the **First** file in the group.
	Hold down the **Shift** key.
	Click the **Last** file in the group.
	Release the **Shift** key.
	Follow any of these sets of directions when all files to be copied are selected.
Copy nonadjacent files	Hold down the **Ctrl** key.
	Click **on each** file to be copied.
	Release the **Ctrl** key.
	Follow any of these sets of directions when all files to be copied are selected.

A box may be dragged around the files to select a group of files. Go to the top left of the group of files. Hold down the left mouse button. Drag the mouse to the opposite corner, and release the mouse button. Once the files are highlighted, follow any of these sets of directions to copy them.

Moving Files and Folders

Moving files and folders is similar to copying. The move command takes a file or folder from one place and puts it in another. It does not duplicate it. There are several ways to move files and folders: use menu systems, use drag and drop, or use the shortcut menu. When moving a file from one drive to another drive, use the right drag option and select move from the pop-up menu. Remember that the default for dragging and dropping a file between different storage devices is copy. When moving from one place on the same storage drive to another on the same storage drive, the default is move. These directions work in both My Computer and Windows Explorer, except for the task pane. Windows Explorer has no task pane option.

Function	Directions
Move one file—menu bar	Click the **File** to be moved.
	Select **Edit, Cut** from the menu bar.
	Go to the **new location** and **Click**.
	Select **Edit, Paste**.
Move one file—task pane	Click the **File** to be moved.
	Click **Move this File** from the task pane.
	Select the **Storage** location from the dialog window.
	Click **Move**.
Move one file—drag and drop	*This only works when going from A to A, C to C, etc.*
	Both the file and destination must be visible.
	Select the **File**.
	Drag to the **new location** on the same drive.
	Release the mouse button.
	If going to a different storage drive:
	Both the file and the destination must be visible.
	Right drag the **File** to the new location.
	Select **Move here** from the shortcut menu.
Move one file—shortcut menu	**Select** a file.
	Right click the **File**.
	Select **Cut**.
	Go to the **new** location.
	Right click in the **new location**.
	Select **Paste**.
Move adjacent files	Click the **First** file in the group.
	Hold down the **Shift** key.
	Click **Last** file in the group.
	Release **Shift** key.

	Follow any of these sets of directions after all files to be moved are selected.
Move nonadjacent files	Hold down the **Ctrl** key.
	Click **each** file to be moved.
	Release the **Ctrl** key.
	Follow any of these sets of directions after all files to be moved are selected.

Deleting Files and Folders

The delete command removes files from the storage device. Use this command to clean storage devices and discard unneeded files. There are several versions of this command, as noted in this section.

When deleting files from a removable storage device such as a floppy diskette or zip disk, the files are not placed in the recycle bin. They are immediately deleted. Only files from the hard drive are deleted to the recycle bin. If files are accidentally deleted from the hard drive, they may be recovered if the recycle bin has not been emptied. Folders deleted to the recycle bin appear as empty folders but actually contain the files in the folder. When restoring a folder in the recycle bin, all of the original files are also restored. These directions work for both My Computer and Windows Explorer, except for the task pane. Windows Explorer has no task pane option.

Function	Directions
Delete—menu bar	Select the **File**.
	Select **File**, **Delete** from the menu.
	Click **Yes** to confirm sending it to Recycle Bin.
Delete—task pane	Select the **File**.
	Click **Delete this File** on the Task pane.
	Click **Yes** to confirm deleting the file or sending it to the Recycle Bin.
Delete—drag and drop	Make both the **File** or **Folder** and the **Recycle Bin** visible.
	Drag the **File** or **Folder** on top of the **Recycle Bin** icon.
	When the icon turns blue, release the **Left** mouse button.
	Click **Yes** to confirm deletion.
Delete—delete key	Click the **File** or **Folder** to highlight it.
	Press the **Delete** key.

	Click **Yes** to confirm its deletion or its trip to the Recycle Bin.
Delete—shortcut menu	Right click **File** or **Folder** to delete.
	Select **Delete** from shortcut menu
	Click **Yes** to confirm its deletion or its trip to the Recycle Bin.

Multiple files and folders may be selected as noted in the copy and move sections. This same technique may be used to delete multiple files or folders at once.

Once files are sent to the Recycle Bin, the Recycle Bin will need to be emptied periodically. How often it is emptied depends on how often files and folders are deleted and how many are deleted.

▶ To empty the Recycle Bin:

Double click the **Recycle Bin** icon.
Select **Empty Recycle bin** from the task pane.
Click **Yes** to confirm the emptying of the recycle bin.

▶ To restore a deleted file or folder:

Double click the **Recycle Bin** icon.
Select the **File** or **Folder** to restore.
Select **Restore all items** from the task pane.

Renaming Files and Folders

The rename command gives the file or folder a new name. Use this command to reorganize and change the names of files to be consistent with an organizational structure or to clarify the name because of additional files or folders created.

Function	Directions
Rename—menu	Select the **file** or **folder** to rename.
	Select **File, Rename** from the menu bar.
	Type the **new name** and press **Enter**.
Rename—task pane	Select the **file** or **folder** to rename.
	Select **Rename this file or folder** from the File and Folder
task	
	pane.
	Type the **new name** and press **Enter**.
Rename—shortcut	Right click the **file** or **folder** to rename.

	Click **Rename** from the shortcut menu.
	Type the **new file name** and press **Enter**.
Rename—click pause click	Click the **file** or **folder** name.
	Pause, and click **again**.
	Type the **new file name** and press **Enter**.

Organizing Folders

Most users store files on removable storage media (floppy disks, zip disks, or flash keys), on hard drives, and on network file servers. Files must be organized so that they can be located and retrieved easily. Electronic files must be organized for the same reason that filing cabinets need to be organized. Electronic files are organized on the storage media in folders and subfolders.

Root Level	The "root" is the top level on which the folders are made. This level stores files the computer needs to access at startup. A general rule is that a folder or file listing of the root level should not occupy more than one screen worth of information.
Folders	Folders organize programs and data files. Before creating them, think about the work being done and the programs that will be used. Most software programs automatically make a directory for their program files when they are installed. Be careful that these directories "fit" the organizational structure of the work world. Customize them during installation if needed.
Subfolders	These folders are contained within other folders. Subfolders assist in providing further divisions or structure to the organization of files.

Some rules for creating and using the folder and subfolder structure are as follows:

1. Place each application suite in its own folder with subfolders for each application program. This makes installation of new versions, deletions of old versions, and maintenance of files easier. Some suites also create subfolders for shared suite files as well as creating the structure automatically.
2. Place programs not belonging to application suites in the Program Files folder in their own subfolder with an appropriate name representing

the application. For example, Adobe Acrobat Reader should have its own folder. Some users create a folder called downloads and then sub-folders for each program downloaded. These are then backed up and used whenever needed. Others also create a Utility Folder off the root and place each Utility program in its own folder within the Utility folder. For example, Norton Anti-Virus, Norton Utilities, and WinZip would each have a folder in the Utility folder.

3. Create folders for storing data files. Never store data files on the root, as they then get mixed with essential computer files. Instead, create a Data folder off the root. In the Data folder, create folders for each user on the system. Let the users then create the appropriate subfolders in their data folder.

4. Create a Graphic Library folder off the root for storing graphic images. The Graphic Library folder could contain subfolders representing graphic file formats or categories. For example, JPG and GIF graphic files or pets, cities, and computers. Some also create a folder for pictures, as many users exchange pictures of family and friends.

5. Use appropriate folder names. No two folders in the same level can have the same name. It is probably better not to name any folder with the same name as another folder.

► 3.6 SELECTED DISK MANAGEMENT CONCEPTS

This section covers a few disk-management concepts that are critical to working with the computer and the operating system.

Copying a Disk

Once files and folders are created and organized, it is a good idea to make a copy of the disk. The Copy Disk command copies all of the files, folders, and structures from one diskette to another, simultaneously erasing all files on the second or target diskette. Use this command to make backup copies of diskettes. Because this makes an exact duplicate of the disk, it requires using a like medium only. That means HD to HD or zip disk to zip disk. This command is not used to backup the hard drive to diskettes, nor is it used to backup a HD diskette to a zip disk.

Because this command erases all files on the target (backup) diskette, check that diskette to make sure no important files are on the disk. The copy disk command can be used in a one-drive system.

Function	Directions
Copy Disk	Insert a **disk** in the floppy disk drive.
	Double click the **My Computer** icon.
	Right click the 3.5" **disk drive** icon (usually drive *A*).
	Select the **Copy Disk** command.
	Click the **floppy** disk drive.
	Click the **Start** button.
	Follow the directions given on the screen.
	Click **Close** to close the Copy dialog box after the copy is done.

When making a copy of a zip disk, the zip disk utility copy command must be used. The process is the same. If using an Iomega zip drive, the copy disk command will have the letter *i* before it.

Backup

Because of the size of hard drives today, most people no longer backup their hard drives. However, that practice will eventually cause the user problems because of hardware or software failures. The question to ask is this: how important are the data? Although applications for the most part can be re-installed, data can be lost if no backup exists. At the least, users should backup all data files, including documents, images, pictures, and in some cases, downloaded freeware. Backup anything that cannot be quickly rein-stalled or recreated. Data stored on the local drive of a networked computer are not routinely backed up when the network is backed up. Only data on the file server are backed up.

The hardware chapter covered storage devices such as tape drives, optical drives, and removable hard drives that can be used for backing up data. What the user needs to ask are things such as the following:

- What type of data do I have that cannot be replaced easily? How much data can I afford to loose?
- What capacity do I need for the backup device?
- How often do I need to backup?
- How reliable is the backup medium?
- How easy is it to use?
- What will it cost?

Ideally, backup systems for large operations are done automatically and regularly. This does not include the local hard drive. Many organizations require users to store critical data on the network file sever so that it is routinely backed up. No critical data are permitted on local hard drives. Those who store some data on the local hard drive can regularly backup the data to their personal space on the file server or copy that data to a CD flash drive.

For a home computer or a small business, this is more difficult to do without a managed network. Some solutions might include a second hard drive installed internally or one that is connected to the computer via a USB or FireWire port. With this approach, the user must remember to do regular backups or use software such as SmartSync Pro to automate the backup process. Automating the backup process requires the computer to be left on. This approach, however, does not solve the issue unless backup files are stored in a different place from the originals. Some experts suggest having a third backup that is stored in a safety deposit box and recycled monthly.

Another solution is to use one of the online backup services. Several companies (e.g., Connected.com, backup.com, and xdrive.com) now offer backup services for a small monthly fee. Although this might sound like a great solution, some drawbacks to this approach exist. Some services discourage certain types of files such as MP3 (music), and others limit how frequently the backups can occur. This approach requires a high-speed Internet connection, trust in the security of the servers used for backup, and trust that the company will not go out of business. Each user must find a solution for backing up critical data that works.

Creating Shortcuts

Shortcuts are used to save time when working in the Windows environment. Instead of using My Computer or Windows Explorer to try to find files, folders, or programs, shortcuts provide access to frequently used items on the desktop. Files, folders, application programs, and storage devices can all have shortcuts. Remember that shortcuts are pointers to these objects; they are not the actual object. Double clicking the shortcut opens the object it is "pointing to." The shortcut tells the computer where to find the object. The general rule for using shortcuts is to create them for frequently used objects. Many people create shortcuts to their data files, the printer, the floppy drive, and selected applications. Do not create shortcuts to infrequently used items. The desktop will become too cluttered.

A shortcut is denoted with a small curved arrow in the lower left corner of the icon. Because it is only a pointer to an actual object, deleting the shortcut only deletes the shortcut, not the actual object to which it is pointing.

▶ To create a shortcut:

Find the **object** that the shortcut will point to.

Resize the windows to make the desktop visible.

Right drag it to the **desktop**.

Select **Create Shortcut(s) here** from the shortcut menu.

In addition, shortcuts can be created for objects on the left side of the start button menu by right clicking the object, selecting Send to, and then Desktop (Create Shortcut). The objects My Documents, My Computer, and My Network Places from the right side of the start button menu can be placed on the desktop by right clicking the object and selecting the Show on Desktop option from the shortcut menu.

Managing Files with Scan Disk and Defragmenter

Before running either program, use the Disk Cleanup program to remove any unwanted files. These files take space and slow the computer. They include things such as temporary Internet files and downloaded program files. Empty the recycle bin. This will free disk space. This should be done on a weekly basis (see Chapter 9 for more on temporary Internet files and cleanup).

Access the Disk Cleanup program through Start, All Programs, Accessories, System Tools and Disk Cleanup. Select the files to remove from the hard drive, and then run the program (Figure 3.10).

Next, use an error-checking tool (ScanDisk) to check the file system for errors and bad sectors. Some technicians recommend using this tool once a week; others recommend using it once a month. In reality, most users are lucky if they do it once or twice a year. Make sure that all programs are closed before running ScanDisk. This includes any program running in the background. If a program is running, ScanDisk will restart itself over and over. On networked computers, this tool may not be accessible unless the user is logged on as the administrator.

▶ To access this error checking tool:

Close all files.

Open **My Computer**.

Right click the **storage device**.

Select **Properties** and the **Tool** tab.

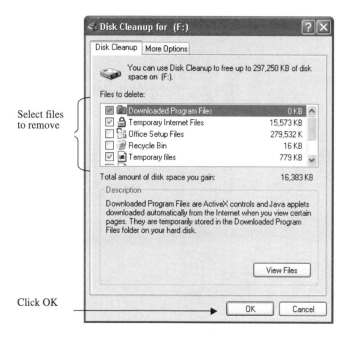

Select files
to remove

Figure 3.10   Click OK

Disk Cleanup

Click the square for **automatically fix file system errors** and **scan for and repair bad sectors**.

Click **Check Now** in the error checking part of the screen (Figure 3.11).

This program takes a while to do its job.

The last file management program is Disk Defragmenter. It consolidates fragmented files and folders on the disk so that each one is stored in a contiguous space. This results in performance improvement in accessing files and folders more efficiently. Once again, all programs must be closed, as this program checks and moves data. This tool should be run about two times per month or more often if programs are loaded and deleted frequently.

▶ **To access Disk Defrag:**

Close all files.

Open **My Computer**.

Right click the **storage device**.

Select **Properties**, and the **Tool** tab.

Click **Defragment Now** in the Defragmentation part of the screen (Figure 3.11).

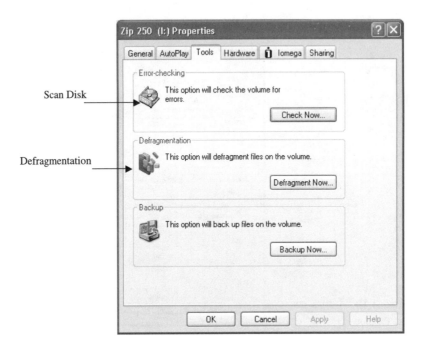

Scan Disk

Defragmentation

Figure 3.11
Scan Disk and
Defragmentation

Updates and Patches

All software, whether programs such as Word, operating systems such as Windows, or device drivers for printers, issue periodic upgrades or patches. Updates are generally enhancements to the software, providing additional features or functions, whereas patches are generally fixes to problems in the software. Many of these deal with blocking security problems inherent in the software that make the user's computer vulnerable to hackers and viruses. The first thing that should be done after installing a software program is to check for updates and patches. After this, every so often the user needs to check for new updates and patches. Some people do this once a month; others do it more frequently.

In Windows XP, the start menu contains an option called Windows Update either on the main menu or under All Programs. Clicking this option takes the user to Microsoft's site. Follow the directions given for updating the computer. When Microsoft scans the computer, a list of updates or patches is presented. These are generally divided into Critical Updates, Windows XP, and Driver Updates. Select the desired updates and download them to the computer. The computer must have an active Internet connection to do this. Note the size of the files before downloading; some of them are quite large and may take substantial time to download, especially over dial-up connections. In addition, a message is displayed periodically on the right side of the taskbar reminding the user to check for updates.

In the Microsoft Office suite, access the updates option by clicking the Help option on the menu bar and selecting Check for Updates.

SUMMARY

This chapter oriented the user to the operating system and the Windows interface. The common objects found on the desktop were presented. Desktop management skills such as setting screensavers, changing desktop colors, moving objects, and managing windows were presented. The chapter ended with file and folder management concepts and commands that teach the user how to create, rename, move, copy, and delete files and folders. Also presented were some basic ideas about organizing files and folders.

Whether the operating system will be proprietary such as Windows or open source like Linux, one thing is certain: there will always be a system for managing the hardware and interfacing with the end user. That system will change to reflect the changes in technology and in user needs.

Exercise 1: Managing a Desktop and Windows
Objectives
1. Identify and describe the desktop.
2. Apply a screensaver.
3. Arrange the desktop to work efficiently and effectively.
4. Change the colors of the desktop.
5. Open, close, minimize, maximize, size, and arrange windows.
6. Switch between windows.

Activity

If necessary, make sure to turn on the computer and monitor and log on.

1. Identify desktop objects using their generic group names, not the specific name of the object the icon represents. Complete these statements:

   An object like this ⬚ is called a(n) _____. It is used for _____.

   An object like this ⬚ is called a(n) _____. It represents _____.

   An object like this ⬚ is called a(n) _____. Use it to _____.

An object like this ![PDF icon] is called a(n) _____ . Use it for _____ .

The bar below is called the _____ . It is used for _____ .

![Windows taskbar: start, icons, Chapter 3, Figure 3.10, My Computer, Microsoft Po..., CaptureEze P..., 12:09 PM]

2. Apply a screensaver.

Right click a **blank area** of the desktop.

Choose **Properties** from the shortcut menu.

Click the **Screensaver** tab.

Click the screensaver **down arrow** ![down arrow] , and then click **Marquee** (Figures 3.12 and 3.13).

Click the **Settings button**. *The screen in Figure 3.12 appears.*

Select position **Random** and background color **Blue**.

Highlight Text, type **Out to lunch, back at 1 PM.**

Click the **Format Text** [Format Text...] button, select **Times New Roman, 72 points, yellow.**

Click **OK, OK.**

Click the **Preview button**, and then click **Apply** and **OK.**

3. Move and arrange objects on the desktop.

Drag the **Internet Explorer** ![IE icon] icon to the right bottom of the desktop.

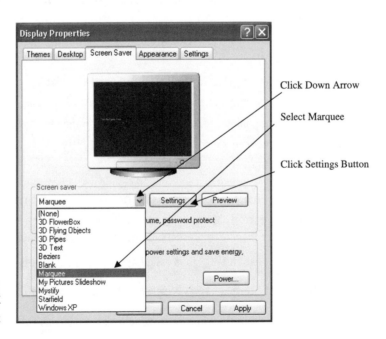

Figure 3.12

Screensaver
Dialog Box

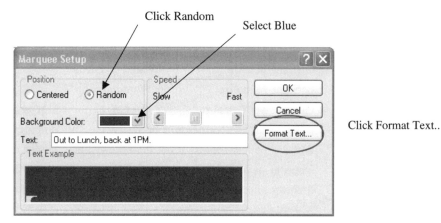

Click Random

Select Blue

Click Format Text..

Figure 3.13
Marquee Setup
Dialog Box

Drag the **Recycle Bin** icon to right bottom of the desktop.

Right click a **blank area** of the desktop. Select **Arrange icons by**, and then select **Name**.

What happened to the icons? _____

Now, drag the **Internet Explorer** icon to the top right of the desktop.

Drag the **Recycle Bin** icon to the top right of the desktop.

Right click a **blank area** of the desktop. Select **Arrange Icons by**, **Align to Grid**.

What happened? _____

Drag the **Taskbar** to the top of the screen.

If the icons snap back into place, right click a blank area of the desktop, select **Arrange Icons by**, and then select **AutoArrange**. This removes the check next to the AutoArrange feature and permits the icons to be moved.

4. Change desktop colors.

Right click a **blank area** of the desktop and choose **Properties**.

Click the **Appearance tab**. Click the **Color Scheme** down arrow button, and then select **Silver**.

Click **Apply**.

To change the setup back to the default colors, right click a blank area of the desktop. Choose properties, appearance tab, and then click the color scheme down arrow. Then select Default (blue).

5. Open, browse, and manage windows.

Open the **My Computer** window.

Drag, using the title bar, the **My Computer** window to the right approximately 3 inches.

Click the **Maximize** ⬜ button. What happened to the window?

Click the **Restore** ⬒ button. What happened?

Click the **Minimize** ▬ button. What happened?

Click the **My Computer** [🖥 My Computer] button on the task bar.

Place the pointer on the **right border** of the My Computer window.

With the double-headed arrow, drag the **Window border** to the right two inches.

Place the pointer on the **bottom right corner** of the My Computer window.

Drag the window border **up and to the left**, making the window approximately 3" square.

What additional bars appeared? _____

Why might you need to know how to open and manage windows? _____

_____

Drag to **enlarge** the My Computer window, making it approximately 6" square.

Double click the **Local drive** (usually *C*) icon. Double click the **Windows folder**.

Notice that the default in Windows is to open each new folder in the same window.

Click the Back button until the **My Computer** window is open.

6. Change the Default Folder Option and Switch between windows.

In the My Computer window, select **Tools, Folder options**.

Click the **Open each folder in its own window** option under the Folder options section of the dialog window.

Click **Apply** and **OK**. *Now each folder will open in its own window.*

Click **Start, Control Panel**.

What happened? _____

Click the **My Computer** button on the taskbar.

What happened? _____

Move the **My Computer** window so that the **Control Panel** window is visible.

Click anywhere in the **Control Panel** window.

Now, hold down the **Alt** key and press the **Tab** key. *This brings up a window for switching between open applications.*

Press the **Tab** key again while still holding down the **Alt** key.

Release the **Tab** and **Alt** keys. What happened? _____

Why might you want to switch between windows? _____

Click the **Close** buttons to close all open windows.

Exercise 2: Managing Files and Folders With My Computer

Objectives

1. Format a diskette.
2. Create folders and files.
3. Move, copy, and rename folders and files.
4. Delete files and folders.
5. Empty the recycle bin.

Activity

1. Format a diskette.

   Place a **diskette** in the *A* drive. Open the **My Computer** window.

   Right click the **3.5" drive** 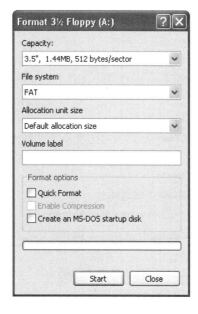 icon. Select **Format** (Figure 3.14).

   Click the **Start button**. If a warning box appears, click **OK**. This may take a while to format.

   Click the **Close** button to close the format dialog window.

   To see the total available space on the diskette,

   Right-click the **3.5" drive** icon. Select **Properties** from the shortcut menu.

   What is the total disk space? _____ What is the available space? _____

   Click the **Close** button to close the properties window.

   A zip disk may also be formatted using the same procedure.

Figure 3.14

Format Dialog Boxes—
Floppy and Zip Drives

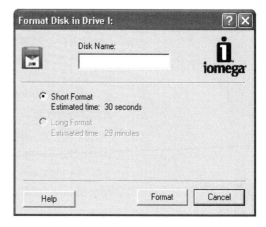

2. Create folders. Use the diskette just formatted for this part of the activity.

   Open the **My Computer** window.

   Double click the **3.5" floppy drive** icon.

   Right click a **blank area** of the 3.5" floppy drive window.

   Select **New, Folder.**

   Type **A&P100** and press **Enter.**

   Double click the **A&P100** folder.

   Select **Make a New Folder** in the task pane.

   Type **Class Notes** and press **Enter.**

   A new folder can be created by using the right-click method or the command from the task pane.

3. Create a file.

   Double click the **Class Notes** folder.

   Right click a **blank area** of the **Class Notes** folder. Select **New, Word Document.**

   Type **Respiratory System Notes** and press **Enter.**

   Right click a **blank area** of the **Class Notes** folder. Select **New, Word Document.**

   Type **Nervous System Notes** and press **Enter.**

4. Copy, move, and rename folders and files.

   Close all open windows except the My Computer window.

   Double click the **Local drive** (usually *C*) icon.

   Double click the **Windows** and **System32** folders.

   Scroll around in the **System32 folder** window until the **Calc** file is visible.

   Click **the file** to select it.

   Select **Copy this file** from the task pane.

   In the Copy Item dialog window, select the **3.5" floppy** drive.

   Click the **Copy** button.

   This task can be accomplished by dragging the file to the floppy drive icon if both windows are visible. Remember that the default for dragging and dropping from one storage device to another is to copy. The calculator icon is now in both windows.

   Close the **Local drive** windows.

   Open the floppy drive window if necessary.

   Right drag the **Calc** icon file onto the A&P100 folder.

   Select **Copy here** from the shortcut menu. Notice that the calculator is now in both windows.

   Why do you need to right drag the icon when copying from *A* to *A*?

   Right click the **Calc** icon in the *A* drive window.

Select **Rename**.

Type **Calculator** and press **Enter**. *The icon now has a new name.*

Click on the text of the **Class Notes** folder in the A&P100 window once, and then **click again**. *The text in the folder icon should be highlighted but not the icon.*

Type **Lecture Notes** and press **Enter**.

Two ways are available to rename files and folders, and the process is the same for both files and folders.

To do this next task the My Computer window setting must be set to Show each folder in its own window (click **Tools**, **Folder options**, and check **Show each folder in its own window**).

Drag the **Lecture Notes** folder to the *A* drive window. What did it do? Why?

Right drag the **Lecture Notes** folder to the A&P100 window.

Select **Copy here** from the shortcut menu.

The default copy or move command can be overridden by right dragging the file or folder and by selecting the appropriate command.

5. Delete files and folders.

   Click the **Calc** icon in the A&P100 window. Press the **Delete** key. Click **Yes** to confirm the deletion.

   Close the **A&P100** window. If the window is set to open all folders in the same window, click the **Up** ⬆ button instead of closing the A&P100 folder.

   Move the **Icons** in the *A* drive window to line them up in a row or column.

   If necessary, move the *A* **drive window** so that the recycle bin is visible.

   Click the **First icon** in the row or column. Hold down the **Shift** key, and click on the last icon. *All of the icons are now selected.*

   Drag the **Selected files** onto the recycle bin.

   When the Recycle Bin turns blue, release the **mouse button**.

   Click **Yes** to confirm deletion of files and folders.

   Close **All** windows.

6. Empty the **Recycle Bin**.

   When files are deleted from a diskette in the *A* drive, they are not placed in the recycle bin. They are deleted immediately. In this case, the recycle bin does not need to be emptied. However, when deleting files from internal storage devices such as the *C* drive, the recycle bin needs to be emptied periodically.

   Double click the **Recycle Bin** icon.

   Click the **Empty the Recycle Bin** option in the task pane or select **File**, **Empty Recycle Bin**.

   Click **Yes** to confirm deletion.

Close the **Recycle Bin** window.

How often should the recycle bin be emptied? _____

Exercise 3: Managing Files and Folders With Windows Explorer
Objectives

1. Format a diskette.
2. Create folders and files.
3. Move, copy, and rename folders and files.
4. Delete files and folders.
5. Empty the recycle bin.

Some people place Windows Explorer on the desktop as a shortcut to make it more accessible. Others use the Folders button on My Computer toolbar to switch to the Windows Explorer view of the storage structure in the left task pane.

Activity

1. Format a diskette.

   Place a Diskette in the A drive.

   Click the Start [start] button on the taskbar.

   Select All Programs, Accessories, and Windows Explorer.

   Click the + sign next to My Computer in the left window pane.

   Right click the text 3.5" Floppy (A:).

   Select Format.

   Accept the default settings by clicking the Start Button.

   Click OK to proceed.

   When the computer finishes formatting the diskette, click OK and Close.

   Right click the text 3.5" Floppy (A:).

   Select Properties from the shortcut menu.

   What is the total disk space? _____

   What is the available space? _____

   Click the Close button to close the properties dialog box.

2. Create folders. Use the recently formatted diskette for this part of the activity.

   Click the text 3.5" Floppy (A:) on the left side of the Explorer window.

   Right click a blank area on the right side of the Explorer window.

   Select New, Folder.

   Type A&P100 and press Enter.

   Double click the A&P100 folder.

Right click a blank area on the right side of the Explorer A&P100 window.

Select New, Folder.

Type Class Notes and press Enter.

3. Create a file.

Double click the Class Notes folder.

Right click a blank area on the right side of the Explorer Class Notes window.

Select New, MS Word Document.

Type Respiratory System Notes and press Enter.

Right click a blank area on the right side of the Explorer Class Notes window.

Select New, Word Document.

Type Nervous System Notes and press Enter.

The screen should look similar to the screen shown in Figure 3.15.

4. Copy, move, and rename folders and files.

Click the + sign next to the text Local Drive (C:) on the left side of the Explorer window.

Click the + sign next to the Windows folder on the left side of the Explorer window. This may require using the scroll bar on the left side of the window until the Windows folder appears.

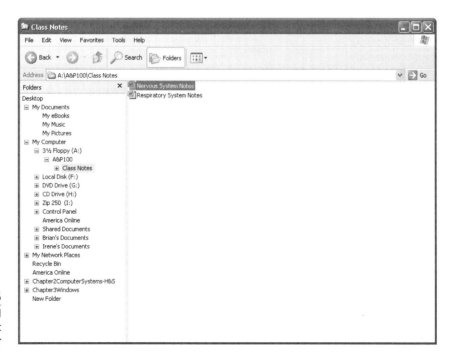

Figure 3.15

Creating Files and Folders with Internet Explorer

Click the + sign next to the System32 folder on the left side of the Explorer window. Use the scroll bar to see all the files and folders in the left pane.

Scroll down on the right side of the Explorer window until the file Calc 🖩 is visible.

Now, scroll on the left side of the Explorer window until the text 3.5" Floppy (A:) appears. DO NOT CLICK THE TEXT.

Drag the Calc 🖩 from the right side of the window and drop it on top of the text 3.5" Floppy (A:) on the left side of the window.

The default for dragging and dropping is to copy when going from one storage device (C:) to another (A:). The calculator icon remains in the right side window while being copied to the floppy diskette.

Click the **3.5" Floppy** (A:) text. *It is now also there.*

Right drag the Calc icon from the right side of the Explorer window and drop it on top of the A&P100 folder on the left side of the Explorer window.

Select Copy here from the shortcut menu. *The calculator remains in the Explorer window.*

Click the A&P100 folder on the left side of the Explorer window. *The calculator is also there.*

Why must the file be right dragged when copying from A to A?

Right click the Calc icon on the right side of the Explorer A&P100 window.

Select Rename.

Type Calculator and press Enter. *The icon now has a new name.*

Click over the text of the Class Notes folder in the A&P100 window once, and then click again. The folder icon text is highlighted but not the icon.

Type Lecture Notes and press Enter.

There are two ways to rename files and folders, and the process is the same for both files and folders.

Drag the Lecture Notes folder from the right side of the Explorer window onto the 3.5" Floppy (A:) text on left side of the screen. What did it do? Why?

Click the Lecture Notes folder on the left side of the Explorer window.

Right drag the Lecture Notes folder onto the A&P100 folder on the left side.

Select Copy here from the shortcut menu.

The default can be overridden by right dragging the file or folder and selecting the appropriate command.

5. Delete files and folders.

Click the **Calculator icon** in the Explorer A&P100 window. Press the **Delete** key.

Click **Yes** to confirm the deletion.

Click the text 3.5" Floppy (A:) on the left side of the screen.

If necessary, move the Icons on the right side of the window to line them up in a row or column.

Click the – sign next to the text Local Drive (C:) on the left side of the screen to collapse the branch.

Click the first icon in the row or column in the right side of the window.

Hold down the **Shift** key, and click the last icon. *All icons are now selected.*

Drag the selected files onto the recycle bin on the left side of the screen.

When the recycle bin turns blue, release the mouse button.

Click Yes to confirm the deletion of files and folders.

Close the Explorer window.

Look at how similar My Computer and Windows Explorer are. Windows Explorer has the advantage of having all the storage spaces accessible through the one window, making it very easy to manage files and folders.

6. Empty the recycle bin.

When files are deleted from the diskette in the floppy drive, they are not placed in the recycle bin. They are immediately deleted. The recycle bin will not need to be emptied. However, when files are deleted from internal storage devices such as the local drive, the recycle bin needs to be emptied periodically.

Double click the Recycle Bin icon.

Click the Empty the Recycle Bin option in the task pane or select File, Empty Recycle Bin.

Click Yes to confirm the deletion.

Close the Recycle Bin window.

How often do you empty the recycle bin? _____

Exercise 4: Software Decisions and Organization Skills
Objectives

1. Begin to select appropriate software and justify its purchase.
2. Appropriately organize a hard drive or floppy diskette with folders and subfolders.
3. Identify appropriate filenames for documents given.

Activity A

1. You are the manager on Unit 93, a 40-bed general medical-surgical unit. You received approval for a new computer for managing the unit's information needs but now need to specify what software is needed. List the software needed and why

(see Chapter 2 for brief descriptions of software categories or look in computer advertisements for specific software programs). Make sure the software complies with the facility's default standards. For example, does your facility require everyone to use Word for word processing or Excel for spreadsheets? Do they let the user determine whether WordPerfect or Microsoft Word better meets their word processing needs? Include an operating system in your request. Some examples of common categories are

    Word Processing

    Spreadsheet

    Database

    Presentation graphics

    Browsers and HTML editors

    Utilities such as Anti-Virus, Norton Utilities, WinZip, and Acrobat Reader

2. You must organize the hard drive so that things are orderly and easy to maintain. Describe the organization of the hard drive. Remember that each program should have its own folder and similar programs, and data should be in the same folders or subfolders.

3. Using your removable storage device, create the previously mentioned folders and subfolders on that diskette.

4. It will take the information systems people 3 weeks before they can install your software. If you decide to do it yourself, how will you go about installing the software?

Activity B

1. You are storing data files on the hard drive so that you will not have to deal with floppy diskettes. You create the appropriate folders and subfolders as follows:

Memos:	Memos folder in the data folder: C:\data\memos
Evaluations:	Jones folder in the evaluation folder under the data folder: c:\data\evaluation\Jones
Teaching materials:	Patient teaching folder in the data folder: c:\data\Patient Teaching
Budget:	Fiscal 2005 folder in the Budget folder c:\budget\Fiscal 2005
Web pages:	Web folder for the unit's web pages.

How will you name the following documents for each of the folders?

<u>Memos</u>	Filename
Request for more staff	_____
Request for communication software	_____
Response to procedure change	_____
Response to vacation request	_____

Evaluations	Filename
Patient Associate Jones	_____
Unit Clerk Quincy	_____
Staff Nurse Walker	_____

Teaching Materials	Filename
AIDS: What you should know	_____
Orientation to our unit	_____
So you are going to have surgery	_____

Budget	Filename
Unit budget for 2005	_____
Unit budget for 2006	_____
Proposed budget for new furniture	_____

Web Pages	Filename
Introducing our Staff	_____
Services provided on our unit	_____
Contact information	_____

Exercise 5: Customizing the Start Menu and Taskbar
Objectives
1. Alter the Start Menu and Taskbar.
2. Change a few default settings.

   Some of these tasks may not be available in computer laboratories or the work environment unless you are logged on as the administrator.

Directions
1. Taskbar.

   Right click on a **blank** area of the taskbar and select **Properties**. *The Taskbar and Start Menu Properties dialog box appears.*

   Click the **square** to the left of Show Quick Launch text. *This will display Internet Explorer, Media Player, and Desktop icons, which can be clicked to start the programs.*

   Remove the **Hide inactive icons check** (if present) by **clicking the square** to the left of the text.

   Click the **Apply** and **OK** buttons.

   Add a few Microsoft Office icons to the quick launch area of the toolbar. With the 2003 version of Office, the separate Microsoft Office toolbar that could be placed on the top right of the desktop is no longer available. Instead, add the icons to the quick launch area of the taskbar.

Click the **Start** button, and select **All Programs, MS Office**. Right click **MS Office Word 2003** and select **Send to, Desktop (shortcut)**.

Now, drag the **MS Office Word** shortcut icon over the quick launch area of the taskbar. *The Word icon appears in the quick launch area ready for you to start the program.*

Delete the **Word shortcut** on the desktop. There is no reason to keep both. Because the taskbar is always visible, Word can be launched at anytime without having to minimize other windows or go through the menu.

Repeat this to add frequently used Microsoft Office programs.

2. Alter the start menu.

Click the **Start menu** tab in the Taskbar and the Start Menu Properties dialog box. *If you do not like the new start menu, you can change it to the old, classic one. Let us leave it alone for now.*

Click the **Customize** button.

Click to show **Small icons** and increase the number to show on the start menu to **10**. Note the clear list button. If you do not want someone to see what programs were recently accessed on the computer, click the clear list button.

Click the **Advanced** tab.

In the Start menu items area, change My Documents to **not show on the menu**.

Click **OK, Apply,** and **OK**.

Check the start menu. *My Documents should not be an item on the list. The number of recently used programs should now be 10.*

In the Advanced tab is another clear list button. This one removes the history of the most recently opened documents. Clearing this will not delete the actual documents, just the file that holds the history of those documents recently accessed.

Add an item to the start menu.

Find **MS Office Outlook 2003** in the All programs menu. Right click the text and select **Pin to the start menu**. *The program now appears in the top left pane of the start menu, making it easier to access than going through several layers. Use this feature for programs used regularly but not daily.*

Some users like to control the All Programs menu so that it does not become too unmanageable. To do this requires thinking about how to organize the programs into appropriate categories. Here is one suggestion. Place all like programs together. For example, create a folder called Multimedia, and place all multimedia programs in that folder. Create a utilities folder, and place all utilities in that folder.

Right click the **Start** button and then **Explore**.

Select **All users, Start menu, Programs** options.

Now, right click a blank area of the right window. Select **New**, **Folder**, and type **Multimedia**.

Repeat the process to create a **Utilities** folder.

Drag the appropriate programs into the folders. For example, move QuickTime and Real Player into the multimedia folder and Norton Anti-virus and WinZip into the Utilities folder.

Close all open windows, and look at the start menu.

Next, place all the folders in order by dragging and dropping them into the correct order. They will be placed wherever the black line is when releasing the mouse button.

Assignment 1: Working With the Desktop

Directions

1. Create the following objects on the desktop. Refer to the appropriate chapter discussions if you cannot remember how to create these objects.

   A shortcut to the printer and to the 3.5" floppy drive

   A folder for your downloaded graphics files

   A Word file titled All About Viruses

2. Explain the terms icon, folder, file, and shortcut.

3. Rearrange the desktop.

   Place the Shortcut to the printer and 3.5" Floppy drive on the top right of the desktop.

   Place the Graphics folder on the bottom right of the desktop.

   Place the All About Viruses file on the top center of the desktop.

   Keep all of the other objects except the taskbar on the left side of the desktop.

4. Change the theme of the desktop to Windows Classic with peace desktop background.

5. Move the Taskbar to the left side of the desktop.

6. Press the Print Screen button to place the desktop image on the clipboard.

   Start WordPad or a word processing program.

   Click the Paste icon on the toolbar.

   Print the File with the new desktop image.

7. Restore the desktop.

   Close All windows.

   Reset the Defaults—Windows XP default and Bliss background.

   Place Taskbar at bottom edge of desktop.

   Delete objects created in number 1 (shown previously).

   Turn in the Print Screen copy of the restored settings.

Assignment 2: Working With Files and Folders
Directions

1. Create folders.

   Create a folder on a diskette titled **Learning 1**.

   In the Learning 1 folder, create a **Graphics** folder, a **Word** folder, an **Excel** folder, and a **PowerPoint** folder.

2. Find and copy files.

   Find a **bmp** file on the hard drive. Click the **Start** button. Select **Search**. Click **All Files & Folders**. Type ***.bmp**, and press **Enter**.

   Copy it to the folder **Learning 1** on the diskette.

3. Create data files

   Create a Word file titled **Word Review Guide**.

   Create an Excel file titled **Unit 93 Budget-2005**.

   Create a PowerPoint file titled **Health Habits**.

4. Move files.

   Move the **bmp** file into the **Graphics** folder.

   Move the **Word Review Guide** file into the **Word** folder.

   Move the **Unit 93 Budget-2005** file into the **Excel** folder.

   Move the **Health Habits** file into the **PowerPoint** folder.

5. Rename a file.

   Rename the **Health Habits** file **My A&P100 Presentation**.

   Place your name on the diskette and turn it in to the professor.

Assignment 3: File and Hard Drive Management
Directions

1. Using the system properties dialog box, identify the following information:

   Operating system _____   Version _____

   Service Pak _____

   To whom is it registered? _____

   What processor is running on the computer? _____

   At what speed? _____ With what amount of RAM? _____

2. Using either your workplace or class material, develop an organizational scheme for storing your work. This means to create folders and subfolders that represent the work that you are doing this semester. Create those folders and subfolders on a disk.

3. Move some of your files into the appropriate folders. Explain the difference between folders and files.

4. List and describe the three main tools available to maintain the files on your storage medium.

5. Using the help system, explain how you would make a file read-only so that others can read it but not change it unless they rename it.

6. Make a backup folder on your disk, and copy all of the current files and folders into the backup folder. Now, rename the original files and folders (not the ones in the backup folder).

7. You no longer need some of these files. List two ways to delete files and folders. Where do the files go that are deleted from a removable storage device?

Submit this sheet and your diskette with this assignment.

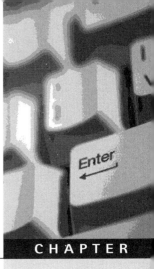

Software Applications: Common Tasks

CHAPTER

4

OBJECTIVES

1. Identify standards common to applications running in the Windows environment.
2. Describe and use the online help that the applications provide.
3. Use the common toolbar and menu commands to perform the tasks of opening, creating, closing, saving, finding, and printing files.
4. Describe and use cut/copy/paste functions to move or copy data from within the same file or from one file to another in the same or different application.

The focus of this chapter is to present some common tasks that are used when working with application programs regardless of the application. In the Windows environment, certain standards exist so that applications share a common desktop environment and menus to access commands. For example, menus provide the paths to the action. Commands on the menu followed by three periods (ellipsis) open a special window called a dialog box, where a person can select the appropriate information before the command is executed. Commands on the menu followed by an arrow result in the appearance of a submenu of commands (see Chapter 3 for more details on this point). All applications use this standard or convention, making it possible to anticipate the response after selecting the command.

All windows display a title bar, menu bar, one or more toolbars, and a status bar (Figure 3.5). All of the title bars permit someone to close, minimize, and maximize the window using the same graphical buttons regardless of the application. The menu and standard toolbar are used to open a file, create a new file, save a file, print a file, and obtain help. It is these common tasks and the consistency in how they are accessed that make working in this environment easier. This chapter, therefore, uses Microsoft Office 2003 to explain and demonstrate these tasks.

▶ 4.1 COMMON LAYOUT

Figure 4.1

Sample Menu Bars
from Microsoft
Office 2003

Before discussing the common tasks that are associated with working in Microsoft Office, an overview is presented of the common layout for accessing the commands used for these tasks. As can be seen in Figure 4.1, some of these tasks fall under the commands File, Edit, View, Insert, Format, and Help.

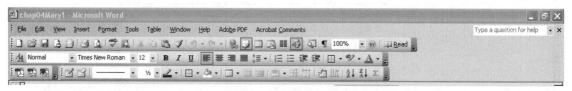

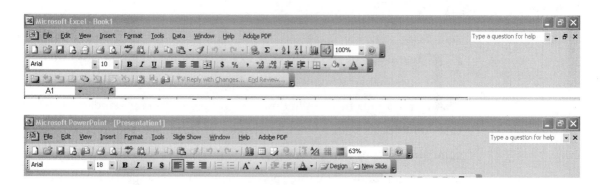

File

File menu commands are represented on the toolbar by the **New** ▯ button, **Open** 📂 button, **Save** 💾 button, **E-mail** 📧 button, **Print preview** 🔍 button, and **Printer** 🖨 button. The **Close document** ✕ button is on the Menu bar.

Edit

Edit accesses commands such as undo, cut, copy and paste, find and replace, and go to. Each application may also add additional commands to this menu. For example, Word includes the commands Select All and Clear, whereas Excel uses the Fill and Clear commands. Selected commands from this menu are represented on the standard toolbar as left pointed arrow (**Undo**) ↺ , scissors (**Cut**) ✂ , double paper (**Copy**) 📋 , and clipboard (**Paste**) 📋 .

View

View permits a person to alter the view of the screen and/or document through such commands as layouts, toolbars, and zoom. Layouts change the appearance of the document showing or hiding specific features such as zoom, margins, and headers and footers. The Toolbars command is used to display or hide specific toolbars such as Formatting, Standard, Web, and Email. Additional commands for altering the view of the screen and/or document are added as appropriate by each application.

Insert

Insert accesses commands such as dates, symbols, footnotes, files, objects, and page breaks. Basically, commands that require inserting an object, code, or special text such as footnotes into the document are located here. Some applications add different commands as appropriate. For example, a button for inserting clip art or a hyperlink is useful if those commands are commonly used in the application.

Format

Most commands related to altering the appearance of the document are located in the format menu. Included are options for altering fonts, paragraphs, bullets, tabs, justification, and inserting columns. Many of these commands are discussed in detail in Chapter 5, "Introduction to Word Processing." Because formatting the look of the document, spreadsheet, database, or slide presentation requires such important and frequently used commands, applications include many of these commands on their own toolbar, called the Formatting toolbar. By default, this toolbar shares the same row as the Standard toolbar.

Tools

The tools option permits access to commands related to additional features available in the application such as spelling checker, thesaurus, merges, sorts, and macros. They are tools that improve efficiency by automating some of the repetitive tasks in the application.

Window

Window accesses commands that let the user switch between different documents in the same application and then display those documents by dividing the screen into different sections.

Help

Opening the Help Menu provides access to the application's help system (Figure 4.2). Other ways

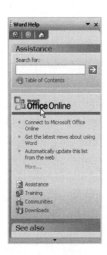

Figure 4.2
Microsoft Office
Word 2003 Help
Dialog Box

to access Help include clicking the blue question mark 🔵 on the standard toolbar, pressing the F1 key, or typing a question in the Search box under Assistance. The Office Assistant or Office Online provides more extensive help.

Additional commands are added to the menu bar depending on the application. For example, in Word there is access to the Table command, in Excel to Data function, and in Power Point to Slide Show tasks. It is important to remember that there are common threads and organizational themes running through all Windows/Office programs. Each program tries to keep a consistent look to each application within it for ease of use and learning. The most commonly used commands are generally also represented on toolbars. However, subtle differences may exist in the toolbar command and menu command. Certain assumptions are made with some of the commands. For example, the diskette represents the File, Save command and not the File, Save As command. The printer button may print one copy of the current document to the default printer as it does in Word and not show the print dialog box.

► 4.2 COMMON TASKS

Familiarity with the common Windows layout for accessing commands provides the basis for this section. It covers some of the common tasks that one does in all applications.

Obtaining Help
Help command
Access this Help through the menu toolbar or the blue question mark on the standard toolbar (Figure 4.2). The Table of Contents provides access to help screens based on commonly used functions or tasks such as opening, creating, and saving documents. This approach is most effective for new users when they are not familiar with the terminology and concepts related to this application.

► To select a help topic:
Click the help 🔵 Button.
Click **Table of Contents**.
Click the **Book** beside "Creating Documents."

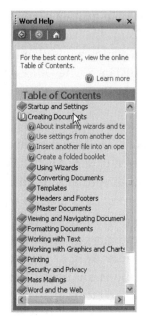

Figure 4.3

Table of Contents
Window with
Creating Documents
Selected

Options appear in blue type with a question mark (?) next to them. These options, when selected, result in the display of a help screen as shown in Figure 4.3.

The Search for box works well when a person is not sure how to find the problem in the Table of Contents. This locates topics about the word entered in the Search Box.

▶ **To select a help topic using the Search for box:**

Click the **question mark**.

In the Search for box, type the **word or topic** about which there is a question and press the **Enter** key.

Click on the result that best matches the question. Questions will be shown in the Results box.

Obtaining online help

All applications designed for the Windows environment provide online help to users. Very few application programs are sold with detailed user manuals. It is therefore important to learn to use the online help.

► **To obtain Microsoft Office Online Help:**

Click the question mark. *"Office Online" appears in the Word Help task pane. When pointing to Connect to Microsoft Office Online, the arrow turns to a hand, and "Connect to Microsoft Office Online" is underlined.*

Click **Connect to Microsoft Office Online**. Internet access is necessary to connect to Office Online.

Figure 4.4 shows the Home Page help screen for Microsoft Office. Many choices are offered such as Assistance, Training, Download, Template, Marketplace, and Product Info. Most of these screens are updated daily so that the one that comes up may look slightly different from Figure 4.4.

Click **Assistance** under Home. *The next screen, Figure 4.5, offers choices such as Office Tips, Helpful Hints, and Browse Assistance.*

► **To access online help in an application program:**

Connect to the **Microsoft Online help** and select **Assistance**.

Click on **the name of the application** under Browse Assistance. *Figure 4.6 shows the results when one clicks on Word 2003.*

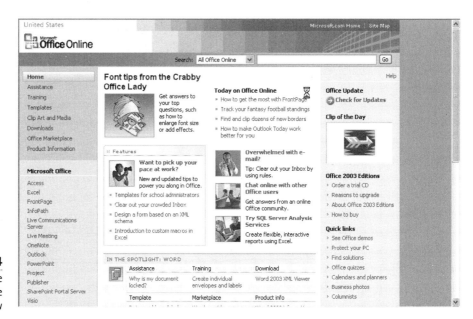

Figure 4.4
Microsoft Office
Online Home Page
Window

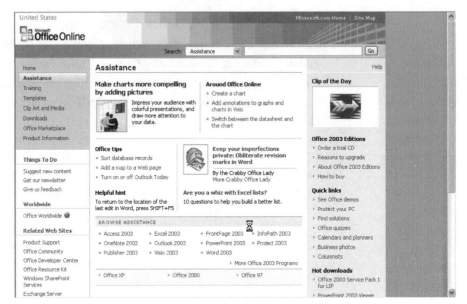

Figure 4.5

The Assistance Window in Office Online

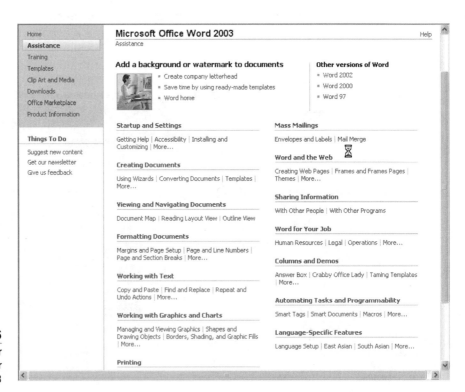

Figure 4.6

Online Browser Assistance for Microsoft Word 2003

► **To access Windows XP Help and Support Center:**

Click **Start**, and select **Help and Support**.

Choices include Pick a Topic, Ask for Assistance, Pick a Task, or find answers to various questions regarding the Operating System (Figure 4.7).

When using the Online Help and Support Center, the home button returns the user back to the home screen.

Using the office assistant

Most applications now provide access to intelligent help called different things in different applications. In Microsoft Office, it is the Office Assistant. This help assistant is available through the menu Help command. Sometimes it pops up while working in a document. To use this "expert," type a question in English phrases. The expert then tries to match the question to a selection of help screens.

ScreenTips/ToolTips

ScreenTips or ToolTips provide the new user with a word that describes the icon command. For example, placing the pointer over the printer icon on

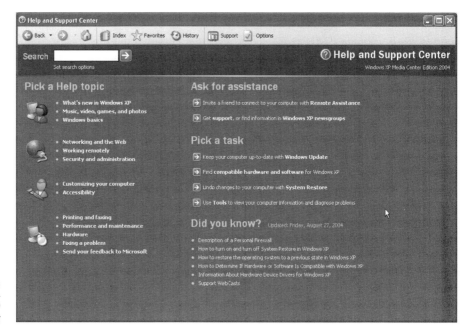

Figure 4.7

Windows XP Help and Support Center

the standard toolbar results in a word dropping down that says print. The new user can then learn what each icon on the toolbar represents.

Creating a New File (Document)

In order to start working in most applications, one must first create a new document, spreadsheet, database, or presentation. Most applications open to a new, blank document or spreadsheet or present a series of dialog boxes asking the user to respond to questions. When Word is started, a new blank document opens. When PowerPoint is started, a blank title slide appears. The word *document* is used here to represent a text document, a spreadsheet, a database, or a presentation.

When the computer is turned on, an application must be selected. For Microsoft Office, click **Start**, and select **All Programs**, **Microsoft Office** in the next menu that appears; then select the correct **application**. A new document will open (Figure 4.8).

One can also go to **Start** and open **Microsoft Office** from the Start Menu if it appears above Start, as shown in Figure 4.9. Microsoft Office icons may

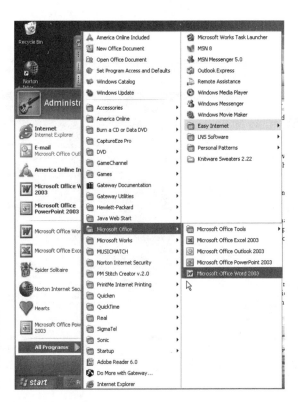

Figure 4.8

Menu for Opening Microsoft Office Word 2003 from Start and All Programs

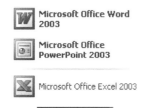

Figure 4.9
Microsoft Office
Icons above the
Start Button

also be placed on the Quick Launch area of the taskbar. Using this approach, the user clicks the correct button on the taskbar to launch the program.

▶ **To start another document once the application is opened:**

Click the **new button** 🗋 on the standard toolbar. *Now there are two documents opened. All documents remain open and accessible through the Window menu command until the user closes them.*

To use the keyboard, press **Ctrl + N**. This is the same command as the new button.

A template is a predesigned style—a document that is already formatted with fonts, colors, layout, and so forth. A wizard is a step-by-step process for developing the document. A series of questions are asked, and based on the answers, the document is developed.

▶ **To start another document using a template or wizard:**

Select **File**, **New**.

From the Task pane on the right side of the screen in the templates area, click on **My Computer**. *A dialog box appears with various tabs.*

Select the **Correct tab** for the type of document.

Select the **Correct template** or the **wizard** if one exists. *The new template or wizard opens.*

Opening/Closing Files

Common to all applications is the function of opening and closing files. Once a document is created, it is saved and often reopened later for additions and corrections.

Open files

In the Windows world, a file can be opened in many ways. Because the focus here is the menu and toolbars, they are demonstrated.

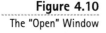

Figure 4.10

The "Open" Window

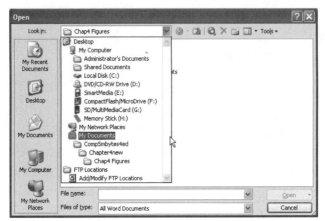

Select **File**, **Open** from the menu bar or click on the **open** button on the standard toolbar.

Clicking on the **down arrow** button to the right of "Look in:" to produce a list of items that are similar to those in Figure 4.10. *Included is a list of locations where the files can be stored—the storage device (drive letter) and folder. In this example, the My Documents folder is stored under My Computer.*

Click on **My Documents** or the **correct storage** device to see a list of files.

Once the file is found, double click the **File** or select the **File** and click the **Open** button.

Files can be opened in many ways. Here are a few more ways:

- In a window or on the desktop, double click the file.
- Select the Start button on the taskbar. Select My Recent Documents, and click on the one desired. The last 15 files that were opened are on the menu list regardless of file type.
- In an application, press Ctrl + O.
- In an application, select File from the menu bar, and select from one of the Files listed at the bottom of the menu, which represent the last few files opened in this application.

Close files
▶ To close a file:

Select **File** from the menu bar; select **Close**.

Click on the **close** ✖ **window** button on the document menu bar. Be careful to close the document and not the application window, whose orange–red close 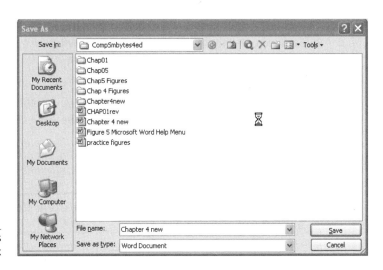 button is just above it. If changes were made to the file and it was not saved, there is a prompt to save the file before closing it.

To use the keyboard to close a file, press **Ctrl + F4**.

Save Files

Once work begins on a file or document, it will need to be saved for future reference or revisions. The first time that a file is saved a location and name must be specified (see Chapter 3 for file naming conventions). If a location is not specified, the file is saved in the default location. In Microsoft Office, the default location is the My Documents folder on the hard drive (C:). Once the file has a name and location, the **File**, **Save** command updates the file by saving any changes to it. The **Save As** dialog window does not appear.

▶ **To access the Save command:**

Click the **save** button on the toolbar, or select **File**, **Save** from the menu bar.

If the file has not been saved before, the **Save as** dialog box appears asking the user to choose the location and name of the file.

If the file was previously saved, the file is updated without displaying the Save as dialog box.

The **File**, **Save As** command is used to change the location or name of the file. The File, Save As command always brings up the Save As dialog window (see Figure 4.11 for the Save As dialog box). This dialog box works like the

Figure 4.11

The Save As
Dialogue Box

open dialog window. Select the location from the Save in drop down arrow, and type the file name in the file name text box. To use the keyboard to save a file, press **Ctrl + S**. This acts like the File, Save command. The computer can be set to automatically save a document every 1 to 120 minutes.

▶ To set the automatic save feature:

Select **Tools** from the menu bar.

Choose **Options** and the **Save** tab.

In the Save options area of the dialog box, click **Save Auto Recover info every . . .** to place a check in the square to the left.

Select the amount of time desired—such as 5 or 10 minutes—and click **OK**.

Use the File Location tab to see where the auto recover files are being stored. The location may be changed.

Printing Files

Once the file is ready for use, it will need to be printed for distribution to others or for a hard copy record. A general rule is to use the print preview feature most programs have before sending the document to the printer. The print preview feature shows the document as it will look when printed. Time and money are saved if changes are made before the document is printed.

To access the print preview command, use the **print preview** [image] button in Microsoft Office, or choose **File**, **Print preview** from the menu. If the full menu does not display, click the File command, and hold the mouse button still for a few seconds. The full menu will display. Another option to display the full menu is to click the double arrows [image] at the end of the short menu.

Some applications make a distinction between the File, Print command and the printer icon on the toolbar. For example, Word sends one copy of the current document to the default printer with the printer icon but brings up the printer dialog box with the File, Print command from the menu bar. The entire document can be printed or just the page or pages necessary.

▶ To print a file:

Click the **printer** [image] **icon** or select **File**, **Print**.

▶ To bring up the printer dialog box (Figure 4.12):

Select **File**, **Print** in the Office Suite.

Adjust the available **options** as needed. Choices available from the printer dialog box are changing the printer; choosing the number of copies to

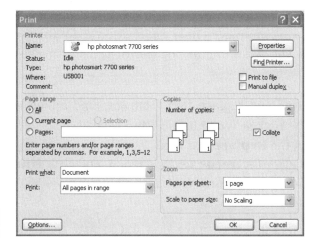

Figure 4.12
Printer Dialog Box

print; printing the total document, the current page, the selection, or selected pages; or collating multiple page documents.

Pressing **Ctrl + P** also brings up the printer dialog box.

Finding Files or Words

Another common task that computer users perform is the finding or finding and replacing of specific files or words within a folder or document. Suppose it is necessary to use a document that was previously created and now must be altered to fit the current situation. It could also be a file or e-mail that must be forwarded to someone else. Instead of manually searching for these files or replacing these words, let the computer do it.

▶ **To access this feature:**

In an application, select **Edit**, **Find**.
In Windows, select **Start**, **Search** and then **All Files** and **Folders**.

▶ **Once in the dialog window to find a word:**

Type the **word** in the find text box and click **Find Next**. *This will find the next occurrence of the word and highlight it. Keep clicking Find next until all instances of the word or file are found.*

▶ **Once in the dialog window to find a file:**

Type all or part of the **file name** in the text box or type words or a phrase in the file.
Click **Search**. *All files matching the description will be displayed in the right window.*

Use the Index headings on the top of the dialog box to give further directions to the computer. Other information about the file such as when it was created, the size of the file, or specific text within the file can also be used in the search.

▶ **To find and replace text from the Find dialog window:**

Type the **text** or **word** in the "Find what" box.

Click in the **Replace** text box.

Type the **replacement text or word**, and click **Find Next**.

Continue clicking **Find Next** until all of the episodes of the word are either left alone or replaced.

Figure 4.13 shows a sample Find and Replace Dialog Box. In this example, the word to find was *school*, and the replacement word is *college*. Be careful with the Replace, All button. This button results in the program automatically finding all incidents of the text "school" and replacing it with "college." This means that schoolbook will be replaced with collegebook. The find feature is not case sensitive, although the option exists to change this default.

Selecting Text or Objects

Selecting text or objects means to highlight the text or object such as a word or the cell in a spreadsheet. This is a common task when editing documents. Although it is fine to use the delete and backspace keys to complete minor editing tasks, it is not efficient for editing lines, sentences, paragraphs, columns, rows, cells, or the entire document. This feature is also used when formatting documents (word processing, spreadsheets, etc.). Once again, each item can be formatted separately, but this is very time consuming.

Each application has some minor variations for selecting or highlighting text and cells. Described here are some of the most common techniques for selecting them. Additional ones are presented in the applications chapters as appropriate.

Figure 4.13

Find and Replace
Dialog Box

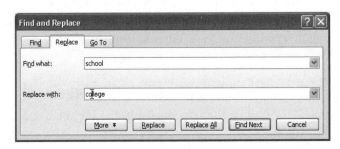

Select	Mouse Action
A word	Double click the word.
Several words	Click and drag the mouse over the words or select the **first** word. Hold down the **shift** key, and click the **last** word.
A sentence	Hold down the **Ctrl** key and click on the sentence.
A line	Click in the quick select area (the margin on the left side of the line; the cursor turns into a right slanted arrow.
Entire document	Triple click the quick select area. Use **Ctrl + A**.
A cell	Click the cell.
Multiple cells	Drag over the cells.

In addition to the mouse strokes, the keyboard can be used to select text. This is especially helpful when what must be selected spans greater distances or is on the edge of the document. For example, to select text that spans several pages, place the cursor at the beginning of the text to be selected. Hold down the shift key, and use the arrow keys to move down the document. As the cursor is moved, all of the text is being highlighted. This technique also works in spreadsheets to select multiple cells.

If the entire document must be selected, press Ctrl + A. The entire document is now selected.

Editing Text

Three basic editing features are used in applications: inserting, deleting, and replacing items.

Insert means to add new text, slides, rows, columns, and so forth. In word processing programs, insert is the default. When the user starts typing, the characters are placed at the insertion point. In applications for spreadsheets and graphics, commands must be used to insert rows, columns, or new slides. These commands are covered in the appropriate applications chapters.

Delete means to remove some text, row, column, or slide from the document. Select what must be deleted and press the **Delete** key. If a mistake is made, go to **Edit** and Choose the **Undo Typing** command or click the **undo** button on the standard toolbar. In some applications, additional features are available for deleting, and they are covered in the appropriate applications chapters. Note the difference between the Delete key and

Backspace key. The delete key deletes text to the right of the insertion point, whereas the backspace key deletes text to the left of the insertion point.

Replace means to substitute one thing for another. In most cases it is not necessary to first delete the text and then type the new. By highlighting or selecting the text it changes to the replace mode. This means typing the replacement will delete what was highlighted. It is not necessary to delete it before typing.

Copying or Moving Text

The last of the common tasks presented in this chapter deals with copying or moving text from one place to another in the same document, from one document to another, or from one application to another. The most common method for doing this is using the cut/copy/paste commands; these use the concept of a clipboard as a temporary holding place for the cut or copied material. Another method for doing this is the drag and drop method. This method relies on selecting data and using the mouse to drag it to the new spot. The general rule for selecting the method to use is based on distance to move or copy the material and how many times you want to paste the item. For short distances in the same document, use drag and drop. To copy or move data longer distances (to another page), to another document, or to another application, use the clipboard strategy. To paste items multiple times, use the clipboard.

The clipboard

▶ **To copy data using the clipboard:**

Select the **data** to be copied.

Click the **copy** button.

Place the **insertion point** (cursor) where the data are to be copied.

Click the **paste** button.

▶ **To move data using the clipboard:**

Select the **data** to be moved.

Click the **cut** button.

Place the **insertion point** where the data are to be moved.

Click the **paste** button.

It is important to know where the insertion point is because that is where **paste** will place the data. The mouse pointer (I-beam) does not reflect where the data will go. If the data are moved to another document or application, it must be switched using either the **window**, **filename** to access the other document in the application or by clicking on the application button from the Start Menu (refer to Chapter 3 if you are unsure about how to do this).

To collect items in the Office clipboard, the Office clipboard must be displayed.

To display the Office Clipboard task pane, select **Edit**, **Office Clipboard**.
The Clipboard task pane appears on the right side of the screen.

Multiple data may be placed on the Office clipboard at one time and may be used in any other documents. The Office Clipboard icon will display in the status area of the taskbar (bottom right). The Clipboard task pane will show how many items are on the clipboard. The user has the choice of pasting one or more of these items into a new document or clearing the clipboard. The clipboard can hold 24 items at one time. When the 25th item is added, the first one is deleted. The last item added to the Office clipboard is also sent to the system clipboard.

▶ To paste the contents of the office clipboard into a new document,

Open a **new** document.

Display the **Office Clipboard**.

Click the **items** to add to the new document. *A new document can be created from multiple items on the office clipboard. When using the paste function, the system clipboard is used, not the Office clipboard.*

Data stay in the Office clipboard until the user exits Microsoft Office or clicks the Clear All button in the clipboard task pane. When clearing the Office clipboard, the system clipboard is also cleared.

The menu and keyboard

The cut/copy/paste commands can be accessed through the file menu, but not as quickly or as efficiently. These commands can also be initiated from the keyboard. Press Ctrl + X for cut, Ctrl + C for copy, and Ctrl + V for paste. The keys for these commands are in the same order on the bottom row of keys on the keyboard as the icons are on the toolbar.

Drag and drop

▶ **To move data using the drag and drop method:**

Highlight the data to be moved.

Place the pointer on the **selected area**.

Hold down the **left mouse** button.

Move the mouse so the insertion point (broken vertical bar) is in the new place.

Release the mouse button.

Notice the changing look of the mouse pointer when using drag and drop. The mouse pointer turns to a left slanted arrow with a box below it, and the insertion point turns to a broken vertical bar. Cut is the default option when using the drag and drop method.

▶ **To copy data using the drag and drop method:**

Select the **data** to be moved.

Place the pointer on the **selected area**.

Hold down the **Ctrl** key.

Hold down the **left mouse** button.

Move the mouse so the insertion point (broken vertical bar) is in the new place.

Release the mouse button and then the **Ctrl** key.

It is important not to release the Ctrl key after releasing the mouse button or else the selected data will be moved, not copied. When copying, the pointer appears the same as when cutting, except that there is a plus sign in the box below the pointer.

SUMMARY

This chapter presented some standard commands that are used in applications in the Windows/Office environment. It described the online help provided in applications. Common toolbar and menu commands were also presented that show how to perform such tasks as opening, creating, closing, saving, finding, and printing files. In addition, the cut/copy/paste and drag and drop functions to move or copy data from one file to another in the same and different applications were presented. These commands and tasks cross applications and provide some consistency in working in this environment.

Exercise 1: Using Online Help in an Application

Objectives

1. Use the various forms of Help available in application programs.

2. Navigate through the help screens.

3. Compare different ways of using offline and online Help.

Activity

1. Find help in Microsoft Office Word 2003.

   Start **Word**.

   Click **Help** on the menu bar and then **Microsoft Office Word Help**.

   Click the **Table of Contents** hypertext object.

   Look for an option about **Creating Documents**.

   Open the Creating Documents help screen. Read the help screen. Close the help screen.

   Click the **Back** button on the Word Help task pane.

   Type **open document** in lower case under Search for textbox.

   Click the **Start searching** button.

   Click **Open a file**. *The help screen opens.*

   Close the **Help screen**. *The task pane is now back at the search results task pane.*

   Look for help on opening a document using the **Type a question for help** textbox on the far right of the menu bar.

   Click the **Box**.

   Type **open document** in lower case and press **Enter**.

   Click **Open an earlier version of the document**.

   Close the **Help** screen.

   Which one of these Help methods did you like best and why?

2. Find help in Excel.

   Start Excel.

   Click **Help** on the menu bar and then **Microsoft Excel Help**.

   Click the **Table of Contents** hypertext object.

   Click **StartUp and Settings**.

   Next, choose **Managing Files** and then **Creating and Opening Workbooks**.

   Click **Create a new workbook**.

   Read the Help screen on opening workbooks. Close the **Help** screen.

   Click the **Back** button.

   Type **create a workbook** in lower case in the Search for textbox.

Click the help topic for **create a new workbook**. Close the **Help** screen.

Look for help on opening a document using the **Type a question for help box** on the far right of the Menu bar.

Click the **Box.**

Type **open workbook** in lower case and press **Enter.**

Select **Create a new workbook**. Read the help screen and then close it.

What were the similarities between this help command and the one from Activity 1?

3. Place the mouse pointer on the diskette on the standard toolbar. Do not click. What happens after a few seconds? What is this called? Under what conditions might this feature be used?

4. Use Microsoft Office Online.

Click on **Connect** to **Microsoft Office Online**. *Make sure there is an active Internet connection.*

Type in lower case **how do I format a document** and press **Enter**. *Your results are displayed.*

Click **Page and Line Numbers.**

How are page numbers formatted?

Why might this be helpful to know?

5. Use Office Online for Training (Figure 4.4).

Click **Training.**

Click **Word** under Browse Training Courses.

Find "See what you can do with the Research Service."

Click on it.

Listen to the Introduction.

Click the **Quick Reference Card**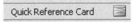

Review the contents.

Exercise 2: Common Tasks: Create, Open, Close, Find, Print, Save
Objectives

1. Create a new document using both the File, New command and the New button on Standard Toolbar.

2. Use the commands from both the menu bar and toolbar to open, close, print, and save a file.

3. Use the Find and replace command to replace text and the Find command to locate a file.

Activity

1. Start an application.

   Click **Start, All Programs, Microsoft Office**, and **Microsoft Office Word 2003**. *There may be other ways to start Word in the school's laboratory. Use the technique that is appropriate for the computer being used.*

   Type **I'm learning how to create a new word processing document.**

   Click the **Save** button.

   Click the **Save in down arrow** button.

   Select **My documents** or whatever folder and storage device used for this class.

   In the File name textbox, type **LearningWord**.

   Click the **Save button**.

2. Open and save another document.

   Click the **New** button.

   Type **I'm creating this second document to tell you about why I entered the health care field.**

   Select **File, Save**.

   Click the **down arrow** button. Select the appropriate folder and storage device as directed by the professor.

   In the File name textbox, type **Choosing a Health Care Profession.**

   Click the **Save** button or press **Enter**.

3. Open an "old" document, edit, and save it.

   Select **File, Open**.

   Double-click on **LearningWord**. *If the file is not visible, make sure that the correct storage device and folder are selected.*

   Add a sentence or two about what you want to learn about Word.

   Click the **Save** button. Notice the Save As dialog box did not appear because the file has a name and location. The file was just updated.

4. Print the document.

   Click the **Printer** button. What happened?

   Select **File, Print** from the menu.

   What happened now?

   Click **OK**.

5. Open and edit the second document.

   Click the **Open** button.

Double click the **Choosing a Health Care Profession** file. *If the file is not visible, make sure the correct storage device and folder are selected.*

Select **File, Save as**.

Type **Nursing** or your health care major and press **Enter**.

6. Find and replace.

Select **Edit, Replace**.

Type the words **health care field** in the "Find what" text box.

Tab to the **Replace with** box.

Type the lower case word **nursing** or your health care major in the replace with text box.

Click the **Find next** button in the dialog window.

Click the **Replace** button. *Be very careful when using the replace all button. Funny things can happen to the document.*

Click **OK** and the **Close** ☒ button in the dialog window.

Notice what happened to the word document.

Click the **Save** 🖫 button to save the file.

7. Close.

Select **File, Close** from the menu bar to close the document.

Select **File, Exit** to close the document and exit Word.

8. Find a file through the Windows find feature.

Select **Start** and then **Search**.

Click on **All Files and Folders**.

Type **LearningWord** in the first box (all or part of the file name). *Make sure the correct storage device is selected.*

Click the **Search** button in the dialog window.

Double click the **LearningWord** document in the results window. *The document opens.*

If necessary, display the Search dialog windows and click the Stop Search button.

Close the Search dialog window and the application.

Exercise 3: Copy and Move Data Using Cut/Copy/Paste and Drag and Drop

Objectives

1. Copy and move text from one place in the document to another using the clipboard.

2. Copy and move text from one place in the document to another using drag and drop.

3. Copy text from one document to another.

Activity

1. Start Microsoft Office Word 2003.

   Select **Start**, **Programs**, **Microsoft Office**, and then **Microsoft Office Word**.

2. Enter text.

   Type **Understanding how to copy and move data is an important skill that can save the user time**.

   Press the **Enter key twice**.

   Type the following text pressing the **Tab** key between items and the **Enter** key at the end of the row.

   Below is a list of physicians and their associated specialty. Please use the beeper number to access these physicians during off hours.

Dr. M. Smith	**Orthopedics*4567**	**Monday/Wednesday/Friday**
Dr. K. Bones	**Orthopedics*4512**	**Tuesdays/Thursdays/Saturday**
Dr. P. Roberts	**Surgery*5678**	**Sunday**
Dr. Z. White	**Internal Med*3489**	**all week**

3. Save the document.

   Click the **save** 🖫 icon.

   Save the document using the filename **Practice-CMwithDrag**.

4. Move text using drag and drop.

   Select the **Dr. Smith line**. (The quickest way to do this is to place the pointer in the quick select area. Place the pointer out at the margin across from Dr. M. Smith; when the pointer is a right slanted arrow, click.)

   Place the pointer on the **highlighted** area. **Hold down the left** mouse button, and **drag** the selection to the blank line below the **D** in Dr. Z. White. **Release** the mouse button. If the enter key was not pressed after the last line, you will not be able to go to the line below Dr. White. Go to the right of k in week and place text there. Click to left of D in Dr. M. Smith, and press Enter.

   Dr. M. Smith is now at the end of the list.

5. Move text using clipboard.

   Select the **second line** of text in the list.

   Click the **cut** ✂ button.

   Move the pointer so the blinking **vertical** bar is to the left of **Dr. M. Smith**. Do not select the entire line.

   With the insertion point to the left of D in Dr. M. Smith, click the **paste** button.

Your list should now look like this:

Dr. K. Bones	Orthopedics	*4512	Tuesdays/Thursdays/Saturday
Dr. Z. White	Internal Med	*3489	all week
Dr. P. Roberts	Surgery	*5678	Sunday
Dr. M. Smith	Orthopedics	*4567	Monday/Wednesday/Friday

6. Copy text using drag and drop

   Go to the **end of the document**.

   Press the **Enter key twice** to create a blank line or two.

   Type the following information remembering to use the Tab key between items and the enter key to go to the next line.

Chris Walker	**Nursing Assistant**
Mary Robb	**Registered Nurse**
Lee Dock	**Nurse Practitioner**

   Click the **save** 💾 button.

   Select the **first line of text** in this list (Chris Walker through Assistant).

   Place the **pointer** over the selected text. Hold down the **Ctrl** key. Hold down the **left mouse button**, and **drag** the text so the broken vertical bar is to the **left of Mary**. Release the **mouse button** and then the **Ctrl** key. *The text is copied.*

   Highlight **Chris** in the second row, and type **Brian**.

7. Copy text using the clipboard.

   Select the text **Mary Robb through registered nurse**.

   Click the **copy** 📋 button.

   Move the pointer to the **left of L** in Lee Dock and **click**. Do not highlight the text.

   Click the **paste** 📋 button.

   Highlight **Mary** and type **Nancy**.

   Click the **save** 💾 button to save the document.

8. Copy text from one document to another.

   Select all the text from **Chris through Practitioner**.

   Click the **copy** 📋 button.

   Click the **new document** 📄 button.

   Click the **paste** 📋 button. *The text is now inserted into a new word document.*

   Save the document as **Practice-CMwithClipboard**.

9. Copy text from one application to another.

Click **Start, All Programs, Microsoft Office, Excel** (or use one of the shortcut techniques to open Excel).

Click the **paste** button. *The contents of the clipboard are now inserted into an Excel worksheet.*

10. Close all files and programs. There is no need to save anything again unless requested to do so by your professor.

Assignment 1: Using Help

Directions

1. Use the Excel online help feature to find out how to create formulas and functions in Excel and what you need to remember in terms of order of precedence.

2. Print and place in logical sequence the appropriate help screens for future reference.

3. Using any application, select a task that you want to learn. Use the online help to learn how to complete that task in that application.

4. Submit the help prints from numbers 2 and 3.

Assignment 2: Copy and Move Text

Directions

1. Create a one-page document describing how to do the following tasks. Each description is to be its own paragraph.

   Save a document.

   Print a document.

   Create a new document.

   Move text in a document.

2. Print the original document.

3. Now, using the move text feature of the program, rearrange the text as follows:

   Create a new document.

   Move text in a document.

   Save a document.

   Print a document.

4. Print the revised document. Submit both documents.

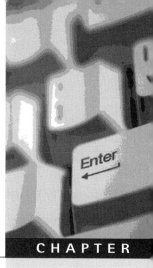

Introduction to Word Processing

5

OBJECTIVES

1. Define common terms related to word processing.
2. Create, format, edit, save, and print Microsoft Word documents.

Word processing is used to create text—letters, memos, reports, proposals, newsletters, and even books! Computers act like smart typewriters when using word processing software. They make any job easier once a few of the possibilities are revealed. This chapter provides the basics of word processing using Microsoft Word 2003.

▶ 5.1 COMMON TERMS IN WORD PROCESSING

Block

A block is a selected (highlighted) section of text that is treated as a unit. Use it to perform formatting and editing functions. Most individual formatting functions, such as bold and underline, also work with blocks of text.

Clipboard   A clipboard is an invisible holding area or buffer for copied or cut data for later use. Users put the data onto the clipboard and can then paste it into another document, another application, or another location within the original document. With the new version of Office, an Office Clipboard holds up to 25 items at a time (see Chapter 4 for details).

Font   A font defines a descriptive look or shape (font face or typeface), size, style, and weight of a group of characters or symbols. For example, one font is Times Roman, 12 point, bold, italic. Another font is Times Roman, 10 point, italic. This term is frequently misunderstood. Several of these terms are important to understanding fonts.

Pitch   Number of characters printed in 1 inch (cpi).

Point size   Height of the font given in printing language, 72 points per inch of height.

Spacing   Proportional or fixed pitch. Proportional means allotting a variable amount of space for each character depending on the character width. Fixed- or mono-spaced means a set space for each character regardless of the character width. For example, an *I* is allowed the same amount of space as a *W*.

Style   Style refers to the vertical slant of the character—normal (upright), condensed, or italic (oblique). Many word processing programs also include bold and other effects.

Symbol set   The characters and symbols that make up the font.

Typeface   This is the specific design of a character or symbol, commonly referred to as the font face. For example, Helvetica, Courier, Times Roman, Times Roman Bold, and Times Roman Italic are all different typefaces.

Footer
The footer is an information area that is placed consistently at the bottom of each page of a document. It can hold the name of the document, the page number, the date, or any information that is helpful.

Format
Format is the process of editing the appearance of a document by using indentations, margins, tabs, justification, and pagination; format conditions affect the document appearance. In Word, format features vary depending on whether someone is formatting characters (font, size, emphasis, and/or special effects such as highlight, or superscript and subscript), paragraph formatting (alignment, indentation, line spacing, and line breaks), or page formatting such as margins, paper size, and orientation.

Grammar Checker
A grammar checker is software that often comes with word processing programs. This software provides feedback to the user regarding errors in grammar. For example, using *there* when *their* is appropriate or using subjects and verbs that do not agree will cause a green wavy line to appear under the offending sentence or phrase. Within the grammar checker are several settings and styles that can be selected. In Word 2003, grammar and spelling appear together under the Tools menu. This feature shows the errors as the user types.

Hard Return
The hard return is a code inserted in the document by pressing the enter key. This is usually done at the end of a paragraph. In Word, the paragraph mark is ¶. The user may toggle the paragraph markers on to show marks on the doc-

ument when typing or toggle them off by clicking the paragraph mark in the Standard Toolbar.

Header
The header is an information area that is placed consistently at the top of each page of a document and that can hold the name of the document, page number, date, or other identifying information.

Indent
Indent refers to tab settings that place subsequent lines of text the same number of spaces from the margin until the next hard return.

Insert
Insert means to add characters in the text at the point of the cursor, thereby moving all other text to the right. It is the opposite of overtype mode and is the default in most word processing programs.

Justified
Justified is alignment of text relative to the left and right margins.

Center   Center places the text line equidistant from both margins.

Full   Full justification is alignment of text flush against both the left and right margins.

Left   Left justification is alignment of text flush against the left margin and staggered on the right.

Right   Right justification is alignment of text flush against the right margin and staggered on the left.

Move
Move is a function in word processing programs that permits the user to relocate text or graphics to another place in the document or to another document.

Outliner
Outliner is a feature of many word processing programs that enables the user to plan and rearrange large documents in an outline form.

Overtype
Overtype means to replace the character under the cursor by the character typed. To turn it off, go to the **Tools** menu, click **Options**, click the

Page Break

Edit tab, and then clear the **Overtype mode** check box.

This is the place where Word ends the text on one page before it continues text on the next page. Insert a page break by going to the **Insert** menu and selecting **Break** or by pressing Ctrl + Enter. The software then places the break at the point where the cursor is. It is a good idea to review the document when it is finished to determine where a page break is needed. Use it cautiously until all revisions of the document have been completed. A page break can also be inserted from the Format menu: choose **Paragraph**, and then click on **Line and Page Breaks**. The user may also alter the appearance of page breaks here.

Pagination

Pagination is the numbers or marks that are used to indicate the sequence of the pages. It is a process of determining when there is sufficient text on one page and then starting the next page. Word processing programs automatically do this if this feature is turned on. Most programs permit the variation of placement and style of the page number.

Scrolling

Scrolling is the process of moving around a document to view a specific portion of a page of text within a document. (All of the document may not fit on the screen.) This does not change the location of the insertion point until the user clicks in the document.

Smart Tags

Smart tag marks (purple dotted underlines) appear when Word recognizes certain types of data and places a mark in the document.

When a smart tag appears, move the insertion point over the underlined text until the Smart Tag Actions button appears. Click the button to see the menu of actions that the user can take.

Soft Return	A soft return is the code inserted in the document automatically when the typed line reaches the right margin.
Spell Checker	Most programs come with an embedded spell checker. This program checks the words for correct spelling. Word combines the spelling and grammar checker. A wavy red line under a word means that it is misspelled or that it is not in Word's dictionary.
Tab	A tab is a setting that places the subsequent text on that line a certain number of spaces or inches in from the left margin. Tab settings by default are five spaces or 0.5 inches. The settings are changeable. There are five styles of tabs—left, right, center, decimal, and bar. All deal with the alignment of the text around the tab mark.
Thesaurus	A thesaurus is a built-in feature that helps the user search for alternative words.
Toggle	Toggle means to switch from one mode of operation to another mode: on or off—such as to insert or replace/overtype.
Word Wrap	This feature automatically carries words over to the next line if they extend beyond the margin.

► 5.2 DATA EXCHANGE

Word processing software saves documents in file formats that are unique to that software program. Many word processing programs allow the option of saving documents under another file format by using the Save As feature. For example, a Microsoft Word 2003 document can be saved in several ways such as in rich text, XML, Word 97–2003, Word Perfect, or Works. This feature permits the user to exchange a file with others who are using different word processing programs, versions, or systems. It also permits saving the file as a Web page.

► 5.3 SAVING WORK

Every person has horror stories that he or she can tell related to lost data or documents. To avoid accidental loss of data, a few tips are in order.

1. Periodically save all work. When a document is being typed, the computer holds it temporarily in random access memory (RAM). Once the program is instructed to save the document on a storage device, the document exists in both RAM and on the storage device. If power is lost, even temporarily, all of the data in RAM are lost except for that stored on the removable storage device, in temporary backup files, or on the hard disk.

2. Pay attention to warnings that the software gives. These warnings are hints to remind the user that doing some things will have a certain result. For example, saving a document with the same name as another one results in a message asking whether the file is to be replaced (Figure 5.1). Do not respond with "Replace existing file" unless there is no need for the original document.

3. Always keep a backup or duplicate copy of a document. That backup could be a diskette, zip disk, memory stick, or another hard drive. Store the backup in a different place. If something happens to the original document or the computer, the backup copy will be available. A particularly valuable document, such as a thesis or research paper, should have a backup that is kept in a different location than the primary document.

► 5.4 INTRODUCTION TO MICROSOFT WORD 2003

Examples in this text use Microsoft Office Word 2003 for Windows XP. Using Microsoft Office Word 2004 for the Macintosh, however, is essentially the same. The menu and toolbars include most of the same headings and

Figure 5.1

Task Pane for Saving a Document When the Name Already Exists

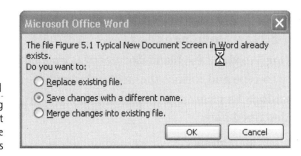

icons, and the windows are remarkably similar in all Office applications. Therefore, both Macintosh and Windows users can use the chapters in this book on word processing, spreadsheets, and graphics presentation with very few changes between operating systems.

Using Keyboard Commands

Most word processing programs are menu driven, with the user carrying out commands by selecting icons or choosing from a menu of options. Menu-driven programs provide users with two options—to select from the menus and icons with the mouse or to use keystroke combinations to issue the command. Some programs are faster when the user issues commands through a series of keystroke combinations. When one clicks on a menu item in Word, the keystroke combination will appear on the right if there is one. For example, when one clicks on File, the keyboard command Ctrl + O appears opposite Open. This keystroke can be used instead of File, Open to open a new document. In the Macintosh operating system, the Apple key (or command key), next to the space bar, acts like the Ctrl key on the Windows system.

Starting Word

As with all Windows programs, there are many ways to start Word. A few ways are presented here. Several ways of opening a new or existing Word document were described in Chapter 4 (see the sections on creating, opening, closing, and saving files).

Click **Start**, **All Programs**. Select **Microsoft Office**, and then choose **MS Office Word** from the available options.

Double click the MS Office **Word** icon if it appears above the Start button or on the desktop.

Click the **Word** icon on the quick launch area of the Taskbar if it appears there.

Creating a New Document

After starting Word, a new blank document is opened by default. A person needs only to type and format the text as desired.

Two methods to create a new document once the Word application is open are described here:

1. Click the **New** button on the standard toolbar under the Word File. This opens a blank new document using the normal template (Figure 5.2).

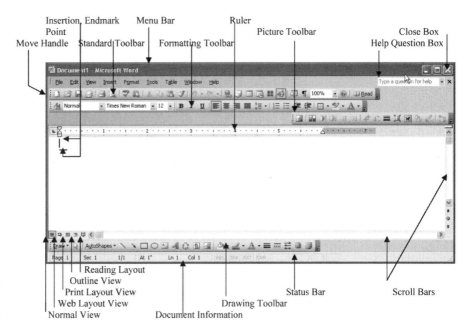

Figure 5.2

Typical New
Document Screen
in Word

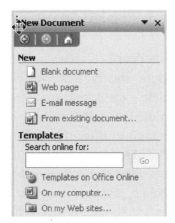

Figure 5.3

New Document
Task Pane

2. Select **File**, **New** from the menu bar. This opens a task pane on the new
    document where the appropriate template can be selected (Figure 5.3).

For each document, Word presents a screen with the menu bar at the top, a
blank window or workplace in the center, and scroll bars on the right side
and bottom right corner. A blinking vertical bar, or insertion point marker,
represents the position in the document. A dark horizontal line marks the

end of the document. In Figure 5.2, the cursor and end mark appear together because nothing has been typed.

Opening a Previously Saved Document in Word

When changes or additions are necessary in a document, several options are available for opening the document again after it is saved (see Chapter 4 for additional ways to open existing documents).

▶ **If the application is not running:**

Start **Word** and choose the **Open** icon. Then select the **location** of the file and **file name**.

Start **Word** and choose **File**, **Open**, and then select **location** of file and **file name**.

▶ **To open an existing document once the application is running:**

Click the **Open** icon. Select the **location** of the file and **file name**. If the document was open recently, it may appear as one of four choices at the bottom of the File Menu.

The user may open recently used files from the Start menu. Select **Start**, **My Recent Documents**, and then select the **file**.

The Menu and Toolbars in Word

Much of the menu bar in Word is the same as in any Office 2003 program (Excel, PowerPoint, Access, etc.) for Windows or Office 2004 for the Macintosh. One difference in the Office Word menu bar is a **Table** option next to **Tools**. Each menu contains a different drop-down list of commands that help one to use Word. The **Standard Toolbar** and the **Formatting Toolbar** appear below the menu bar and share one row by default. Several icons are in the Standard toolbar, the row of icons (or buttons) directly under the menu bar. The Standard Toolbar is shown in Figure 5.4.

These same icons appear under the different drop-down menus when the user clicks on a menu item. For example, the first five icons all appear under File beside the appropriate command. Clicking on the new document button at the left in the standard toolbar opens a new document, on the open folder button opens an existing folder, on the save button saves the document, on the printer button sends one copy of the current document to the printer, on the magnifying glass button a print

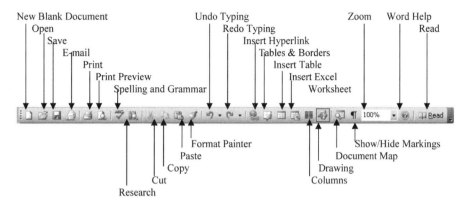

Standard Toolbar in
Word 2003

preview window, on the spelling and grammar checker 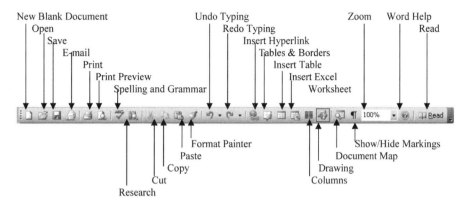 suggestions for
spelling or grammar, and so on.

The Formatting Toolbar (Figure 5.5) shares the same row as the Standard
Toolbar. It is used mainly for font style and size and for bolding **B** , itali-
cizing _I_ , or underlining <u>U</u> text. In addition, the justification and outlining options appear here. Adding borders , adding highlighting color
, or changing font color **A** can also be done from this toolbar.

▶ **To display each toolbar on its own row:**
Click the **Toolbar Options** button at the far right of the toolbar.
Select **Show Buttons on Two Rows** option. *Now the toolbars appear on
two rows.*

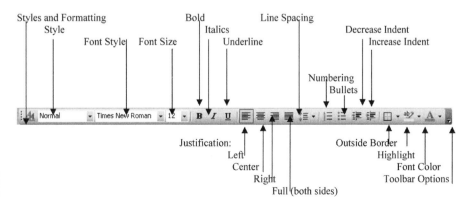

Figure 5.5
Formatting Toolbar

Another option to show them on two rows is to select **View**, **Toolbars**, **Customize**, and check **Show Standard and Formatting Toolbars on Two Rows**. From this dialog box, the user may also show the full menu instead of the default short menu.

In the menu bar, a click on a menu heading (the top row) results in a drop-down menu below the heading (see Common Layout in Chapter 4 also). Next to the command are keyboard commands that can be used instead of the mouse. If the command is gray, it is unavailable. Clicking on a command followed by an arrow causes another menu to appear. A command followed by an ellipsis (...) causes a dialog box to appear. Dialog boxes communicate ways to set up the document. The more that one works on a computer, the more useful the keyboard commands become. Familiarity with the program helps the user decide which method is preferred. This book uses the mouse because beginners usually find it the easiest. A brief description of each drop-down menu appears here.

File

The file commands help in document handling and printing as well as provide a list of the Word documents most recently opened. The user can select a **New Document** here or **Open** a previously prepared document that may reside on a diskette or in a folder. Page formatting commands appear under **Page Setup**. Figure 5.6 shows the Page Setup Dialog Box. Here a person can set margins, page orientation, page size, header and footer location, and add line numbers or borders.

Also under File are the commands for **Web preview** and **Print Preview**, to **Close** the document, and options for **Sending** the document via e-mail or fax.

Edit

These commands allow a person to copy and move text. The **Undo** and **Repeat** commands are at the top of the menu. **Undo** reverses a recent delete, cut, paste, or typing change. If one hits the wrong key and something disappears that should be kept, click the **Undo** command before doing anything else. If a section of the document is accidentally deleted and then discovered after

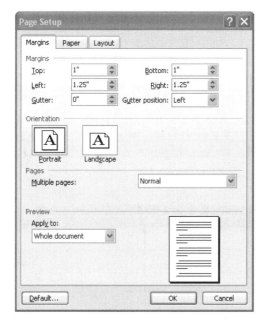

Figure 5.6

Page Setup
Dialog Box

new typing occurs, keep clicking the **Undo** button (or icon in the toolbar) until it reappears. A
list of the actions that one can undo is available if
one clicks on the down arrow next to the **Undo**
button on the **Standard Toolbar**. The
Find and Replace commands were discussed in
Chapter 4 (see Figure 4.13).

View

Under the View option are the commands that
allow one to view the document's layout in
Normal, **Web**, **Print**, **Reading**, or **Outline**.
Icons for these commands appear in the bottom
left corner of the document as well (Figure 5.2).
View also contains commands that allow access
to the **Toolbars** or **Ruler**. Toolbars can be customized to show the Word drawing toolbar or to
hide toolbars that are not used frequently by
clicking to select or deselect. This is also the
menu that brings up the **Header** or **Footer Bars**
(Figure 5.7).

Change font size here by highlighting header and choosing smaller size.

Type in this box for header. Use tab key to move to middle and right side.

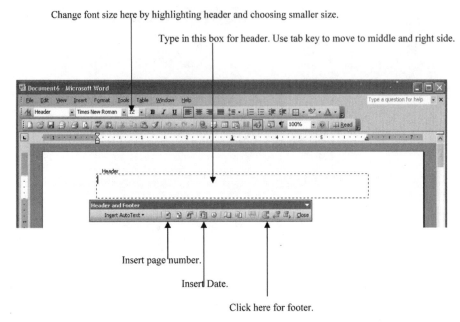

Insert page number.

Insert Date.

Click here for footer.

Figure 5.7

Screen for adding a
Header or Footer

Insert

This menu helps one to insert a **Break**, **Page Numbers**, the **Date** and **Time**, **Reference**, **Picture**, or a **Hyperlink**. Use Section breaks to create different formatting within a document. Two common uses are to create a different section or to create two or more columns.

Format

These commands allow a person to define the style of a document and the appearance of text or picture. Select the **Font** header, and choose the size, color, and style of type. Here one can add **Bullets** or **Numbers** to lists, **Borders** or **Backgrounds**, and **Change case**. This dialog window available under **Paragraph** provides indents and line spacing and break choices.

Tools

Under **Tools**, one finds **Spelling and Grammar**, **Language** (thesaurus), **Word Count**, and **Letters and Mailings** commands. Word count is helpful when a 250-word abstract or a paper of a certain length is needed. This menu also allows one to customize the layout of

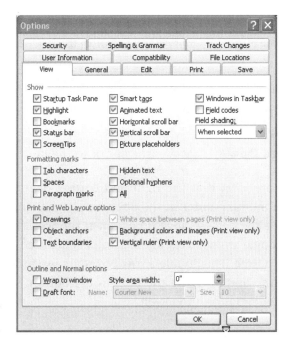

Figure 5.8

Options Dialog
Window under Tools

	Word's toolbars, menus, and editing features using the Options Dialog Window (Figure 5.8).
Table	Under **Table** are the commands for creating and modifying tables.
Window	Here one can move between document windows, split a document into two parts if one needs to see one section while working on another, and see a list of all active documents.
Help	Help provides access to Word Help, Online Help, the Office Assistant and other Help items (see Figures 4.2 and 4.3).

Moving Around the Document

There are several ways to move around a document.

Arrow keys	Move the insertion point or cursor a line or letter at a time.
Ctrl + arrow keys	Move one word or paragraph at a time.
Home key	Moves the cursor to the beginning of the line.

End key	Moves the cursor to the end of the line.
Ctrl + Home	Moves the cursor to the beginning of the document.
Ctrl + End	Moves the cursor to the end of the document.
Page Up and Page Down	Moves the cursor quickly through the document one screen at a time.
Ctrl + Page Up	Moves the cursor to previous printed page.
Ctrl + Page Down	Moves the cursor to the next printed page.

Scroll bars are located at the right and bottom of the screen (Figure 5.2). Placing the mouse pointer in the open box in the scroll line allows one to click or drag the box to move up or down the scroll line as quickly as desired. The single arrow boxes in the scroll bar are used to move up or down one line at a time. The double arrow boxes are used to move up or down a page. Clicking and dragging the box on the bottom scroll line moves the document sideways on the screen.

Formatting the Document
Page formatting
Described here are the options for changing page formats:

1. Open a new document and choose **File**, **Page Setup** from the menu bar. *The Page Setup Dialog Box appears* (Figure 5.6). Use it to adjust margins and decide on paper orientation (portrait or landscape), paper size, and layout. Usually margins are set 1 inch at the top and bottom and 1.25 inches at the left and right side. Vertically centering is also set in this dialog box. Use it to center the title page.
2. Set a Page break by pressing the **Ctrl + Enter** keys or selecting the **Insert**, **Break**, **Page** from the menu bar.
3. Use **Headers and Footers** to have text appear on each page of the document.

▶ **To add a header or footer to a document:**
Choose **View** and select **Header and Footer**.
Type the **text** wanted in the **header or footer** box and/or
Select Options such as page number, date, or filename, from the header/footer toolbar.
Click the **Close** button.

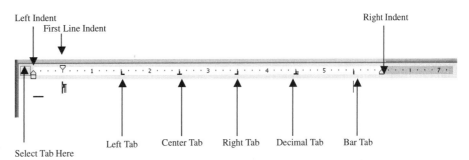

Figure 5.9
Ruler and Tabs

In Figure 5.7, the header is shown. The header is the default box that appears first. The title of the document could appear in the left corner, the page number in the middle, and the date on the right. To open the footer, click in the footer box [icon] in the dialog bar. Click on the # sign to add a page number. The calendar gives the date, and the clock gives the time. A running head can be placed in the header by putting the insertion point where the header should appear and typing it. The tab key moves the cursor from the left side to the middle and then to the right side of the box. Choose the appropriate spot for inserting the name of the document, the date, or page number.

Paragraph formatting—indents

Word has three indents: First, Left, and Right (Figure 5.9).

These indent markers are displayed on the Rule Bar. Dragging the top indent marker [icon] to the right (first line indent) indents the first line of a paragraph. Pressing the **Tab** key does the same thing. The middle marker [icon] is the left-indent marker. Use it to indent all lines of the paragraph except the first one. The top and middle markers will move together when the bottom marker [icon] is selected and moved. The middle marker is the hanging indent. To get a negative indent (to the right of the first line), drag the middle marker to the right of the first-line indent marker. A hanging indent is an indentation of all of a paragraph except the first line. If the **Format** and then **Paragraph** menus are selected, the hanging indent will appear under **Special** by clicking on the down arrow.

▶ **To set the indents:**

Place the **insertion** point in the paragraph that will be indented or highlight multiple paragraphs.

Drag the appropriate marker to the chosen tick mark on the ruler bar.

These features may also be accessed through the **Format**, **Paragraph** menu.

Paragraph formatting—tabs

Word has default tabs every 0.5 inches along the ruler. It also offers the standard four tab types from left to right: left tab, center tab, decimal tab, and right tab (Figure 5.9). The tabs can be placed in the ruler using the mouse.

Click the **Left Corner** tab icon until the correct tab mark appears.
Click the **Ruler setting** where the tab should be.

To remove a tab, click on it and drag it off the ruler into the document.

Tabs settings may also be adjusted and additional features applied through the **Format**, **Tabs** menu dialog box. For example, set the tab dot leaders here.

Paragraph formatting—alignment, numbering, bullets, and borders

The icons for justification, numbering, and adding bullets or borders are in the Formatting Toolbar (Figure 5.5). The first icons after font style involve text alignment or justification: left, centered, right, and full (both right and left, respectively). Next, a line spacing icon ⬆☰▾, the numbering icon ☰, and then the add bullets icon ⦙☰ appear. The next two icons move numbered or bulleted text to the left (decrease) or right (increase). The next icons bring up the border tool, which allows for a partial or complete border around selected text.

Character formatting—font size and style

As in previous examples, several ways are available to choose the font size and style.

1. Click **Format**, **Font**. Choose a **Font**, **Font Style**, and **Size** from the Dialog Box.
2. Use the Font Style and Size menu boxes in the beginning of the Formatting Toolbar. Business default size is 10 to 12 points. A larger size can be chosen that can be read easily on the screen. Later, the font can be changed. Highlight the document by choosing Select All under Edit (or Ctrl A) and reduce the print size before printing by choosing another font size or print style or both. Clicking on **Font** under the Format Menu opens a dialog box in which a font style and size can be

chosen that can then be set as the default style for all documents. The font size and style are shown in the beginning of the Formatting Toolbar (Figure 5.5).

3. Style buttons are available in the Formatting Toolbar for bold, italics, and underline.

> **To use the Formatting Toolbar for bold, italics, and underline:**

Highlight a **word** or section of text.
Click the desired **style** button.

Clicking the button again changes the style back to normal. These attributes can also be turned on or off by pressing Ctrl + B, Ctrl + I, or Ctrl + U. When Font is selected under the Format menu, the same commands appear in the Font Dialog Box.

4. Click on the **Styles and Formatting** button. The Styles and Formatting Task Pane opens on the right of the document. Use it to select style and size of text. This is especially important when creating a table of contents.

Preparing a Document

Two ways are available to prepare the formatting for a document. The first is to set the formatting before beginning to type the text; the other is to type the text and then format the document. Whichever way it is done is a personal preference; remember, however, that the idea is to create and format the document efficiently and effectively. A process is described here for setting the formats before creating the document.

Although the formatting features can be accessed from the Format menu, many of the settings are also available under the File menu as discussed previously here in Page Formatting. If the product will be bound, a left-hand margin is needed of at least 1.5 inches. If using a letterhead, measure its height. As much as 2.4 inches may be needed to make sure that the body of the letter begins below the letterhead. If the margins of a section of the document need to be changed, go into Page Setup again, and change the margins to what is needed; then select "this point forward" under "Apply to" (Figure 5.6).

Next go to **Format** and choose **Font**. Select the type and size of font desired from the Font Dialog Box. Often the Word font and size default is Times New Roman, 10 points. This can be changed by (1) selecting the desired font and size in the Font dialog box, (2) clicking the Default button in the lower left of the window, and (3) responding "Yes" to change the Normal template. This means that Word will always open to this font and size for any future documents. If the settings are changed for this document only, then change the settings and click OK.

Next choose **Format** and then **Paragraph**. The Paragraph Dialog Box appears as shown in Figure 5.10. Besides alignment options, single-, 1.5-, or double-spacing options can be chosen under Line Spacing. One can also choose line spacing by clicking on the arrow next to the line spacing button in the Formatting Toolbar.

It may be easier to work on a document using 1.5 or single spacing. Later it can be changed to whatever spacing is required or preferred. The document can also be highlighted and its spacing changed by pressing:

Ctrl + 1 to create single spacing
Ctrl + 5 to create 1.5-spaced lines
Ctrl + 2 to create double-spaced lines

In the same Paragraph Dialog Box (Figure 5.10), there is a tab for Line and Page Breaks. Clicking the Widow/Orphan Control box adjusts page breaks so that two or more paragraph lines always begin or end a page. A page break can also be inserted by going to the Insert menu and choosing **Break**.

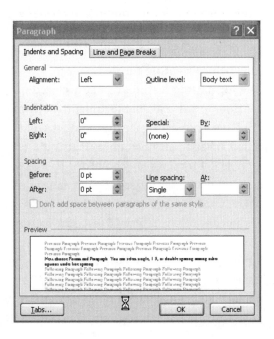

Figure 5.10

Paragraph Dialog Box

Simply highlighting a Page Break dotted line and pressing the Backspace key will delete it.

Clicking on the Paragraph (¶) sign in the Standard Toolbar (Figure 5.4) will result in the addition of formatting marks for spaces, indents, and ends of paragraphs to the document. The marks are helpful if a document needs to be reformatted or if one is not sure why the document looks the way it does. Remember that it is always better to use tabs instead of spaces when formatting a document.

Viewing a Document

Word provides several ways to view a document on the screen. The best view for preparing a document is usually Normal.

▶ **To change a view:**

Select **View** and click the **View Option** desired from the choices or click the **button** on the left bottom corner of the screen that corresponds to the view desired (Figure 5.2).

The first View Option is Normal. The next View is the Web Layout—a view that is designed to be used to read documents online. This view provides an outline view of the document on the screen's left side in a scroll box with the text on the right screen. Print Layout shows the document as it will look when printed. It can help when arranging pictures or columns and so on. A space is shown between each page. The Outline view displays the document in outline form using Word's Standard Headings style. The Reading layout shows the document on facing pages. This view can help one to organize thoughts and ideas when writing or reorganizing a paper.

Numbers and Bullets

Automatic bulleting and numbering can be helpful—and frustrating!

▶ **To create a numbered list:**

Put the cursor where the list will begin.

Click the Numbering button ⊟ in the Formatting Toolbar (Figure 5.5).

Type the **list** pressing the **Enter** key at the end of each item.

When finished, press the **Enter** key twice or click the numbering button to turn off the numbers.

One can also type the first number, press the Enter key, and for the next item, Word will add the 2. If the list is ended, simply backspace to get rid of the next number, or press the Enter key twice.

▶ **To create a bullet list:**

Type the **list**.

Highlight the **list**.

Click the Bullets ⁝☰ button on the Formatting Toolbar (Figure 5.5).

To modify the appearance of Numbers and Bullets, go to **Format**, and choose **Bullets and Numbering**; then select the tab for **Bulleted**, **Numbered**, or **Outline Numbered** and choose an appropriate style.

Spelling and Grammar Checks

Spelling and grammar checks, readability statistics, and a thesaurus are tools included in Word 2003 to help with proofreading. Word automatically checks spelling and grammar as one types. If a word is misspelled, a wavy red line appears under the word. If it is a grammar error, the wavy line is green.

▶ **To correct the error:**

Right click over the error.

Select a correction. Choose to ignore it, or add the word to the spelling dictionary.

When adding a word to the dictionary, be sure that it is correct. The spelling dictionary is stored on the hard drive, and thus, it is only available on the computer to which it was added. Other ways to correct spelling and grammar are to choose **Spelling** and **Grammar** under the Tools menu or by clicking the **ABC** button on the Standard Toolbar (Figure 5.4).

Because some people are distracted by the wavy lines, Word provides an option to turn this feature off.

▶ **To turn the spelling and grammar checker off:**

Select **Tools** and then **Spelling and Grammar**.

Click on **Options** in the Dialog Box that appears.

Uncheck the boxes that "Check spelling as you type" and "Check grammar as you type."

Click **OK**.

After this is done, in order to check spelling and grammar:

Click the **Spelling and Grammar** button in the Standard Toolbar, or select **Tools**, **Spelling and Grammar** from the Menu Bar.

Usually one keeps the spelling and grammar checks turned on as the document is typed. When text is entered into the document, the Spelling and Grammar 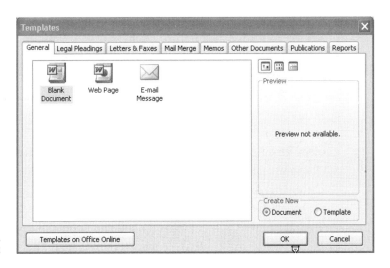 Icon appears in the lower Status Bar (Figure 5.2). When a red X appears on the icon, Word has detected a possible spelling or grammar error.

It is best to do grammar, spelling, and readability checks after the document is finished and the cursor is at the beginning of the document. It will still be necessary, however, to read the document over, as Word will not find all of the misspellings or grammar problems that might exist.

Using Word Templates

Word provides several templates that can be applied to a new document. Choose **New** under **File** (Figure 5.3). The first screen shows the blank document icon as well as Web page and e-mail message. Under **Templates**, choose **On my computer**.

Figure 5.11 shows the Template Dialog Box.

Templates for such things as Letters and Faxes, Mail Merge, Publications, and Reports are included. Here one can choose a preset style or create a new special document. The Wizard helps in this process. For example go to

Figure 5.11

Template Dialog Box

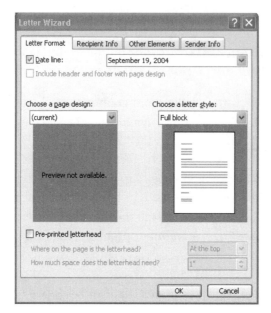

Figure 5.12
Letter Wizard
Dialog Box

Tools, and choose **Letters and Mailing**; then click on **Letter Wizard**. The Letter Wizard Dialog Box appears (Figure 5.12).

If one modifies a certain style and wants to save it as a template, choose **Save As** from the File menu. In the Save as type box choose **Document Type**. Then name the document template. Choose the appropriate template folder in which to save it.

Creating a Table

The table feature is used in many ways. It helps set columns when recording minutes or when organizing any kind of information. Tables are also essential to research reports. It is a good idea to plot out the kind of table needed in terms of number of rows and columns before selecting them. Among the choices for a new table in the Table menu are **Draw Table** or **Insert**. Figure 5.13 shows the dialog box that appears when **Insert** is selected.

Choosing **Auto Format** from the dialog box allows customization of the table with predesigned styles, as shown in Figure 5.14.

To draw a table, select **Draw Table** from the Table Menu. The Tables and Borders Formatting Toolbar appears (Figure 5.15). This toolbar can be added below the other Toolbars.

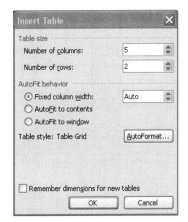

Figure 5.13
Insert Table
Dialog Box

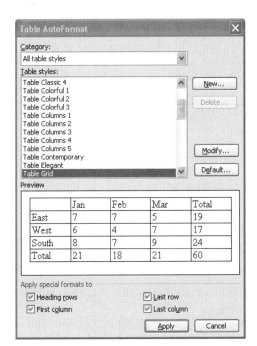

Figure 5.14
Table AutoFormat
Dialog Box

Clicking on the Insert Table ▦ Button in DrawToolbar will bring up the same Dialog Box as shown in Figure 5.13. There is also a Table ▦ Button in the Standard Toolbar. Figure 5.16 shows the box that appears when it is selected. Clicking over the squares highlights the number of rows and columns needed for the table. This method used to be limited, but now is not. Just keep dragging until the correct size is reached and the drop-down window will expand.

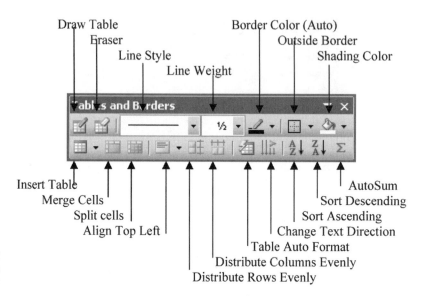

Figure 5.15

Table and Borders
Formatting Bar

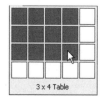

Figure 5.16

Method for Drawing
a Table Using the
Standard Toolbar Icon

▶ **To create a table:**

Place the **insertion** point where the table should appear in the document.

Select **Table**, **Insert** from the menu or click and hold the **Table button**.

Select the **Number of Rows** and **Columns** and click **OK**, or if using the table button, drag over the cells for the **Number of Rows and Columns** desired.

Remember that a row is needed for headers. Another row or column can be inserted if necessary.

▶ **To insert a row:**

Click in a **Row**.

Select **Table**, **Insert Rows**. Choose whether to add the row above or below the row where the cursor is. Columns are inserted the same way.

Many more commands are available under the Table menu, as well as in the Tables and Borders Formatting Bar, that allow one to change the width or height of a row or column, alter the style, or delete grid lines. To delete the table, highlight it, and choose Backspace or Cut.

Creating Merged Documents

Word will create envelopes and form letters and print a personalized copy for each person on a list. Word replaces merge fields from a main document with information from a data source. Like many other Word functions, more than one way is possible to send a form letter to a list of people. One method is described in this section.

Two documents will be created:

1. A *data source* contains the name and addresses (and whatever else must be individualized) for each letter. A series of subdocuments can also be set up that Word will merge into a main document. The data source can be an Outlook address book, an Access database, an Excel spreadsheet with column headings, or a Word table. For this exercise, a Word table will be the data source. Every data document consists of three parts: records, fields, and field headers. Each paragraph in a data document is a record, and each column is a field. One must plan the data source carefully so that it does what is expected.

2. A *main document* contains the same text that will appear in each letter and the field code from which to insert the personalized data from the data source.

Creating the main document

Open a new document.

Select **Tools**, **Letters and Mailings**, and then **Mail Merge**. *The Mail Merge Task Pane appears on the right of the document* (Figure 5.17).

Click on **Letters** if there is no green dot in it.

Choose **Next**.

Choose **Start from a template**, and then click on **Select Template . . .**

Choose **Plain Merge Letter**, and click **OK**.

If the letter template is hard to see, click **Normal** under View. Then write the body of the letter below the Greeting Line. Double chevrons mark the data source fields. Add your name and title next.

Click on **Next** in the Task Pane.

Choose **Type a new list**, and then click on **Create**.

Figure 5.18 shows the New Address List Entry Box.

Type in two or three entries.

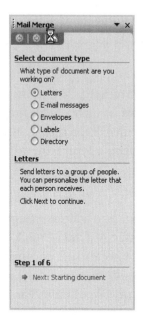

Figure 5.17

Mail Merge Task Pane

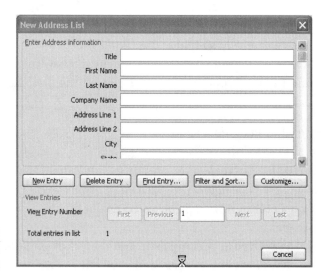

Figure 5.18

New Address List
Entry Box

When finished click on **Close**. *The Save Address List Dialog Box appears.*

Name the List and save it in My Data Sources. *Next, the Mail Merge Recipient Box will appear* (Figure 5.19).

Click **OK**.

In the Task Pane, click on **Next: Write your letter**.

Then click on **Next: Preview your letter**. *The letter to the first recipient appears.*

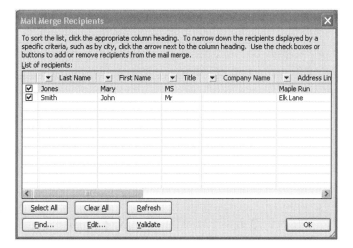

Figure 5.19

Mail Merge
Recipients List

Another letter can be previewed or the recipient list changed (Figure 5.20).

Choose **Next: Complete the Merge**. *At this point, Mail Merge is ready to complete the Merge.*

Click on **Print**. Choose to print all of the letters, the current record, or records between selected numbers.

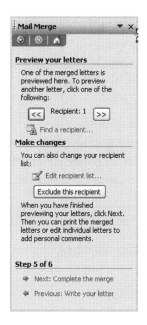

Figure 5.20

Task Pane for
Previewing Letters or
Recipient List

SUMMARY

The possibilities are unlimited for creating documents in Word. Described here are only a few of the basics. Some of the possibilities include outlining, creating an index, generating a table of contents, inserting clip art, making newsletters, addressing envelopes, and customizing and optimizing Word. Use the documentation from the software company or go online to Microsoft Office and take advantage of the many assistance and training opportunities available. It will take time and diligent work to take advantage of all of the program's features.

Exercise 1: Basic Microsoft Word Functions
Objectives
1. Perform selected word processing functions.
2. Explain basic word processing terms and functions.

Activity
1. Start Word. (This exercise can be done using any word processing program.)
2. Create a document. Type the following text as fast as possible. Do not correct mistakes, and do not hit the enter key. Do not pay attention to spelling errors.

   Using word processing software can save many hours and much pain. It can also be very exasperating. It is important to follow a few simple rules. If the rules are ignored, disaster can strike. These are a few of the simple rules: (1) Save all work periodically. (2) Pay attention to the warnings given. (3) Always keep a second copy of the document or project on another disk or hard drive in another place.

3. Save the document.

   Select **File**, **Save**, or press **Ctrl + S**.

   Type **Rules for wp** in the highlighted File Name Box. Then go to the Save in Text box at the top of the Save As Box. Select the correct storage device by clicking the **down arrow** button and selecting the option (see Figure 4.11 for further help).

   The document can also be saved by clicking on the **Save** button on the Standard Toolbar (next to the Open icon). Once the document has a name and location, clicking on Save will just update the file and not display the Save As dialog window.

4. Move around the document.

   Practice moving around the document.

   Use the **arrow** keys and **Page Up** and **Page Down** keys.

5. Edit text.

Highlight the **text** (press **Ctrl + A**).

Select **Edit** and **Copy** (or press Ctrl + C).

Position the **insertion point** two or three lines below the original paragraph. Press **Ctrl + End**, and press **Enter** twice.

Select **Edit** and **Paste** (or press Ctrl + V). *Now there are two copies of the text.*

Select **Edit** and **Undo Paste**.

Try doing the same things using the **Cut** , **Copy** , and **Paste** buttons on the Formatting Toolbar.

Finish with one copy of the text on the page.

Go back to **Edit** and choose **Repeat Paste**; the text returns.

If one copies a different text, the first text that was saved will be gone from the clipboard unless the Office clipboard is active. The last few commands can be undone, however, by choosing Undo Paste or Undo Cut. Keyboard commands can also be used to cut (**Ctrl + X**), copy (**Ctrl + C**), and paste (**Ctrl + V**). End this task with two of the same paragraphs.

6. Align text.

Highlight the **second copy** of the text.

Click the **Align Right** button.

Note what happens. To get both right and left justification, click on the **Justify** button. All sentences are flush at both margins except for the last sentence.

Click the **Align Left** button.

7. Edit the document.

One copy of the text can be deleted if desired.

Use the tab and enter keys to create a document that looks like this:

Using word processing software can save many hours and much pain. It can also be very exasperating. It is important to follow a few simple rules. If the rules are ignored, disaster can strike.

These are a few of the simple rules:

1. Periodically save all work.

2. Pay attention to the warnings given.

3. Always keep a second copy of the document or project on another disk or hard drive, and keep it in another place.

Press **Ctrl + Home** to place the insertion bar at the beginning of the paragraph.

Select **Tools**, **Spelling and Grammar** to correct any errors. *When the dialog window appears, it will highlight misspelled words and offer corrections.*

Click the **Change** button if the highlighted selection is correct and the **Ignore** button to ignore a correctly spelled word.

Word will announce the completion of the spelling and grammar check.

8. Format the document.

   Type a **title** above the text. (Press **Ctrl + Home**. Type **Word Processing Rules**, and press the **Enter** key twice.)

   Highlight the **title**. Click the **Bold** **B** button, and click the **Center** ≡ button.

   Click in the text to deselect the title.

9. Print the document.

   Press the **Ctrl + P** keys, or click the **Printer** button.

10. Close and save the document.

    Click the **Save** button to save the document. This will update the file saved earlier.

    Click the **Close** button on the Word application or go on to Exercise 2.

Exercise 2: Find, Replace, and Paragraph Borders

Objectives

1. Use a find and replace function.
2. Create a document with a paragraph border.

Activity

1. Create the document.

   Type the following text in the new document window:

   A descriptive survey was used to elicit information concerns of new moms as part of an evaluation of single room maternity care (SRMC) at a small Mid-western hospital. The investigators developed a list of concerns common to new moms. New moms were asked to check as many of the 16 concerns listed that they would like the nurse to help with or discuss after the birth of their baby. After a pilot study of 10 new moms, the survey was mailed to all new moms who delivered a live infant during a 12–month period.

2. Search and replace all occurrences of moms with mothers.

   Press **Ctrl + Home** to go to the top of the document.

   Select **Edit** and then **Replace** from the menu bar.

   In the **Find what** box, type **moms**.

   Press the **Tab** key, or click on the **Replace with** text box.

   Type **mothers.**

Click the **Replace All** button. What happens?

Click **OK** button.

Make sure to use the Replace All with caution, as it will change all words that have the sequence of letters *moms* in them.

Change dialog boxes again and reverse the directions.

Type **mothers** in the Find what box and **moms** in the replace with box.

Click the **Replace All** button. *The document will return to normal.*

Click the **Close** button to close the replace dialog window.

3. Create paragraph borders.

   Go to the end of the document, and press **Enter** four times.

   Select the **above** paragraph.

   Copy it and **paste** it below the first paragraph.

   Highlight the first paragraph.

   Click the **Outside Border** ⊞ ▾ button on the Toolbar.

   Now highlight the **new paragraph**.

   Select **Format** and **Borders and Shading**.

   Click the **3-D border box**.

   From **Style**, choose the **double line**.

   From **Width**, choose $1^1/_2$ **pt**. Click **OK**.

   Put the cursor inside the box, and add a line at the top and one at the bottom.

   Then **highlight** the text and choose **Justify** ▤ from the Formatting Toolbar.

   The box should look like this box:

> A descriptive survey was used to elicit information concerns of new moms as part of an evaluation of single room maternity care (SRMC) at a small Midwestern hospital. The investigators developed a list of concerns common to new moms. New moms were asked to check as many of the 16 concerns listed that they would like the nurse to help with or discuss after the birth of their baby. After a pilot study of 10 new moms, the survey was mailed to all new moms who delivered a live infant during a 12-month period.

4. **Save** the document, and **print** it.

   Tip: Always leave a paragraph mark (press **Enter**) below the text that will be boxed or below a table to enable titles or text to be added. If the last paragraph mark is within the box, pressing **Enter** will only enlarge the box or table.

Exercise 3: Merge and Find Functions
Objectives

1. Create main, data source, and merged documents.
2. Use the find and replace function.
3. Print created letters.

Activity

1. Create the documents.

   Create the main and data source documents like those at the end of this exercise. Use the directions earlier in this chapter on creating the Mail Merge documents.

2. Use the Find and Replace function and replace all occurrences of:

   DM with diabetes mellitus

   April 25, 2005, with April 25, 2006

   medications with insulin

3. Merge the documents.

   Use the merge (mail merge) feature to generate and print the individual letters. Check them for accuracy.

   The appearance of the fields depends on the word processor. They may be the name of the field, a number with a -, etc.

Main Document

<<Title>> <<FirstName>> <<LastName>>

<<Address>>

<<City> <<State>> <<PostalCode>>

(Use the automatic date function to place date with this style: Month Day, Year.)

Dear <<FirstName>>:

We invite you to attend a patient education program on adult-onset DM. The date of the program is September 25, 2005. The program time takes place from 1 to 3 p.m. in the Patient Education Conference Room, 4th floor, Computerville Hospital.

We designed this program for newly diagnosed diabetics. The program will address adjusting to diabetes, diet and exercise, and medications. The guest speaker is Nellie Netscape, Nurse Practitioner.

Please notify us at 624-3333 if you plan to attend. There is no charge for this program. We look forward to seeing you.

Sincerely,

Mary Data, PhD, RN

Data Source

Title	FirstName	LastName	Address	City	ST	ZIP
Ms.	Mary	Jones	325 First Street	Carnegie	PA	15102
Mr.	Robert	Tutor	45 Software Ave.	Milford	PA	15102
Dr.	Susan	Master	8997 Default Lane	Eagan	MN	55123

Assignment 1: Preparing a Resume

This assignment can be done with any word processing program.

Directions

A resume that summarizes educational and professional accomplishments is necessary when applying for a new job.

1. Obtain a want ad from the paper (preferably in the health field).
2. Compose a resume using Word's Resume Template.

   Choose **New** under File.

   Then Click on 🔲 On my computer... under Templates.

   Go to the **Other Documents** tab

   Choose **Professional Resume**.

   Make sure the resume includes

   a. Information about the person

      Name

      Address (city, state, zip)

      Telephone, fax, and e-mail address

   b. Job/work objective (not always included)

   c. Summary of qualifications (use the job description in the advertisement as a guide)

   d. Education (school, degree, date, major)

   e. Professional experience as a nurse.

      Begin with most recent and include year, name of position, and type of unit.

   f. Other information—licensure, honors, professional organizations, publications, grants, special skills, projects, etc.

   Use uppercase and lowercase.

   Use the spell checker as appropriate.

3. Compose a cover letter applying for the position.

   a. Run the cover letter through a spell and grammar checker.

   b. Make appropriate revisions in the cover letter based on results of the spell and grammar checker (if available).

4. Submit an advertisement, a letter of application (original and revised), and a resume.

Assignment 2: Merge Function
Directions

1. Write a procedure or policy for some aspect of your practice. It can be something that exists but requires revision, or it can be a new one that requires development.

   Use the following document format:

Margins:	Left	2"
	Right	1.5"
	Top	2"
	Bottom	1"
Header	Flush right, procedure/policy number on each page	
Footer	Pagination centered	
Last page	Add your initials	

2. Merge function. Create a form letter to send to the five procedure/policy members that includes an explanation of the attached, a due date for review, and the person to contact if they have questions. Set it up to use the merge function. Embed the field codes in the form letter. Create the data source with the following information: name (first and last), title, and hospital location.

3. Turn in the procedure/policy, letter with merge fields, and a copy of the merged letter.

Assignment 3: Announcement
Directions

1. Prepare an announcement of a special function or party for a class.

2. Go to Office Online. Choose Clip Art, and then select **Academic** under **Browse Clip Art**. If there is not an appropriate one under Academic, choose another topic, and select something that matches the announcement purpose.

3. Look at the possibilities, and pick one for the announcement.

4. Click on the clip that will work. Make sure that a document is open to receive the clip art.

5. Construct the announcement around the clip art. Make sure all of the relevant information is included in the announcement.

6. Turn in the announcement.

Introduction to Presentation Graphics

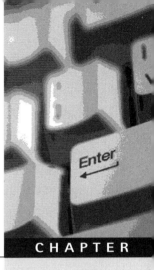

CHAPTER

6

OBJECTIVES

1. Define basic terminology related to presentation graphics.
2. Describe selective uses of presentation graphics software.
3. Recognize components of a quality slide presentation.
4. Develop a PowerPoint presentation.

Presentation graphics software programs are among the fastest growing applications used by computer consumers, and Microsoft PowerPoint is one of the most commonly used. Many software programs contain some graphics capabilities. For example, word processing packages, with a wide variety of fonts, now permit creation of overheads and limited graphics. Spreadsheets permit the creation of pie, line, and bar graphs. Some database programs can also be used to create limited graphs.

Graphic programs include presentation software, draw programs, and computer-aided design programs. Most presentation programs include text handling, outlining, drawing, graphing, clip art, and special effects. They allow the production of high-quality presentation slides, transparencies, handouts, or electronic slide shows. Draw programs help to produce clip art and images used in presentation programs or other applications where images enhance the message. Computer-aided design programs assist draftsmen, engineers, and architects to produce their design plans and drawings.

The focus of this chapter is presentation graphics using PowerPoint. The main use of presentation graphic programs is to present information in a pleasing visual fashion to facilitate decision making and to communicate a message. Visuals that sustain interest, highlight content, and disseminate information enhance presentations by creating an impression.

► 6.1 SLIDE LAYOUTS AND CHART TYPES

Slide layout and chart types refer to the appearance of the content or how the content on the slide is displayed. PowerPoint has 14 types of charts with many variations and many types of slide layouts. Listed here are those most commonly used:

Slide Layout

Described here are some of the slide layout schemes.

Combination	Combination layouts include more than one style. For example, there may be a clip art with text, a title with text, and a chart with a bulleted list.
Drawing	Drawing graphs can create a diagram, map, or flow chart. For example, if one wants to show the process or flow of a procedure, use the drawing features to create the boxes and arrows to show the direction or flow of the process. Use the draw options to import clip art.
List	Lists help to organize the presentation content to cover the main points of the topic. Often a bullet or number precedes each item on the list.
Organization Structure	Organization structure graphs show relationships of people or positions within an organization.

Table	A table presents text information in column form. Use it to display two or three items and some related information about those items (e.g., when showing the elements of three concepts).
Title	Title charts are used to introduce the presentation and to separate sections within the presentation. It is a helpful tool to orient the audience to the topic and its parts.
Text	Text charts contain textual information and sometimes clip art. Use it to show the main points of the presentation and to help orient the audience to the topic.

Chart Types

Described here are some chart types.

Area	Area charts present or emphasize total quantities (volume) of several items over time.
Bar	Bar graphs compare data against some value at a specific point in time. The categories (similar to types of antibiotics) are arranged vertically in a column on the y axis, whereas the values (rating effectiveness) are arranged vertically. The emphasis is on the comparison, not time.
Column	Column graphs show data changes over time or illustrate comparisons. The charts (data or values) are vertical (y axis), whereas the categories are horizontal (x axis), the reverse of bar charts. Many variations of column charts exist.
Doughnuts	Doughnuts are variations of pie charts. They compare parts to the whole but can combine more than one data series.
High/Low	High/low graphs show changes for data within a specific time period or show the changing nature of data over time. They can be used to show temperature changes.

Line	Line graphs present a large amount of data to show trends over time.
Pie	Pie graphs compare parts to a whole or several values at one point in time. They also help to emphasize a particular part or to show relationships between sets of items.
Scatter	Scatter graphs show trends or statistics, such as average frequency, regression, or distribution.

► 6.2 PRESENTATIONS

The first step in preparing a presentation is to define the purpose or message clearly. The second step is to outline or organize the content. Many presentation programs offer an outliner feature to help with this step. Be careful when using this feature to prevent all of the slides from containing just text or bulleted lists. Next, decide the best medium to present the message given the time allowed. This requires knowledge of both the environment where the presentation will occur and the equipment that will be available. Some common media used for presentations are as follows:

Handouts	Sometimes handouts are provided to the audience to outline the presentation, define selected terms, or present complex information. Use the presentation program's handout feature to prepare the handouts when copies of the slides or speaker notes are desired. It is easy to develop appropriate handouts and notes that go with the presentation. To prepare details not covered in the presentation or reference lists, use a word processing program.
Slides	Some presenters use 35-mm slides when the appropriate graphic presentation equipment is not available or when the environment is more conducive to slides. Slides focus the audience on key points and present data in a pleasing and helpful manner. Depending on the slide projector, a dark room may be required. The slides need to project the text with large enough letters to be seen by all.

Slide Shows

Connecting the computer to a data projector enables PowerPoint slides to be projected on a large screen. Slides are created in PowerPoint, and then special effects that control how the slide content appears are added. Adding sound makes the experience truly a multimedia event.

Save the presentation as a slide show to the secondary storage device. This makes it easy to adapt this presentation to different audiences and time slots without going to the expense of making new 35-mm slides. Data projection systems are increasingly available in educational and health care institutions as well as at convention centers. Newer models are portable and project high-quality images that are easily seen in regular lighting.

Transparencies

Some presenters opt for transparencies because they are easy to prepare and use, and the equipment is readily available. In some environments, the overhead projector is being replaced by a document camera, which can also show transparencies. An advantage of transparencies is that they can be used in rooms with normal lighting, which facilitates note taking. Transparencies can be easier and cheaper to produce than slides and may work better in less technologically developed places. Laser and color printers also add to the effectiveness of transparencies. Transparencies, however, are not as easily revised as electronic slide shows.

▶ 6.3 KEY POINTS IN CREATING GRAPHIC PRESENTATIONS

Nothing is worse than a speaker using a graphics presentation that detracts from the message that the speaker is trying to convey or presents nothing but text on the screen. When the slides are complete sentences, the tendency for the speaker is to read the slides. Using a program such as PowerPoint does not substitute for a good speaker who is organized, prepared, speaks well, and can adjust to the needs of the audience. PowerPoint will not make the speaker a great speaker. Remember that the program is a tool to aid in the presentation; do not read the slides or pay more attention to the slides and the technology than the audience. The technology, in this case the PowerPoint presentation, should be transparent to the audience.

Outlined here are some basic guidelines for preparing the graphic presentation.

- Begin the presentation with a title slide. The content of the slide should orient the audience to the title of the presentation and the presenter and/or company. Many presenters also include some form of clip art or a picture. Optional items for a title slide are a subtitle and date.
- Select a design theme and apply it to the presentation. PowerPoint comes with many design templates; additional ones are available online from Microsoft. Others are available for purchase from independent providers.
- Use an easy to read font. This means a simple upright font without swirls and scripts. Good fonts to use are Times New Roman, Arial, and Garamond.
- Obey the 44/32 guideline. Titles should be between 40 and 44 points, whereas text should be between 28 to 32 points. It is better to err by making the font too large than having people unable to read slides from the back of the room.
- Use a maximum of three different fonts in a presentation. Using too many different fonts is distracting to the audience.
- Use uppercase and lowercase letters. All capital letters are more difficult to read.
- Use no more than five to seven words across and five to seven lines down. This means to use phrases and not complete sentences. Break the slide into two if there are more than seven items.
- Limit the use of italics. Slides in italics are more difficult to read.
- Boldface and shadow text. The boldface increases the stroke weight and projects the words better. Shadowing fonts puts a crisp edge around the text.
- Use bulleted lists to organize the points for the audience, but use no more than three bulleted list slides in a row. It becomes very boring if all slides are bulleted list slides.
- Use clip art and AutoShapes to add interest to the slides. Make sure that they "fit" into the message being conveyed by the slide and that they are

an integral part of the slide. For example, place a definition in the "call-out" AutoShape or list of items in a pyramid.

- Use diagrams instead of complete sentences to describe processes. One can use the AutoShapes to lay out the process being described. People tend to remember things when visuals are added.

- Use an interesting image to serve as a break for questions and answers during the presentation.

- Keep special effects to a minimum unless they add to the presentation.

▶ 6.4 PRESENTATION GRAPHICS TERMINOLOGY

General Terms

Described here are general terms used when discussing presentation graphics software.

Analytic	Analytic graphics present data in graph form for analysis, understanding, and decision making. Presentation graphics, spreadsheet, or statistic programs can be used to create these graphs.
DPIs	DPIs (density per inch) represent pixel density or the number of dots (pixels) per inch. The larger the DPIs the better the resolution.
File Formats	File format is how the program stores the graphic or image. The file format is important for importing data and developing slides. PowerPoint permits inserting some popular graphic file formats, such as enhanced metafile (.emf), graphics interchange format (.gif), joint photographic experts group (.jpg), portable network graphics (.png), and Windows bitmap (.bmp). Additional file formats may be imported using a separate filter.
Handles	This term is used to describe the squares that surround a selected image or block of text. Use them to move, enlarge, or shrink the image or text block.
Landscape	Landscape refers to the orientation of the slide in a wide or horizontal view. Use this orientation for on-screen presentations and to produce 35-mm slides.

Pixels	Pixels are tiny dots or picture elements (the more pixels used, the sharper the image or resolution).
Portrait	Portrait is the orientation of the slide in an upright or vertical view. Use this view for overhead transparencies.
Presentation	Presentation is the group of slides or charts that make up the actual material to present. A presentation may consist of an unlimited number of slides from one to many. Remember that more slides are not necessarily better. The general guideline is to use one slide for every 1 to 3 minutes of a presentation.
Resolution	Resolution is the number of pixels on the screen.
Slides	Slides are the individual screens that make up a presentation.
Slide Layout	Slide layout refers to how the placeholder for the text and images are arranged on the slide. Many different slide layouts are available in PowerPoint.

Graphics Terms

The basic concepts in this section deal with terms used to describe and work with graphics or clip art.

AutoShapes	AutoShapes are predesigned forms used to enhance the look of the slide. Use them in place of bulleted lists or to show processes. They include rectangles, circles, arrows, callouts, and so forth.
Bullet	A bullet is a graphic to the left of a text list. Different symbols can be used as the bullets such as a dot, arrow, block, or check.
Bitmapped	Bitmapped refers to graphics images stored and represented by pixels or tiny dots. It is a common form for clip art images. Examples are GIF, PCX, and TIF.
Clip Art	Clip art is a library of symbols (images) prepared by others for use with specific graphics programs. Additional clip art may be obtained online at the Microsoft website or at other image sites. When

	downloading clip art from websites, make sure to obey copyright laws.
Pictures	Pictures are digital photographs that can be imported and used in a graphic presentation.
Symbols	Symbols are the clip art or images that are available or importable into the presentation program.
Template	The template is a professionally designed format and color scheme for a presentation. Some programs call this the presentation style.
Vector graphics	Vector graphics are images created with lines, arcs, circles, and squares. This file format stores images as vector points. Some examples are CGM and PGL.

Chart Terms

Chart terms describe components used when creating charts. Charts are used to visually represent data in a more meaningful fashion.

Labels	Labels refer to the groups that represent the content of graph slides. They help the user to understand the graph (e.g., the names given to each pie wedge or bar).
X-axis	X-axis refers to the horizontal reference lines or coordinates of a graph.
Y-axis	Y-axis refers to the vertical reference lines or coordinates of a graph.

► 6.5 INTRODUCTION TO POWERPOINT

PowerPoint is the graphic presentation program that is grouped with the Office suite. It provides the user with the ability to design, create, and edit presentations. These presentations can be presented to the target audience in several ways: as transparencies, using computer screens, as web pages, as 35-mm slides, as handouts or notes, and even as a workbook.

PowerPoint screens have many similarities to Word and Excel, especially when using the menu and toolbars. For a quick overview in creating presentations, click Help from the menu bar, Microsoft PowerPoint help, and then Creating a presentation.

▶ **To start PowerPoint:**

Click the **Start** button on the Taskbar. Select **All Programs**, and then highlight **Microsoft PowerPoint** or some systems place PowerPoint in the Microsoft Office menu option.

Click the **PowerPoint** 🔲 icon on the quick launch area of the taskbar or Double click on a previously prepared **PowerPoint** presentation.

The main PowerPoint menu and toolbars are shown in Figure 6.1. In addition, PowerPoint places a Draw toolbar at the bottom of the screen. This toolbar is covered later in this chapter.

As in Word and Excel, the toolbars can be customized. Comparing Figure 6.1 with the figures from the Word and Excel chapters demonstrates how similar the menus and toolbars are. When the pointer is positioned over one of the toolbar buttons, a box appears with the name of the command the button represents. These floating toolbar button descriptions are called ToolTips or ScreenTips.

PowerPoint has a Slide Show Menu, instead of a Table Menu (Word) or a Chart Menu (Excel). The menu commands are similar to Word and Excel, except many involve *Slides* in PowerPoint instead of documents and spreadsheets. *Slide* refers to an overhead or a slide(s). Here is a brief description of the PowerPoint menu options.

PowerPoint Menu Options

The icon to the far left contains some windows controls such as restore, minimize, and close.

File   The file menu contains commands that are similar to those in other Microsoft applications. They include the commands New, Open, Save, Close, Send to, and Print.

Menu Bar - PowerPoint
↓

Standard Toolbar - PowerPoint
↓

Formatting Toolbar - PowerPoint
↓

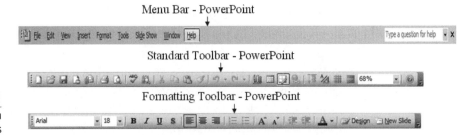

Figure 6.1

PowerPoint Menu and Toolbars

Edit	Edit contains the Select, Undo, Cut, Copy, Paste, Clear, Duplicate text or objects, Find, and Replace commands. It is also similar to the other applications.
View	From the View menu, choose how the slide appears on the screen (Normal, Slide Sorter, Notes Pages, and Slideshow). In addition, these menu options provide access to the Master slide function as well as commands for the Toolbars and Zoom.
Insert	Insert provides options for adding new slides, a Date and Time, a Slide Number, or other objects like Pictures, Sounds, Diagrams, Charts, and Tables.
Format	The format menu has options for changing fonts and font sizes, adding bullets and numbers, and aligning text. In addition, options for adjusting the look of the presentation are found here. These include the slide design, layout, and background.
Tools	The tool option contains commands for spelling and style and dialog boxes for customizing the presentation with macros, altering the autocorrect options, and altering the look of PowerPoint through customization and options features.
Slide Show	Contained here are options for designing how the presentation will run if displayed on the computer screen. It provides for inserting sounds, animation, and special effects for transition between slides.

The Window and Help options are similar to the menus in other Office programs.

Create a New Presentation

Before creating a new presentation, do some thinking about what information is being presented and how it might be shown. Create an outline of the major points that need to be made.

Start **PowerPoint**. *The PowerPoint main screen opens. By default, the user is presented with a title slide layout screen using a Blank presentation template* (Figure 6.2).

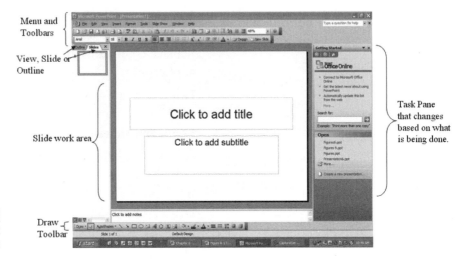

Menu and Toolbars

View, Slide or Outline

Slide work area

Task Pane that changes based on what is being done.

Draw Toolbar

Figure 6.2

Main PowerPoint Screen

Click the **Title place holder**, and type the **Title of the presentation**.

Click the **Subtitle place holder**, and type the **Subtitle for the presentation**.

Now click the **New slide** New Slide button on the toolbar.

Select a **Layout** from the layout task pane. *By default, the next slide will be a title and bulleted slide unless it is changed.*

Type the text and continue adding new slides until the presentation is complete.

When the "Create a new presentation text" at the bottom of the task pane is selected, the following options are then presented in the top of the task pane. These options may also be obtained through the menu bar by selecting **File, New**.

Blank Presentation   This is the default template used when opening PowerPoint. The slides have minimal design and no color applied to them. The user types the title and subtitle and then clicks the new slide button to continue adding slides. The menu and toolbars provide the option to change the design, layout, and background of the presentation and/or slides.

Design Template   This option presents the user with a variety of templates to apply to the presentation. The user simply clicks a design template from the slide design task pane. Other options are presented to pick a color scheme and an animation scheme. Slide layouts can be changed from the format menu. Additional slides are then added as the presentation is developed.

AutoContent Wizard
This option functions like the wizards in Word and Excel. Follow the screen directions, and a presentation based on the options chosen will appear. The user than replaces the content generated at the completion of the wizard with his or her own content.

Existing Presentation
This option creates a copy of an existing presentation so that it can be changed without altering the original. The user is free to change the design, delete or add new slides, or change the content of existing slides.

New slides can be inserted into a current presentation from another presentation. With the current presentation open, click **Insert** on the menu bar. Click **Slides from Files**. Browse to the presentation from which the slides will come, and select the slides to insert.

Template–Website
Find and use a template located on a Website. Many businesses create templates that can be used for free or for a small price.

Template–Microsoft.com
Microsoft Office Template Gallery provides additional PowerPoint templates. They are arranged according to the type of presentation needed.

Developing a Presentation

Most users will start with either a Blank Presentation or Template. If starting with a template, the design templates task pane appears (see Figure 6.3 for sample templates).

After clicking the template desired, the user can also choose to change the color scheme of that template or add an animation scheme. Most users select the template and then move to the slide layout. First, complete the title slide information, and then click new slide. The task pane now displays the slide layout options (Figure 6.4). Pick one.

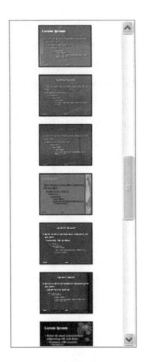

Figure 6.3
Design Templates

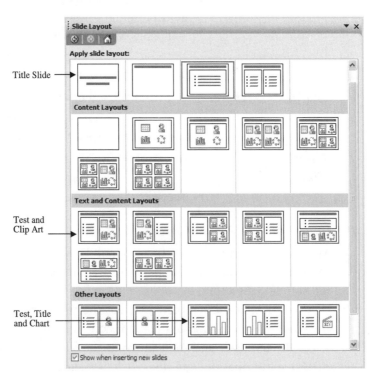

Figure 6.4
Slide Layout Options

Now begin typing the presentation. Typing can be done directly on the actual slide or can be done in Outline View, which works well for organizing the presentation and ensuring a logical flow of ideas. It is easy to add or delete parts of the outline. If working in the outline mode, an outline toolbar can be used to arrange the content (Figure 6.5). The arrow buttons help to promote bulleted items to titles or to demote something to a lesser part of the outline. Objects on the slide do not appear in Outline View; text created as an object or with TextArt does not show in Outline View. The only text that shows in this view is text in text place holders. Also, outline view may lead the presenter to use all text slides; this violates good design guidelines.

As the presentation develops, there may be a need to use the table, chart, or graphic slide layouts.

▶ **To change or select a new slide layout:**

Click the **New Slide** button, and then select the correct **Slide Layout** from the task pane or

Select **Format**, **Slide Layout**, and then select the correct **Slide Layout** from the task pane.

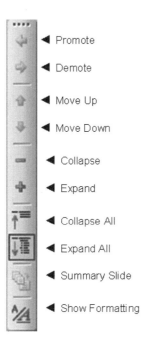

Figure 6.5
Outline Toolbar

The screen shown in Figure 6.4 appears, and the correct slide layout is chosen.

The user can also move back and forth between the outline and slide. In fact, after typing an outline segment, go to the slide show and review the slide. View buttons make it easy to do this.

View Buttons

Figure 6.6 shows the View buttons located at the bottom of the screen that are used to scroll through the different views of the slide presentation. The View buttons are located just above the draw toolbar at the bottom of the screen. These choices can also be found under the View option on the menu bar. Use these to move between different views of the presentation.

Normal	The normal view shows by default. It contains three parts: the slide, the notes pane at the bottom, and the left pane for seeing all of the slides or outline view. The user works on one slide at a time in this view. The double-arrow keys at the bottom of the right scroll bar allow moving between slides by going back and forth.
Slide Sorter	Slide sorter displays the entire presentation so that slides may be easily rearranged. This view gives the presenter an opportunity to view the presentation in total. To move a slide, simply click on it and drag it to a new location. Slides may also be selected and easily duplicated in this view. Some people use this view to add transition effects.
Slide Show	This is the best way to view the slide show. Transitions from one slide to another or any special effects or sounds can easily be seen in this view. Press the Esc key or right click the mouse to end the Slide Show.

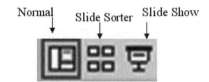

Figure 6.6
Slide Views

In earlier versions of PowerPoint, the view included the notes page view and outline view. These views are now part of the normal view. The outline view can be accessed by clicking the outline tab in the left pane of the window, and the notes page view can be accessed at the bottom part of the screen. The notes section of the normal view is used to create and edit the presentation speaker's notes. To see the total notes page and to edit it, select the **View**, **Notes** page option from the menu. At this point, the slide may be made smaller, and thus, more room is available for the notes. The notes may also be enlarged, and thus, the speaker can easily refer to them.

The master view is accessed through the View menu options. Use it to alter the master slide. This includes both a title and subsequent slides. Altering the master affects all of the slides in the presentation. If wanting to alter all of the notes pages or handout pages, use the master option from the view menu.

Adding Clip Art, Pictures, and Sound

More than 500 clip art pictures are included with PowerPoint as well as some sounds and movies. A Search feature is available that helps locate a particular piece of clip art. Pictures may also be added to the Art Gallery from CD collections, from the Web, or even from a scanned photo.

Click the **New slide** New Slide button.
Select a **Slide with a graphic** on it from the Slide layout task pane.
Click the **Insert clip art image** on the insert object placeholder (Figure 6.7) and the Clip Art Gallery opens.
Type the word that represents the clip art category, and click **Go**.

Clip art and pictures may also be inserted from the normal view when they are not to be placed in an object place holder or from the toolbars. From the

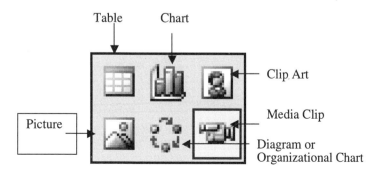

Figure 6.7
Inserting Objects

normal view, select **Insert**, **Picture** from the menu bar, and choose **Picture from Clip Art** or a picture from a file. When using the Clip Art Gallery for the first time, PowerPoint must create a clip art database, and thus, click **Yes** in the dialog box if it comes up. This will take some time. Figure 6.8 shows the location of icons on two toolbars that may also be used to insert objects.

When looking for clip art, the user has several choices. First, the user may search for a specific type of clip art by typing a name. All clip art meeting the name will then be returned. Second, the user may locate clip art by using the organize clip art option on the task pane. This provides the ability to look for clip art by categories such as business, technology, and health. Clip art may also be located by file. This means that clip art from any file can be inserted into PowerPoint as long as it is a compatible graphic file format. Finally, clip art may be found on the Internet either at Microsoft's site (by selecting clips online) or by going to other Internet sites and saving the images found. Please be aware of copyright issues when finding and using clip art online.

Digital pictures may also be inserted into PowerPoint presentations. Follow the same procedure used to insert clip art. Be aware that digital pictures can dramatically increase the size of the presentation and may require a storage medium beyond a floppy diskette.

▶ **To Display the slide to which the picture is to be added.**
Select **Insert**, **Picture**, **From File**.
Select the **Location** and **File name** for the picture. *It is now an object on the slide that can be sized and moved.*

Movies and sounds may also be inserted and played from a PowerPoint presentation. Movies are video files with extensions like .avi, .mov, and .mpeg.

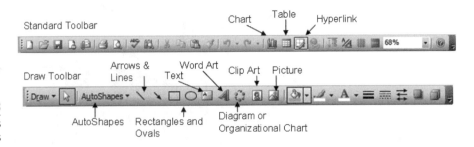

Figure 6.8
Inserting Objects
from Toolbars

An animated .gif file includes motion and has a .gif file extension. They contain multiple images that are streamed together to produce the effect of animation. They are not technically a movie, but can show a process or motion.

▶ **To add a movie or sound:**

Display the slide to which the sound or movie is to be added.

Select **Insert**, **Movie and Sounds**.

Select the **Location** and **File** that is the movie or sound.

At the prompt, select whether the sound or movie is to play automatically or on a mouse click.

Once inserted, the file can be started in three ways. First, it may start automatically when the slide displays in the Slide show view. Second, it may start on a mouse click. Finally, it can be set to start after a delay and to run for a certain time period.

Movie files are linked files. That means they are linked to the presentation, not embedded in it like clip art or pictures. When the presentation has linked files, they must be copied along with the presentation if using another computer for the presentation.

Adding a Table

Tables are used to summarize data, place information in categories, show research results, or help the reader make comparisons between items.

▶ **To add a table:**

Click the **New Slide** button on the toolbar or **Insert**, **New Slide** from the menu bar.

Click the **Title and Table** option from the Slide layout task pane. *A Table icon and a dialog box appear on the slide* (Figure 6.9).

Double click the **Table** icon and a dialog box appears to choose the number of rows and columns wanted (Figure 6.10).

Type the **Number of columns** or use the scroll arrows.

Press **Tab** key, and type the **Number of rows**.

Click **OK** when finished.

Prepare the table like a Word document table. When working in the table, a Table Menu toolbar floats on the screen. Rows and columns can be added as they are in Word.

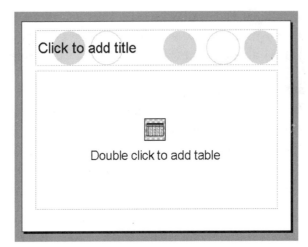

Figure 6.9

Add Table Screen

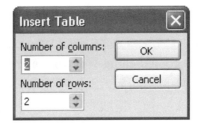

Figure 6.10

Insert Table

When the table contents are completed, click **Outside** the table on the slide. Select the **Title** place holder.
Type the **Title** of the slide.

Remember, however, that there is a limited amount of space on a slide. Too many rows or columns will render the contents unreadable. Tables may also be imported from Word. Select **Insert**, **Object**. In the dialog box, click **Created from file**, **Locate the file**, check **Link to file**, and **OK**. The table is now inserted into the PowerPoint slide.

Adding a Chart (Graph)

Remember that charts are pictorial representations of data.

▶ **To add a chart or graph:**

Select the **New Slide** button.

Click **Chart slide** from the slide layout task pane. *A chart slide presents a chart icon (Figure 6.11). There are several versions of chart layouts—one with a chart to the left of the bullets, one to the right of the bullets, and one full slide chart.*

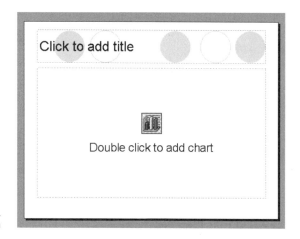

Figure 6.11
Slide with Chart Icon

Double click the **Graph** icon on the slide or click the **Insert**, **Chart** from the menu bar. *The graph application program starts, and a Standard Toolbar is now at the top of the screen. A new datasheet is displayed with a chart object behind it. It has a set of default values with a three-dimensional default chart behind it.*

Highlight (select) the **Cells** and press the **Delete** key to clear the datasheet or go to **Edit** on the menu bar, and select **Clear**, **All**.

Select **Chart** from the menu and choose **Chart Type**. *A list of chart types on the left with pictures of subtypes on the right appears.*

Choose **One** that fits the data and click **OK**.

Pie charts are good for comparing parts to the whole. Bar and column charts compare different items over time. Line charts show progress over time or multiple data sets.

Filling in the data sheet is much like doing an Excel spreadsheet. Once data are entered, if the data sheet has too many columns, clear the ones not needed. Rows and columns may also be added. Because the sample data sheet was cleared, data need to be typed in the datasheet. Figure 6.12 shows a highlighted data sheet overlaid on a slide.

Type the **Numbers** and **Labels**.

Click the **Slide**. *The data sheet disappears and the graph appears.*

Single click the graph, and it can then be moved or changed as desired. Double click it to make the data sheet return.

Under the Insert menu are commands for inserting a text box if a caption is needed. Even the color of the graph can be changed. Under **Format**,

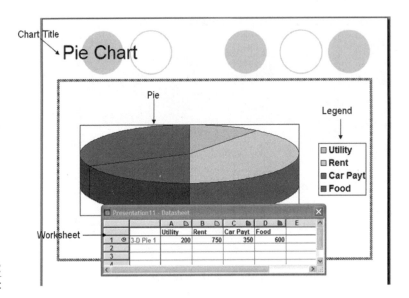

Figure 6.12

Pie Chart

choose **Slide Color Scheme**. A dialog box appears that allows choosing different colors. At this point, the type of graph can also be changed if the type selected is not as clear as it should be. The data sheet can also be prepared in Excel and imported into the slide by using the Insert command.

There is much more to learn about graphs and charts so be sure to look at the documentation that comes with PowerPoint and keep experimenting.

Adding a Hyperlink

Hyperlinks are used to take the user someplace else or to provide additional information about a topic. PowerPoint permits the use of hyperlinks to go directly to a specific slide within the presentation or to go to a place on the Internet.

▶ **To add a hyperlink:**

Select the **Text** or **Object** that will be used to access the linked site or slide. Select **Insert**, **Hyperlink**. *The hyperlink dialog box opens* (Figure 6.13). Make the appropriate selections and click **OK**.

The hyperlink will not work unless in Slide show view.

Adding Transitions to a Slide Show

When graphic presentations are prepared as an electronic slide show, transitions to parts or all of the slide show can be added. Figure 6.14 shows the selection screen for adding transitions to a presentation.

Text that is hyperlinked.

If the link is to an existing file or web page, click this option.

If the link is to an another slide in this presentation, click this option.

Figure 6.13
Hyperlink Dialog Window

If the link is an email address, click this option.

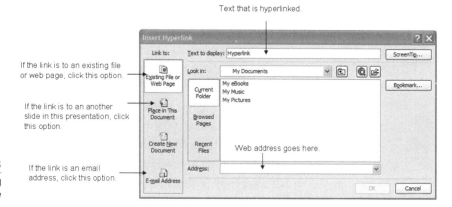

Available transitions

Adjust speed of transition

Adjust how the transition advances

Apply this transition to all the slides

Figure 6.14
Slide Transitions

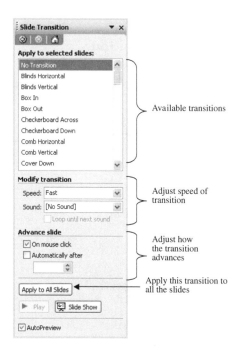

Click the **Slide Show** menu.

Click **Slide Transition**. *The slide transition task pane appears.*

Many different transitions are available. These transitions may be applied to one slide or to the total presentation. Be sure to view the transitions with the Slide Show view. As experience is gained in using transitions, themes for which ones work well together emerge. Practice using different transitions to find ones that work well with the presentation and audience.

Adding Custom Animations

Text, graphics, diagrams, charts, and other objects on the slides can have custom animations added to emphasize key points, control the flow of information, or add interest to the presentation.

Custom animations can be applied using a preset animation scheme, or they can be applied to each item individually on the slide. Be careful that the animation adds clarity to the message and does not detract from it. Most users carefully select items for custom animations and do not apply them to the total presentation. This provides some variety and interest to the presentation without boring the audience.

▶ **To activate the custom animation task pane:**

Select the part of the slide to animate.

Select **Slide Show**, **Custom animation**.

Click the **Add Effect** button.

Select when the animation is to occur—entrance, emphasis, exit, or motion path.

Select the type of **Effect** (Figure 6.15).

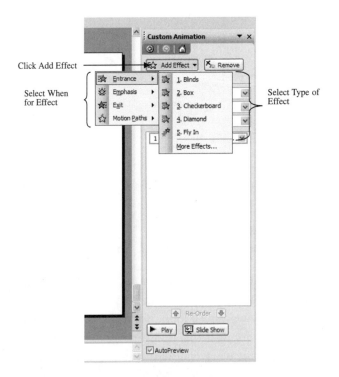

Figure 6.15

Custom Animation

Associated with many animation options are other options for playing a sound, applying one letter at a time, and adjusting the speed of the animation. In addition, previous bullet items may be dimmed as a new one appears (Figure 6.16).

Changing a Presentation Design

The design of a presentation can always be changed. When the presentation is open

Select **Format** and **Slide Design** or click the **Design** 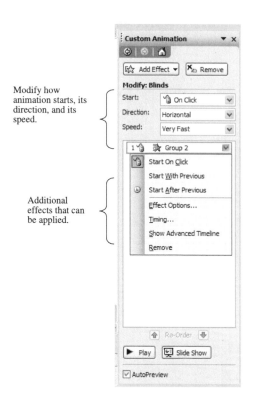 button on the Formatting Toolbar.
Choose **Another** design.

To change text or objects for all the slides in the presentation use the Master Slide. This is the template used for all slides in the presentation and is where things are added such as corporate or university logos to all slides. It is also the place to change the text properties of all slides.

Figure 6.16

Modification of Custom Animation

Select **View**, **Master**, **Slide Master**.
Select the **Text** or **Text holder** on the Slide Master that is to be changed.
Change the **Text** properties (e.g., bold, shadow, 30 points, green).

Sometimes the need is to change the font size on only one slide, not the total presentation.

View the slide in **Slide View**.
Select the **Text** that needs to be changed.
Change the **Text** properties with the format toolbar or through the **Format**, **Font** menu.

Color, style, and other characteristics can be changed with the Format menu command.

Printing with PowerPoint

PowerPoint has many options for printing various parts of the presentation. To print overheads, audience handouts, notes, or a presentation outline:

Click **File**, **Print**. *The Selection Screen appears* (Figure 6.17).
Select **Slides**, **Handouts**, **Notes page**, or **Outline**.
Check the other settings to make sure that they are correct, and click **OK**.

Slides   This option prints the entire presentation, one slide per page, or the current slide on an 8½ × 11 paper. This is the default option.

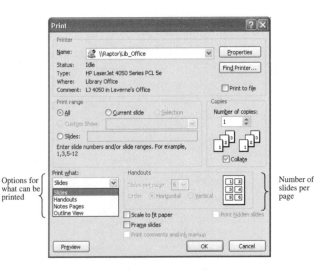

Figure 6.17
Print Screen in
PowerPoint

Handouts	Choosing this option prints a smaller version of the slides, the number selected per page (e.g., three or six slides per page).
Notes Page	Choose this option to print a slide at the top of the page with notes on the bottom half of the page. This option prints one slide per page.
Outline	Make sure the outline is expanded. This option prints all of the text shown in the outline view.

Be sure to choose the correct option before printing so that only what is needed is printed. If printing handouts, print one page of three or six to a page to decide which one will work the best for your audience. Avoid printing handouts before the presentation is complete and all revisions are made. Always run the spell checker and consider using AutoCorrect to handle misspellings along the way.

SUMMARY

PowerPoint is a powerful presentation program that will help produce presentations that are professional and make the appropriate points with the audience. This introduction is only a start in getting acquainted with all of the things that can be done with PowerPoint, such as putting a presentation on the Web. This chapter provides a basic introduction to PowerPoint and should serve as a starting point.

Exercise 1: Creating a Powerpoint Presentation*
Objectives

1. Create slides with the correct information on them.
2. Create a bulleted list slide.
3. Edit slides by altering the formatting and placement of objects.
4. Insert and adjust clip art from the clip organizer and from Microsoft's website.
5. Save the presentation.

Activity

Create a title slide

Start **PowerPoint**.

Click the **Design** ⊞ Design button on the formatting toolbar.

Double click the **Stream** design template from the task pane. It may be necessary to scroll to find it.

Click the **Title text placeholder**.

Type **Health Assessment.**

Click the **Subtitle text placeholder.**

Type **By** and press the **Enter** key.

Type **Your name.**

Add a bulleted list slide

Click the **New slide** New Slide button on the formatting toolbar.

Click the **Title place holder.**

Type **Healthy Habits.**

Click the **Text placeholder.**

Type **Diet.**

Press the **Enter** key, and type **Exercise.**

Press the **Enter** key, and type **Relaxation.**

Click **Outside** of the Bulleted list placeholder.

Edit the title slide

Click the **Title** slide in the left pane.

Click the **Subtitle text placeholder.**

Click the **Border** of the subtitle placeholder.

Select **Garamond** and **20 Points** from the formatting tool bar.

Resize the place holder to make it smaller, and drag it toward the bottom of the slide.

Edit the bulleted list slide

Click the **Bulleted** list slide in the left pane.

Click the **Text placeholder border.**

Drag the **Right text placeholder border** to the left about 2 inches.

Drag the **Text place holder** to the right until the **D in Diet** is under the H in Health.

Insert clip art and pictures

Click the **Title slide** in the slide pane on the left.

Select **Insert** from the menu bar, **Picture**, and then **Clip Art.**

Click the **Organize clips** Organize clips... option at the bottom of the task pane.

If necessary, click the + sign next to the words Office Collection.

Click the + sign next to Healthcare.

Select one of the clip art images by clicking the **Down arrow** on the left side of the image and select **Copy**.

Click the **Title** slide and select the **Paste** button from the toolbar.

Adjust the placement of objects so that they are arranged on the slide nicely.

Change slide layout and insert clip art into placeholder

Click the **Bulleted** slide in the left pane.

Click **Format**, **Slide Layout** from the menu bar.

Scroll to the **Other layouts** area.

Click the **Title, Clip Art and Text** option (clip art on left, bullet list on right).

Double click the **Clip Art** button in the clip art placeholder.

Type **Exercise** in the search text box, and click **Go**. *If this does not work, try another word to find a clip art that is appropriate for the slide.*

Double click a **Clip art**.

Arrange the slide to look attractive by altering the location and size of objects.

Add additional clip art as desired.

Insert clip art from the Microsoft website

Click the **New Slide** New Slide button.

Select **Title only** slide from the Slide layout task pane.

Click the **Title placeholder**, and type **Assessment**.

Select **Insert, Picture, Clip Art**.

Click the **Clip art online** Clip art on Office Online text at the bottom clip art task pane. Make sure that there is an active Internet connection.

In the search textbox, type **Health**, and click the **Go** button.

To add the clip art to the organizer for future use, follow these directions.

Click the **Square** of one of the clip art images desired.

Click the **Download 1 clip** button on the left pane.

Click the **Download Now** button.

Save it to the **Desktop** if asked, and then click the **Open** button. *The image is now in the downloaded section of the clip organizer.*

To use it:

Click the down arrow to the right of the image, and select **Copy**.

Click the **PowerPoint slide** and **Paste**.

If there is no need to add it to the clip organizer, right click the **Image** on the Microsoft web site, and select **Copy. Paste** it in the slide.

Size and move it as necessary.

Save the presentation

Click the Save **button on the toolbar.**

Type a name for the presentation and select a location.

Click the Save **button.**

The slides just created should look like these (Figure 6.18).

*This exercise was modified from one used at La Roche College, CIS105W Online course. It is used with permission of La Roche College and Irene Joos.

Exercise 2: Inserting a Picture and Printing Handouts*
Objectives

1. Add a picture to a slide.
2. Print handouts.

Activity

Inserting a picture

Open the presentation created in Exercise 1, and go to the end of it.

Click the **New Slide** New Slide button.

Select **Format, Slide layout** from the menu bar.

Select the **Title only** layout.

Type a title for the slide: **A Picture with Clip Art**.

Find a clip art that is a map of some part of the world.

Copy it into the fourth slide of the presentation.

Find a digital picture of something related to that part of the world or some aspect of health. For example, students or health professionals working in that part of the world.

Click **Insert, Picture, From File**.

Select the **Drive** and **Folder** where the .jpg picture was placed.

Select the file, and click **Insert**.

Enlarge the picture if necessary.

Click the **Textbox** icon on the draw toolbar. Draw a **Box** on the slide, and type a capital letter **X**.

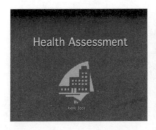
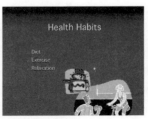
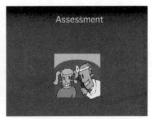

Figure 6.18

Sample Presentation

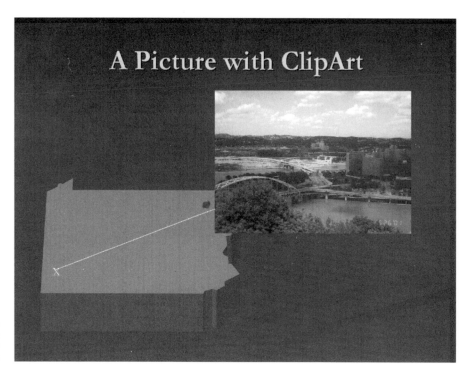

Figure 6.19
Sample Picture and
Clip Art

Click the **Line draw** tool. Draw a line between the **X** and the **Picture**.

Save the file.

The slide should resemble the slide in Figure 6.19.

Print handouts

Select **File**, **Print** from the menu bar.

Select **Handouts** from the Print What option.

Make sure that it says six slides per page. Click **OK**.

Print speaker notes

Select **File**, **Print** from the menu bar.

Select **Notes page** from the Print What option.

Click **OK**.

*This exercise was modified from one used at La Roche College, CIS105W Online. It is used with permission of La Roche College and Irene Joos.

Exercise 3: Table, Line, Pie, and Bar Graphs

This exercise can be done with PowerPoint or Excel, but the preference is to have you practice with PowerPoint. The table can also be done in Word.

Objectives

1. Create a computer-generated table, bar, pie, and line graph for PowerPoint presentations.
2. Save and print the slide.

Activity

Create a line chart and table

Start **PowerPoint** and select **Title and Chart** from the Slide layout task pane.

Select the **Title text** placeholder and type **Projected FTE Requirements and Supply of RNs in the US**.

Double click the **Chart** icon in the middle of the slide.

Type the following data in the datasheet.

Year	Requirements (Column A)	Supply (Column B)
2005	2,095,000	2,128,000
2010	2,232,000	2,214,000
2015	2,391,000	2,277,000
2020	2,575,000	2,284,000
2025	3,450,000	2,110,000

Click the slide, and look at it. Now, change it to a line chart.

Double click the **Chart**, and click the **Chart type** ▨ ▾ button down arrow. Select **3-D line**.

Click the **Slide**, **Save**, and then click **Print** it.

Now create a new slide with the same data in a **Table**.

Which one presents the data in the clearest manner?

Create a pie chart

Follow directions given previously but create a **Pie chart**.

Title: Medicaid/Medicare Expenditures Fiscal Year 2007

Items: Home Care   34%

Physician   18%

Hospital   23%

Skilled Care   24%

Others   1%

Save and **Print** it. What alterations can be done on this pie to enhance it?

Reformat the pie chart.

Right click the pie, and select **Format Data Series**.

Click the **Pattern** tab if needed, and remove the **Border**.

Click the **Data Label** tab, and place checks in **Category name**, **Percent**, and **Show leader lines**.

Click the **Labels** once, and pause and click again. They should separate. Drag each label a little distance from the pie wedge. Each one will need to be done separately.

Now click the pie wedge **Hospital** once; then pause and click it again. Drag the wedge away from the other wedges. (This is called exploding the wedge.)

Now right click the **Hospital wedge**, and select **Format Data Point**.

Select **Yellow**. Change the colors of the other wedges.

Save the changes.

Create a line chart

Title:	Present and Future Sales of Computers	
Data:	X-axis	Y-axis
	2004	4 billion dollars
	2005	5.5 billion dollars
	2006	10.5 billion dollars
	2007	20 billion dollars
	2008	36 billion dollars
	2009	50 billion dollars

Save and Print it.

Exercise 4: Autoshapes and WordArt
Objectives

1. Create a slide using Autoshapes and WordArt.

Directions

Open the **Presentation** created in Exercises 1 and 2.

Go to the end of the presentation and click **New slide** button, **Title only** layout.

In the Title placeholder, type **Using AutoShapes and WordArt**.

Create the autoshape

Click the **AutoShapes** AutoShapes ▾ text on the draw toolbar.

Select **Basic shapes**, **Rectangle**.

Go to the slide area and, with the pointer a + sign, and drag to create a rectangle.

Adjust the autoshape

Right click the rectangle, and select **Format AutoShape**.

In the color area, click the **Fill Color down** ⌄ arrow, and select the **Purple** option.

Click the **Fill color down** ⌄ arrow again, and select **Fill effects, bottom Right Square**, **OK**, and **OK**.

On the draw toolbar, click the **Line color** ⟋⁃ down arrow button, and select **No Line**.

Duplicate the rectangle

Click the **Rectangle**, and then the **Copy** button on the standard toolbar.

Click the **Paste** button three times.

Move the rectangles to place one in the center top, one on the left, one on the right, and the fourth one at the center bottom.

Insert arrows

Click the AutoShapes AutoShapes ▾ text on the draw toolbar, and select Block Arrows.

Select the Bent ⌐➔ arrow (first column, third row).

Draw it on the slide Between the left rectangle and the top center rectangle.

Alter the colors—Yellow, Fill effect, No Line, Shadow (click the shadow ▢ button and select the second column, fourth row).

Click the Arrow and the Copy button. Click the Paste button three times.

Move the arrows between the other rectangles.

Click the arrow, and using the green dot, rotate them so that the tip of the arrow points to the next rectangle.

Insert WordArt

Click the WordArt ◢ button on the draw toolbar.

Select the 2nd **column**, 5th row option, and click OK.

Type Assess and click OK.

Place the WordArt in the top center rectangle.

Repeat the process typing Plan, Implement, and Evaluate.

Place each in the appropriate rectangle.

Now make one more adjustment.

Copy three of the arrows, and add them as shown in Figure 6.20.

Assignment 1: Create Pie, Line, and Bar Charts
Directions

Pie chart

Find research data that provide information about a health care problem or nursing shortage problem. Make sure it compares parts to a whole (e.g., a comparison of the budget for a clinical unit[s]).

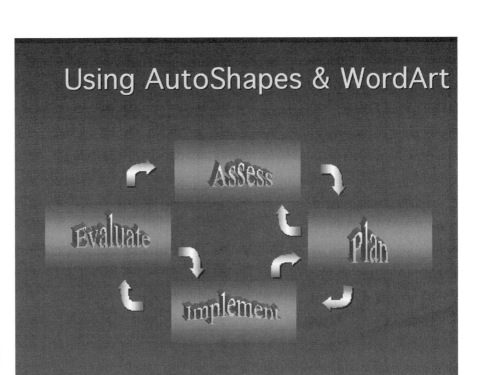

Figure 6.20

AutoShapes and
WordArt

Create a pie chart using PowerPoint.

Move the legend to the bottom of the slide.

Enhance the title of the slide.

Try different styles of the pie charts. Pick the one that most clearly shows the data in the best light.

Save and **Print** the slide.

Under what conditions would a pie chart be used?

Bar chart

Find research data about the educational levels of practicing nurses from 3 different years (e.g., from 2003, 2004, and 2005).

Title: Educational preparation of registered nurses: diploma, associate degree, and baccalaureate.

Use a slide with only a title on it so that there is more room for the bar graphs and legend.

Save and **Print** the slide.

Line chart

Find research data about a clinical trial or clinical problem in your area that lends itself to creating a line chart.

Create a line chart.

Save and **Print** it.

Under what conditions would a line graph be used?

Submit this sheet along with your printouts if instructed. Submit the articles with the data.

Assignment 2: Preparing a PowerPoint Presentation
Directions

Prepare a PowerPoint presentation on a topic related to technology in health care that you will present using a computer and data projector. Use your creativity and knowledge gained from this chapter to produce quality slides following the good design tips given in the chapter.

- Include a minimum of 10 slides with at least one title slide, one table, one chart/graph, and some clip art. Use some variety in the layout of the slides. You should not have more than three bullet list slides in a row. Use some of the shapes to enhance the slide.
- Use a transition between slides.
- Print an outline and a handout with three slides to a page. Prepare at least one "Notes" page. Turn in the papers if instructed.

Introduction to Spreadsheets

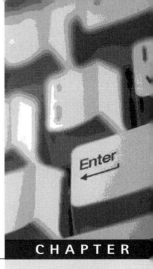

OBJECTIVES

1. Identify uses of the spreadsheet in general as well as for health care applications.
2. Define basic terminology related to spreadsheets.
3. Review selected functions for using Excel 2003.

Spreadsheets do for numbers and charts what word processing does for writing. Although their strength is their function as numeric calculators, most spreadsheets also have a database management component for organizing, sorting, and retrieving information and a chart component for creating and printing graphs. This chapter presents information on how to use the spreadsheet as an electronic calculator. The advantages of computerized spreadsheets include accuracy and speed. Spreadsheets also have the capacity to recalculate formulas automatically when any numbers used in the calculation are changed. Spreadsheets have many uses; they can be used for inventories, tax returns, patient records, grade records, personnel files, budgets, and quality assurance information.

► 7.1 COMMON SPREADSHEET TERMS

Rows
Rows run horizontally across the spreadsheet, numbered beginning with 1 down the left side of the spreadsheet. Although the maximum number of rows varies with different spreadsheets, there are as many as 65,536 rows.

Columns
Columns go vertically down the spreadsheet, labeled from left to right, A to Z. After Z, labeling continues with AA to AZ, BA to BZ, and so on, usually for 256 columns.

Cell
A cell is a place holder for data. Each cell occurs at a specific intersection of a row and column. Cells are labeled by the column letter followed by the row number (e.g., A1 or T112).

Cell Address or Cell Reference
The cell address is the label for each cell. It is used to reference the cell when creating formulas or using functions.

Active Cell
The active cell is the cell currently being used; it is outlined or highlighted so that it can be quickly seen on the spreadsheet. The address of the active cell appears in a designated location on the spreadsheet screen.

Range or Block
A group of cells in a rectangular pattern defined by the top left and bottom right corners is called a range or block of cells. For example, a range of cells from A1 to E6 would include all of the cells in columns A, B, C, D, and E in rows 1, 2, 3, 4, 5, and 6. A block of cells on a spreadsheet is identified as a dark rectangle. Blocks of cells may also be noncontiguous.

Workbook or Notebook
A workbook or notebook is a collection of spread sheet pages. In some spreadsheet programs, pages

in a notebook are numbered; in others, they are labeled by a letter or word. All of the pages are saved together in one file. Worksheet pages are also called worksheets in many programs. In some programs, when the worksheet is blank, they are called sheets. When they contain data, they are called worksheets. Figure 7.1 shows that worksheets are labeled Sheet 1, Sheet 2, and Sheet 3. Spreadsheet programs have a default number of worksheets in each workbook; the user can add more worksheets in a workbook or delete the unused ones if desired.

Template   This is a spreadsheet formatted with labels and formulas but no specific data; it is helpful when multiple uses of the same spreadsheet are needed. Use a template for a yearly personal budget or for

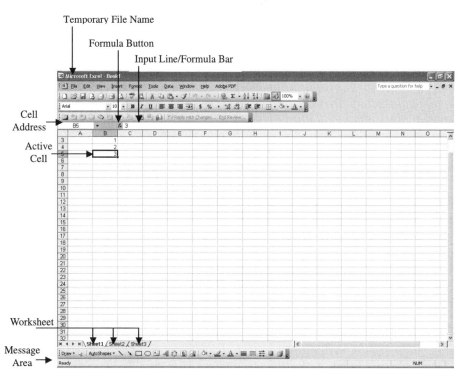

Figure 7.1
Excel Screen Display

a health care unit. The labels used and the calculations remain stable from one year to the next; only the figures change.

▶ 7.2 SPREADSHEET SCREEN DISPLAY

The screen displays for most spreadsheets are similar. Spreadsheets look like a page from an accountant's ledger with many rows and columns. A series of letters, denoting columns, goes horizontally across the screen, and a series of numbers, denoting rows, runs vertically along the left hand side of the screen. As with other Windows programs (previously discussed in Chapters 3 and 4), the menu bar and any additional toolbars are located across the uppermost part of the screen; scroll bars appear along the right and bottom of the screen. Features specific to the spreadsheet screen display include the current cell address, formula bar or input line, and the message area (Figure 7.1).

Current Cell Address	This indicates the active cell and is usually located near the top left of the screen.
Formula Bar or Input line	The data or formula entered appears in this location on the screen.
Message Area	This shows what actions will occur when a function or button is activated. It may also show error messages. It is usually located in the lower left corner of the screen.

▶ 7.3 GETTING READY TO USE A SPREADSHEET

Before beginning spreadsheet use, it is important to consider carefully the goals of the project so that an optimally useful spreadsheet is developed. Consider the following:

1. What type of data is needed in the spreadsheet for example, text such as labels for individuals or inventory supply information or numbers for income or expenses?
2. Are time intervals going to be used for example, monthly, quarterly, or yearly?
3. Is there a need to make comparisons for example, between units or across time periods?

4. How many data are there? Is one worksheet adequate or would it be better to divide data into several?

It is often most logical to place categories of data in columns because the width of columns can be customized to the data. The specific data for each record, situation, or individual can then be entered in each column under the category headings.

Once the goals of the project have been determined, the general process for creating the worksheet includes the following steps:

- Enter spreadsheet-identifying information on the first few rows. This includes data such as name of the organization, department or division, the project (quarterly budget, inventory), and spreadsheet originator.
- Next, enter labels that identify the columns and rows.
- Enter data.
- Enter formulas and functions.
- Format the data and labels (fonts, size, justification, number format, etc.).
- Format the worksheet (borders, shading, etc.).
- Create charts or graphs.
- Print worksheets and/or charts.

▶ 7.4 ACCOMPLISHING TASKS IN THE WORKSHEET

Moving about the worksheet is accomplished by using the mouse or arrow keys alone or in combination with other keys on a keyboard (more details are provided later in the chapter). As the mouse is moved, the active cell is highlighted and noted as the cell address. In order to accomplish a task, select commands from the menu bar, or click on icons. Using the scroll bar to move around the spreadsheet does not change the active cell; it only changes the view of the spreadsheet until a cell is clicked in the worksheet area.

Data Entry

Spreadsheets allow the user to enter two types of data: *constants* and *formulas*. Constants include dates, numbers, text, logical values, and error values. Formulas perform mathematic operations such as calculating the mathematical relationships between the constants on the worksheet. When constants are changed, the formulas are still there, and the results on the spreadsheet are recalculated to keep the spreadsheet up to date.

▶ **To enter data:**

Click the **Cell** in which the data will be entered. *The cell address will be displayed, and the cell will be highlighted or outlined.*

Type the **Data** into the cell.

Press **Enter**. Click in another cell, or press an **Arrow** key.

When data are typed, they appear in the input line. An example of this is shown in Figure 7.1 where data has been typed into B5, the active cell. Although there are a variety of ways to enter data into the cell, the most common is by pressing **Enter** or clicking the mouse. In some programs, data are entered automatically when the cursor is moved to another cell. If new data are entered into a cell that already has data, they will overwrite the original data. Typically, in spreadsheets, text is aligned to the left, and numeric values are aligned to the right.

The numbers 0 to 9 and certain characters are treated like numbers unless otherwise indicated. Other characters that are commonly treated as numbers include the following: – + . ( ) $ % / *. Any number is treated as positive (+) unless a negative sign (-) is placed in front of it. When a % is placed after a number, it may be displayed differently. For example, 45% will appear as .45. Some spreadsheet programs automatically convert any numbers beginning with a $ to a decimal. For example, $12 will be displayed as $12.00. In other spreadsheets, the way percentages and dollars are displayed is controlled through format functions.

The following numeric operators are commonly used in formulas:

Symbol	Meaning	Symbol	Meaning
^	exponentiation	=	equals
*	multiplication	+	addition
/	division	–	subtraction
<	less than	>	greater than

When multiple numeric operators appear in a formula, the formula is calculated using certain ordering rules. Most often the standard rules of precedence are used. The first operator evaluated is exponentiation, followed by multiplication and division, and finally addition and subtraction; if there is a tie, calculation proceeds from left to right. Calculations enclosed in parentheses will always be calculated before other operations.

Example: 5 * 4 + 3 would calculate as 20 + 3 or 23

5 * (4 + 3) would calculate as 5 * 7 or 35

Saving Worksheets

Each spreadsheet program has specific conventions for saving. Similar to word processing programs, spreadsheets replace newer versions of a worksheet or notebook by overwriting older versions. The cautions that relate to saving word processing documents are equally important with worksheets and notebooks. Save often and before trying something new!

Using Charts

Creating charts is another spreadsheet feature. Because the data in a spreadsheet can be more easily understood in graphic form, all spreadsheets come with the ability to create charts. A good chart lets the reader instantly see the point being made by the data. It graphically displays the data.

▶ **To create a chart:**

Select the **Data** to be graphed.

Choose the **Chart** type.

Select and orient the **Data range and series**.

Type the chart options—such as **Title** and **Labels** for X- and Y-axis.

Choose a **Location** for the chart—this worksheet or a new one.

Some new terms related to charts are defined here:

Axis	The horizontal (x) and vertical (y) plane or line on which the data are plotted is the axis. It provides a comparison or measurement point.
Categories	Categories are labels given the X-axis and Y-axis.
Chart Type	This refers to the way the chart will display the data. Some examples are pie or bar charts.
Data Series	A data series is a group of related data points on a chart that originated from rows and columns in the worksheet. These values are used to plot the chart.
Legend	The legend is a box that identifies the pattern or color of a specific data series or category.

Although the Wizard makes it easy to create the charts, only the person knowledgeable about the data knows the best type of chart to use in displaying the data. For example, when comparing parts to a whole, such as the department's budgets to the total budget, a pie chart might be useful. Some questions to ask when creating a chart are as follows:

1. Is this the right chart to convey the data in the worksheet?
2. How would a viewer expect to see this data displayed?
3. Does it add to the understanding of the data and help the audience to make decisions?
4. What questions or solutions does the chart suggest?

▶ 7.5 INTRODUCTION TO EXCEL

A number of spreadsheets are available for use. This chapter focuses on Excel 2003. Excel is available for both the Macintosh and Windows operating systems. Although this chapter provides specific information about the Office 2003 version of Excel for Windows, previous Office versions and versions for the Macintosh are very similar. Because Excel operates in a Windows environment, the features common to Windows outlined in earlier chapters also apply to Excel. Starting Excel is just like starting other Windows programs. Click the **Start** button at the lower left of the screen. Select **All Programs**. Then highlight and click **Microsoft Excel**. Some systems may be set up to display a window where Microsoft Office is highlighted first. Microsoft Excel 2003 did away with the shortcut toolbar, although some systems place the most commonly used programs in the quick launch area of the taskbar. If there is an Excel icon ▨ in the quick launch area, click on this to open Excel immediately. If help is needed, ask a laboratory assistant how to access the program.

The Menu Bar and Commands

Refer to Figure 4.1 to see how similar the menu bar for Excel is to that of Word. Only one menu item is different; Excel has *Data*, whereas Word has *Table*. Many of the icons in the toolbar below the menu bar are also the same. As in Word, the menu bar and mouse can be used to select commands and options. For basic spreadsheet use, File, Edit, View, and Help operate as previously described in Chapter 4. Uses specific to spreadsheets for the other commands on the menu are outlined here.

Insert	Use this for adding rows or columns or page breaks. The chart and function wizards are also located in this menu option.
Format	Use this menu to format cells, rows, columns, and worksheets. Control how numbers are displayed and aligned, such as in currency or percentage using format options. Other options allow selecting the font style (bold or italic), adding a border or pattern, protecting a cell, or making a column width narrower or wider. The AutoFormat command for selecting predesigned spreadsheets and the sheet command for renaming sheets are also located in this menu option.
Tools	Use this menu for spelling, auditing, and sharing the worksheet. The option command is also located here. Use it to customize Excel.
Data	Use this to sort or filter data when using the spreadsheet as a database or to access data from an external source.
Window	Use this to split a window into several parts. When working with long spreadsheets, sometimes selected parts of the spreadsheet need to be viewed as a whole. Use the Freeze Panes with larger spreadsheets to keep the labels displayed on the screen when accessing rows and columns that exceed the width or length of the screen. Remember this is also the command to use when switching from one spreadsheet to another.

The Toolbars

Many icons in the toolbars are similar to those in Word. The menu and toolbars are also essentially the same for the Windows and Macintosh versions of Excel. On the Standard Toolbar, from left to right, icons similar to Word are Open a New Workbook, Open Another Document, Save, E-Mail Document, Print, Print Preview, Check Spelling, Research, Cut, Copy, Paste, Format Painter, Undo, Redo, Add a Hyperlink, and the Drawing Toolbar. At the far right, similar to Word, the last icon is the Help button. Other icons

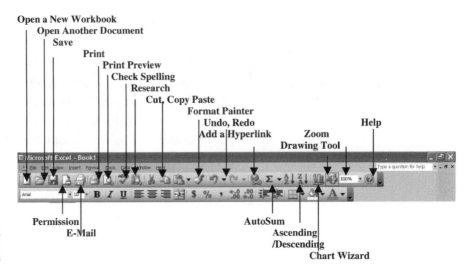

Figure 7.2

Excel Standard
Toolbar and Icons

between these are specific to spreadsheet functions and provide shortcuts for Excel commands. These buttons are Permissions, AutoSum, Sort Ascending, Sort Descending, Chart Wizard, and Zoom control (Figure 7.2). Use the mouse to move the arrow slowly just inside the icon, and Excel will show the command function of the icon. These icons initiate the following functions in Excel.

Permissions

Helps prevent sensitive documents from being forwarded, edited, or copied by unauthorized people.

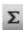

AutoSum

This button automatically sums a selected series of numbers and puts the total in a designated blank space. It looks to the cells above first. If no values are available to sum, it looks to the cells to the left. The user can change the cell range to sum.

Sort Ascending

This button sorts according to ascending numbers or letters, that is, beginning with the letter closest to the beginning of the alphabet or the smallest number used.

Sort Descending

This button sorts according to descending numbers or letters, that is, beginning with the letter closest to the end of the alphabet or the largest number used.

Chart Wizard

This button opens a dialog window presenting commonly used graphs such as bar, line, or pie and helps the user develop the selected graph through a set of questions.

Zoom Control

This button changes the view of the worksheet by increasing or decreasing the magnification; it does not alter the worksheet itself.

Similar to the **Standard Toolbar**, the Formatting Toolbar contains many features that are the same as those in Word (Figure 7.3). Beginning on the far left are Font Style and Size, Bold, Italics, and Underline icons, and Justification options. As in Word, these are used to change the format of text and its placement (left, right, or center) in the cell. Next are icons unique to Excel: Merge and Center, Currency, Percent, Comma, Increase and Decrease

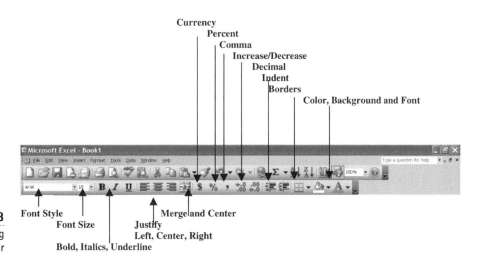

Figure 7.3

Excel Formatting Toolbar

Decimals, Increase and Decrease Indent, Borders, and Cell Color and Text Color icons. To use most of these, merely select the cell or cells to which the command will apply. Click the icon, and where presented with a dialog window, click the selection desired. Clicking the arrow beside the **Cell Border** works as in Word to present a dialog window to select the border desired for the selected cells. **Cell and Text Color** also work like the Word buttons and allow change of color for text or cell background. The first button fills the cell with that color; the second changes the text color. Click the arrow to change the color from the one that is displayed to another.

Merge and Center

When a single cell with data is selected, this button centers the data. When a cell range is selected, it merges the selected cells and centers the data across the columns; if the cells include multiple rows and have data, some data will be lost.

Currency

This button automatically formats selected cells in currency format (e.g., 4 becomes $4.00).

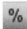

Percent

This button automatically formats selected cells in percent format, (e.g., 5 becomes 500%).

Commas

This button automatically inserts commas in appropriate places and adds two decimal places.

↑ and ↓ Decimals

For selected cells, the first button adds, and the second subtracts one decimal place with each mouse click.

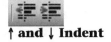

↑ and ↓ Indent

For selected cells, the first button adds and the second subtracts one indentation, usually five spaces.

Additional toolbars can be placed in the spreadsheet and left in place or opened and closed as desired. Access these easily in one of two ways:

1. Click **View** and choose **Toolbars**. Place the cursor on the **desired Toolbar** and click.
2. Place the cursor on any toolbar and right click; when the dialog box of toolbar selections appears, click on the **desired Toolbar**.

To move the toolbar to another location on the screen, move it like any other window. Place the cursor to the far left of the **Title** bar on the vertical dotted line and drag the toolbar to the desired location. To remove the toolbar from the screen, right click on the toolbar; then in the dialog box listing the toolbars, click on the toolbar to be removed.

Underneath the toolbars is the address of the current active cell and the input line or formula bar labeled *fx*. When data are entered into the active cell, those data also appear in the formula bar. As data are entered, two buttons ☒ ✓ appear to the left of the formula bar. Clicking the **X** cancels the data entry. Clicking the ✓ has the same effect as pressing the Enter key; it finalizes the entry.

The Title Bar

The title bar is similar to the one in Word and, as in other Office software, appears at the top of the screen. Files are named using the conventions for Windows. Excel automatically adds an extension so that the file is recognized as a spreadsheet document. The extension for Excel is the three letters *xls* (see an example of this in Figure 7.1 in the title bar). By dragging the title bar, the worksheet window can be moved around the screen. The standard buttons for minimizing, full screen display, and close file are found at the right of the title bar.

Entering Data and Correcting Errors

Notice in Figure 7.1 the message area at the bottom left of the screen. This says "Ready" when data can be entered. After typing the data and before doing anything else, the message area says "Enter." Entering data is accomplished several ways; the most common are to

1. Press **Enter**
2. Use the mouse or an arrow key to move to another cell

When an error is noticed after entering data, it may be changed in one of three ways:

1. **Retype** the data, and press **Enter**. This will automatically overwrite the error.
2. Place the cursor in the **Input** line where the error occurs. Press **Delete**. Type the correction, and press **Enter**.
3. Place the cursor on the **Cell** to be changed. **Double click** and make appropriate **Changes** to the cell.

Moving in the Worksheet

Moving in the worksheet may be done with the mouse, arrow keys, or key combinations. The simplest way to move is to place the mouse in the desired cell and click. Other ways to move include the following:

Arrow Keys	Move one cell in the direction of the arrow key used.
Tab Key	Moves one cell to the right.
Shift+Tab	Moves one cell to the left.
Ctrl+Home	Moves to the beginning of the worksheet, or A1.
Page Up/Down	Moves to the cell one screen up/down in the same column.
Alt+Page Up/Down	Moves left/right one screen in the same row.
Ctrl+End	Moves to the intersection of last row and column containing data.

▶ **To go to a specific cell:**
1. Type the **Address** in the cell address area, and press **Enter** or
2. Press **F5** for the Go To dialog window. Type the desired **Cell address** in the reference box, and press **Enter**.

Viewing the Worksheet

Changing the view of the worksheet is done in several ways. This does not change the location of the cursor, just the part of the worksheet being viewed. Clicking the arrow keys on the scroll bars will move the worksheet one cell at a time in the direction of the arrow. For example, clicking the down arrow on the vertical scroll bar moves one cell down in the worksheet; clicking the right arrow moves one cell to the right. Clicking in the gray area between the scroll bar and the arrow moves the display by an entire screen either vertically or horizontally, depending on the scroll bar selected. The PgUp and PgDn keys move the screen view up or down to the next section that fits onto the screen.

Common Commands

▶ **To create a new worksheet:**

Select **File**, **New** or click **New** 🗋 button. File, New presents a dialog window and templates from which to choose. Selecting the new page icon provides a new blank worksheet.

▶ **To access an existing worksheet:**

Select **File**, **Open** or click **Open** 📂 button, and then access the **Drive** and/or Folder where the file is stored. Click the desired **File**.

▶ **To select cells:**

To clear cells, cut, copy, and change cell formats or to apply formulas to a series of cells, first select the cells.

To Select	Do This
A single cell	Click the **Cell**.
A range of cells	Click a **Cell** at one end of the series and drag the mouse to **Highlight the desired range** of cells. Make sure the pointer is the white plus sign when holding down the mouse button to drag. If it is a four headed arrow or a black plus sign, the data will be moving or autofilling, respectively. In earlier versions, if the pointer is a left slanted arrow, that will move the cell contents where dragged.
Entire rows columns	Click the **Row** or **Column Heading** (the gray or horizontal or vertical area containing row numbers or column letters). Drag to include more than one row or column.

Multiple cells, columns, or rows not contiguous	Hold down the **Ctrl** key while clicking all **Desired cells**, **Columns or Rows**. Then release the **Ctrl** key.
Entire worksheet	Click the **Rectangle** at the left of the columns just under the title bar.

▶ **To clear:**

Clear acts as an eraser and eliminates information or formats from a worksheet. One or more cells may be cleared at one time. The cells are left on the worksheet and retain a value of zero. Select **Edit**, **Clear**, and **All** to clear both format and content, **Formats** to erase cell formatting features, or **Contents** to erase the data.

▶ **To delete:**

The **Del** key erases cell contents.

▶ **To change column size:**

At the top of the worksheet along column letters, place the cursor on the **Vertical** line to the right of the column to be widened or made smaller. The cursor will appear as a vertical line with arrows pointing left and right. Drag the **Column lines** to the size desired. Double click to use the size to fit option. If a column is filled with ####, this means the column needs to be wider to show the numeric data that are there.

▶ **To insert row/column:**

Place the cursor where the new row or column is desired; click **Insert** and then **Row or Column**, or right click on the Row or Column header and select **Insert**. Rows are inserted above the current row and columns to the left of the current column. More than one row or column may be inserted by highlighting the row or column headers equal to the number to be inserted and following the steps mentioned previously here.

▶ **To delete row/column:**

Place the cursor on the row or column heading to be deleted, and click **Edit**, **Delete** or right click the **Row or Column header** and select **Delete**.

Working with Multiple Worksheets

Excel, by default, includes three worksheets in a spreadsheet file. Move between worksheets by clicking on the labeled tab at the bottom left of the worksheet. Worksheets may be added or deleted.

▶ **To add a worksheet:**

Click on **Insert**, **Worksheet**. A worksheet is added to the left of the current worksheet. Worksheets can also be reordered by right clicking on the worksheet tab and selecting **Move or Copy** and then selecting the order desired.

▶ **To delete a worksheet:**

To delete a worksheet from the worksheet to be deleted, click **Edit**, **Delete sheet**. Data may be copied and pasted between these. Any formulas based on data in one worksheet that are not copied to another will result in an error message #REF because the formula will be looking for the reference data in the cells of the new worksheet.

Working with Multiple Spreadsheets

Just like in Word where it is possible to have multiple documents, multiple spreadsheets may be open at the same time; data may be copied and pasted between these as well. Open spreadsheets will be shown in the task bar at the bottom of the screen and selected from there; another way to move between spreadsheets is by clicking on **Window** and the **Name** of the spreadsheet.

▶ **To save, save as, print, cut, copy, and paste:**

These functions work the same as in all Office 2003 programs (see Chapters 3 and 4 for a review of these functions).

Numbers and Formulas

Cell entries are considered as either labels or values. Values can be numbers or formulas. The first character typed determines the type of cell entry. In addition to the numbers 0–9, Excel treats the following characters as values: - + / *. E e ( ) $ and %.

Formatting Numbers

The default for numbers is general numbering. Any numbers entered into Excel appear exactly as typed. Number formatting can be changed to reflect decimals, percentages, currency, or other types of numbers. As different selections are made, examples are presented in the dialog window to allow a view of the effects of the format.

▶ **To format cells:**

Highlight the **Cells** to format first.

Select **Format**, **Cells**.

Click the **Number tab**. The dialog window presents the various numbering formats available.

Select the **Desired format**.

In the formatting toolbar (Figure 7.3) are shortcut icons for changing the format of numbers to currency and percentages, adding commas, and changing the number of decimal places. To make these changes, simply highlight cells to be formatted, and click the desired formatting icon. When formatting currency, use the same method for formatting throughout the spreadsheet. The two formatting methods create a slight difference in placement of the dollar sign ($), and using them both in the same spreadsheet will give an uneven look to currency cells.

Formulas and function

Formulas help analyze the data on a worksheet. With formulas, it is possible to perform operations such as addition, multiplication, and comparison and to enter the calculated value on the worksheet. A function is a preprogrammed formula. An Excel formula or function always begins with an equal sign (=).

▶ **To build a formula:**

- Type an = sign in the cell where the formula will be placed.
- Enter the **Formula** by typing cell addresses or selecting cells by clicking on them with the mouse and including the desired math calculation symbol where appropriate (e.g., + - * /).
- Press **Enter** or click the enter box (green checkmark) in the formula bar.

When using formulas in Excel, the standard rules of precedence listed earlier in the chapter dictate how the mathematic calculation proceeds. In Figure 7.4, the formula to add the cells appears in the formula line.

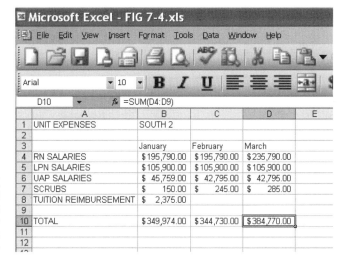

Figure 7.4

Numeric Formulas:
Note formula for the
total in cell D10
appears in the
formula bar

The AutoSum **Σ** function is the most commonly used function. It automatically adds a series of numbers in either rows or columns.

▶ **To use the Sum function:**

  Highlight the cells to be summed and include a blank space at one end
    of the series.
  Click the **AutoSum** icon, and the sum will be displayed.

  Another way to use this function is to do the following:

  Click an **Empty** cell where the sum will be displayed.
  Click the **AutoSum** icon.
  Confirm the **Range of cells** to be added by highlighting them.
  Click the **AutoSum** button again, or press **Enter**.

Some commonly used formulas have been included in numeric functions; this eliminates some of the steps of writing a formula. Several hundred functions are built into Excel, including financial, date and time, and mathematical, statistical, and lookup functions.

▶ **To access these:**

  Click the **Function** *fx* button on the toolbar, or click **Insert**, **Function**.

Commonly used functions include the following:

Function Name (cell/range)	Purpose
=AVERAGE(range)	Averages the values indicated
=COUNT(range)	Counts numbers within a range
=MAX(range)	Returns the largest value within a range
=MIN(range)	Returns the smallest value within a range
=STDEV(range)	Computes the standard deviation for the range
=SUM(range)	Sums the values indicated
=VAR(range)	Determines the variance for the range

Lookup Function

An additional useful function is the lookup function. This can be used with an array of data to find and add information. The VLOOKUP, or vertical lookup function, searches for a value in the leftmost column of a table and then returns a value in the same row from a column specified in the table. The HLOOKUP, or horizontal look up function, searches for information in the top row of an array.

To use the LOOKUP function, the following definitions are useful:

Lookup Value   This is the information to be found in the first column of the lookup table; it may be a numeric value, reference, or text.

Table Array   This is the table address containing the data to be retrieved.

Col Index Num   This is the number of the column in the table array from which information will be obtained; column numbers begin with 1 starting from the left.

Range Lookup   This determines whether the lookup function matches for exact data or the closest match. The default is the closest match, and this can be left blank when this is desired. When matching for exact data, type in **false**.

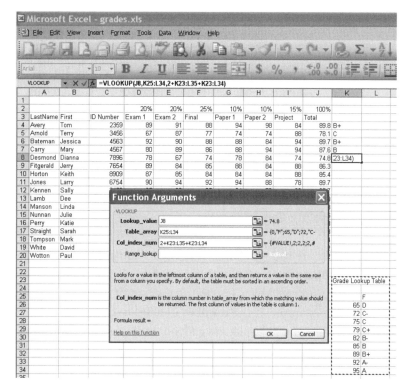

▶ **To use VLOOKUP, do the following:**

1. Build the information array with the look-up values in a column; these can be values, references, or text (see Figure 7.5 for an example of a grade worksheet that uses VLOOKUP to assign the letter grades to the numeric final grade data).

2. Place the values, references, or text to be looked up and the corresponding information that is to match these in an array, placing the values in ascending order. It is possible to put the values in ascending order by choosing the **Sort** command from the **Data** menu and selecting **Ascending**. It is also wise to place this look up table in an area of the worksheet where deleting rows or columns of other data will not delete some of the table data.

3. In the cell where the lookup value is to be placed, build the VLOOKUP formula by clicking *fx* and then typing **vlookup** in the search dialog box and clicking **Go**.

4. In the VLOOKUP dialog areas indicate the lookup value, table array, and column index number by clicking on specific cells or highlighting the ranges for a table. If matching for the closest value to the look up value, as in Figure 7.5, versus matching for an exact value, leave the **Range look up** dialog box blank. If matching for exact values appearing in the table array, type **true** in the range look up box.

5. Use these steps to build a formula for each value to be matched or make the cell addresses for the table array absolute cell addresses for both row and column as described below and copy the formula to other cells where VLOOKUP is to be applied.

Absolute Cell Addresses

Cell addresses in formulas that are designed to change when copied to other cells are called relative addresses. Absolute addresses are cell addresses in formulas, which remain the same despite other changes in the worksheet. These are indicated by a $ prefixing the part of the address that is to remain absolute. For example, if the number in C5 is to be the divisor in a formula, no matter where the formula was moved, indicate that address as C5. The following are various combinations for keeping certain parts of an address constant.

CR   Both the row and column addresses always remain the same.

$CR   The row changes, and the column address always remains the same.

C$R   The column changes, and the row address always remains the same.

Sorting data

Excel allows data to be sorted after it has been entered. It is possible to sort alphabetically or by numerical order. To sort, all data relevant to the sort must be included in the sort.

▶ **To sort:**

1. Using the mouse, highlight all of the data involved.
2. Click **Data**, **Sort**, and designate whether data should be sorted in ascending or descending order; indicate whether a header row is to be included in the sort.
3. Fill in the sort columns; it is possible to use up to three, and each sort will occur after the preceding one. Thus, a sort order might indicate the

last name and first name or department, course, and course number. Once the sort columns are determined, click **OK**.

Scenarios

Scenarios are a type of what-if analysis tools. A scenario is a set of values that Excel saves and can substitute automatically in the worksheet. Scenarios are used to forecast the outcome of a worksheet model. Different groups of values can be created and saved on a worksheet; it is possible to switch to any of these new scenarios to view different results. For example, when creating a budget with uncertain revenues, scenarios can be defined with different values for the revenue. It is then possible to switch between the scenarios to perform what-if analyses. To check a final course grade, different grades can be defined and the various final grades predicted under those different circumstances. Name a scenario worst case, and set the value of the final grade (F 4) to 55. Name the second scenario best case, and change the value of the final grade to 95. This is illustrated in Figure 7.6, where the original scenario has been copied and the changed final grade value and scenario outcome shown.

Creating Charts

Charts or graphs allow data to be visually displayed. Excel has a **Chart Wizard** that guides the user through the procedure to make the graph. First, highlight the data to include in the chart. Include labels for the X-axis and Y-axis as well as the numerical data. Click the Chart Wizard button to access the first page (Figure 7.7), and then follow the four steps.

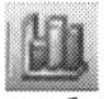

1. Click the **Type of graph** desired (pie, bar, etc.). Select **Next**.

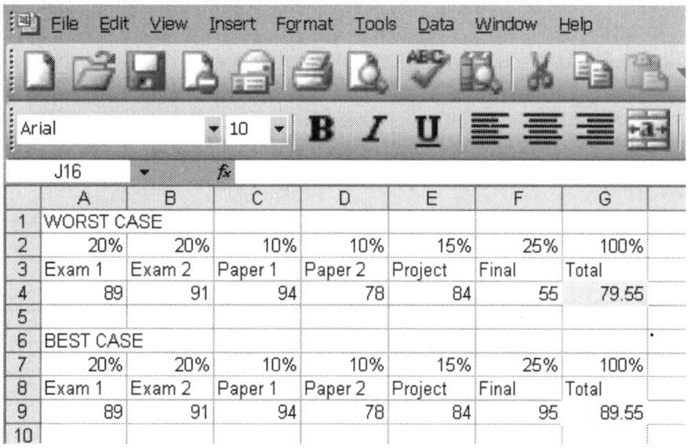

	A	B	C	D	E	F	G
1	WORST CASE						
2	20%	20%	10%	10%	15%	25%	100%
3	Exam 1	Exam 2	Paper 1	Paper 2	Project	Final	Total
4	89	91	94	78	84	55	79.55
5							
6	BEST CASE						
7	20%	20%	10%	10%	15%	25%	100%
8	Exam 1	Exam 2	Paper 1	Paper 2	Project	Final	Total
9	89	91	94	78	84	95	89.55
10							

Figure 7.6
Scenarios Showing how a Grade Affects the Final Grade

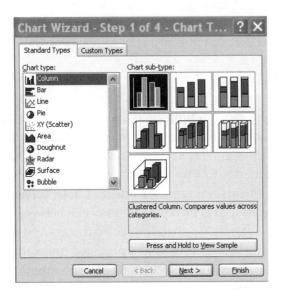

Figure 7.7

Chart Wizard for Selecting Type of Chart

2. Select **How the data are to be displayed** on the X-axis by indicating a series in columns or rows. The variations appear on the screen. Once satisfied, click **Next**. To try a different chart type, go back.
3. Add **Legend** and **Axis Titles** here. Type those in the appropriate dialog window and click **Next**.
4. Select the **Location** for the chart. Select **Finish**.

The graph will be displayed on the screen. If the chart is placed on the spreadsheet, it will have an outline around it that can be moved to the desired location on the spreadsheet.

SUMMARY

Spreadsheets can make things such as budgeting, inventory tracking, quality assurance documentation, and many other tasks involving numeric calculations much easier and more accurate. This chapter provided information about using spreadsheets at a basic level, building simple formulas, using common functions, examining what-if scenarios, and developing charts to represent data visually. Although this chapter focused on Microsoft Excel, other spreadsheets are similar.

Exercise 1: Create and Project Salaries
Objectives
1. Create a simple spreadsheet.

2. Use simple formulas and functions.

3. Format a worksheet.

4. Print, save, and retrieve a spreadsheet.

Activity
1. Access Excel.

   Click **Start**, **Programs**, **Microsoft Office**, and **Microsoft Excel**. An Excel button may be on the quick launch area of your task bar or in another area of the Start menu.

   Once you see the spreadsheet on the screen with "Ready" in the message area, you can begin. Be certain that you are in the correct cell for performing the designated actions that follow.

2. Practice moving the cursor.

   Practice moving from one cell to another using the mouse and the arrow keys.

   Move from cell **A1** to cell **C5**. What happens to cell C5 when you moved the cursor there? _____

   What shape does the pointer assume when it is inside the worksheet? _____

   Look for the current cell address in the top right corner of the screen. What do you see?

3. Practice entering data.

   Type **First Name** in cell C5 using small letters.

   Then place the cursor in cell **C6**, and type **Last Name** and press **Enter**.

   Go to cell **C6, press the space bar**, and then press **Enter**.

   What happens? _____ Now erase the name from cell C5.

4. Enter spreadsheet ID information.

   Click cell **A1**. Type **UNIT BUDGET**, and press **Enter**.

5. Enter labels. Click each cell indicated below, and type the appropriate data. Do not worry about making it look nice at this point. Formatting comes after the labels and data are entered.

   Highlight the range of cells **A3:G3**.

   Press the **Cap Lock** key.

   Type **Last Name** in cell **A3**, and press **Enter**. *A3 will look white, and B3 to G3 will be black.*

Type **First**. Press **Alt + Enter**. Type **Name**, and press **Enter**.

Type **Social**. Press **Alt + Enter**. Type **Security**. Press **Alt + Enter**. Type **Number**, and press **Enter**.

Type **Care**. Press **Alt + Enter**. Type **Level**, and press **Enter**.

Continue typing the labels as shown in Figure 7.8. Be sure to press **Alt + Enter** after each word entered and **Enter** for the last word to move to the next cell.

6. Enter the data.

Press the **Caps Lock** key to turn off caps lock. Click cell **A5**.

Type the following data in the cell as indicated and press enter after each name:

ROW	COLUMN A
5	Henderson
6	Nightingale
7	Barton
8	Wald
9	Dock

Complete the rest of the data as shown here and continuing on Figure 7.8. Do not type numbers for columns **F and G or totals in row 10**. Those are formulas. Enter data for only columns **B** through **E** and rows **5–9**. Do not worry about the $ or commas now; you will format them later.

A	B	C	D	E
5	Veronica	123–45–6789	1	32290
6	Felicity	345–80–6543	4	37654
7	Connie	234–68–6789	1	5412

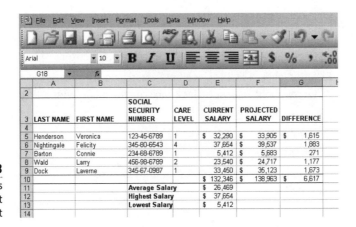

Figure 7.8

Exercise 1 - Labels and Data Unit Budget

7. Create formulas. Project a salary increase of 5% for each health care worker.

   Click cell **F5**. Type **= (E5*1.05)**, and press **Enter**.

   Click cell **F5**.

   Place pointer at bottom right of cell until it turns to a **Black plus** sign. **Drag through cell F9** and release.

   What formula appears in cell **F7**? _____

   Click cell **G5**. Type **=**. Click cell **F5**. Type **–** sign. Click cell **E5**, and click the **Green check** on formula toolbar.

   Place the pointer at bottom right of cell until it turns to a **Black plus sign**. **Drag through cell G9** and release.

8. Use functions. Use the sum function to total the salaries and differences in the budget.

   Click cell **E10**.

   Click **AutoSum** button twice. What total do you get? _____

   Place a sum in cell **F10** and **G10** to total the projected salaries and differences.

   Add the following labels in the designated cells:

   C11 **Average Salary**

   C12 **Highest Salary**

   C13 **Lowest Salary**

   In cell **E11**, type **=average(E5:E9)**.

   In cell **E12**, type **=max(E5:E9)**.

   In cell **E13**, type **=min(E5:E9)**.

   Change Nightingale's salary to 39000 by typing **39000** in cell **E6**. What total do you see now in cell **E12**? _____ Now change it back.

9. Format labels, numbers, and worksheet.

   Click cell **A1**.

   Click **Font down arrow** Arial ▼ 10 ▼ and select **Times New Roman**.

   Click **Size down arrow**, and select **16**. Click the **Bold button**.

   Select the range **A1:G1**. Click the **Merger and Center** button.

   Select the range **A3:G10**. Select **Format, Autoformat, Simple** format from the menu bar.

   Select range **E5:G5**. Hold down the **Ctrl** key, and select range **E10:G10** and **E11:D13**.

   Click the **Currency $** button on the formatting toolbar.

   Click the **Decrease decimal** button twice.

   Select range **E6:G9**, and click the **Comma   ,** button.

Click the **Decrease decimal** button twice.

Drag Columns A:G header, highlighting these columns.

Place the pointer on the Vertical line between F and G, and double click to use the autofit feature. If you still need to make adjustments, use the manual column sizing command.

The last formatting that you need to do is to center the labels. Think about how you do this using Word. What will you do? _____. Do it now.

If all of these steps have been completed correctly, the spreadsheet should look like the one in Figure 7.8.

10. Save the worksheet.

Click **File**, **Save** on the menu bar, or click the **Save** button.

Be sure you have a diskette in drive A if you are in a public laboratory.

Select the correct storage location for the file. This may be the A drive, hard drive, network file server, or other storage device drive. If needed, place the storage medium in the drive.

If needed, select the correct folder on the storage location.

In the **File name** box at the bottom of the screen, type the initials followed by budget and click the **Save** button.

11. Sort the information by last name.

Highlight cells A3 to G9. Click **Data**, **Sort** on the menu bar. What do you notice in the column letters and the row numbers? _____

Make sure that you indicate the data range has a header row by clicking in the appropriate box (see Figure 7.9 for a view of this dialog box).

Select Last Name for the first sort and first name for the second sort.

12. Save the worksheet again as in step 10 giving it a different **File name**.

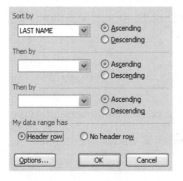

Figure 7.9

Exercise 1 – Sorting
the Unit Budget

13. Exit Excel.

Click **File**, **Exit** on the menu bar or click the **Close** ✕ button in the upper right of the screen.

14. Reopen Excel and find the sorted file.

What steps will you use to see where you stored the budget file?
_____

What is the full filename of the sorted budget file? _____

Retrieve the worksheet. Click **File**, **Open**.

Make sure the Look in text box points to the correct storage location, for example, A drive for a floppy disk. If not, correct it.

Highlight the **Budget file** with the mouse, and click the **Open** button.

Click the **Printer** 🖨 button, or select **File**, **Print** to print the spreadsheet.

Be sure that you have access to a printer and that it is turned on.

Exit the program. Be sure to exit windows fully, and turn off the equipment as instructed.

Exercise 2: Create a 6-Month Budget

Objectives

1. Create a 6-month budget using selected spreadsheet commands.
2. Use selected functions and simple formulas.
3. Add color to highlight selected information.

Activity

1. Create the identifying information.

   In row 1, type the heading for the spreadsheet: **6-MONTH BUDGET**.

   In row 2, column B type **BUDGET**. In column C, type **ACTUAL**. In column D, type **DIFFERENCE**.

2. Add the labels.

   Type **JAN** in cell **A3**.

   Use autofill to fill the labels through cell **A8**. (Place the cursor in the lower right corner of cell **A3**. With the black plus sign, drag through cell **A8**.)

A3	A4	A5	A6	A7	A8
JAN	FEB	MAR	APR	MAY	JUN

3. Enter the data. For each month, under the headings, enter the data as indicated here:

MONTH	BUDGET	ACTUAL
JAN	850	743
FEB	850	695
MAR	825	789
APR	875	849
MAY	850	778
JUN	875	834

4. Add functions. Use the sum function for finding sums in row 9, columns B and C.

5. What formulas would you use to compute the differences between the budgeted amounts and the actual amounts for JAN?

   BUDGET: _____

   ACTUAL: _____

   Enter this in column D.

6. What feature would you use to copy the formula to compute differences for each month? _____ Copy the formulas to the appropriate cells.

7. How would you write the function to determine the average for the 6-month BUDGET and ACTUAL amounts? _____ In row 11 column A type **Averages**, and then enter that function to determine those averages in B11 and C11.

8. Format the spreadsheet by using AutoFormat and selecting the **Classic 1** style.

9. Highlight cell B9, and click on the down arrow beside the color icon ![color icon] and highlight yellow. Highlight cell C9, and add a color fill of your choice.

10. Save and Print the spreadsheet.

Exercise 3: Create a Chart

Objectives

1. Use the Chart Wizard to create several chart styles.

2. Print several chart styles.

Activity

1. Create a spreadsheet representing the expenses for 3 months. Include the following categories: utilities, rent, food, car expenses, and personal expenses, and use the figures below or fill in your own.

Expense	JAN	FEB	MAR
Utilities	175	145	124
Rent	350	350	350
Food	234	245	275
Car Expenses	45	85	75
Personal Expenses	145	176	143

2. Using the Chart Wizard, create a chart showing how the expenses are divided for the month of January. What standard chart type would work most effectively for this? _____ (If you are not sure what chart would be best, open the Chart Wizard using step b. Click each type of chart and read the description provided under each pictured version of the chart.)

a. On the spreadsheet, highlight the **Labels and Data** for expenses for the month of January.

b. Click the **Chart Wizard** button on the standard toolbar.

c. *Step 1.* The first step in the Wizard allows you to select the chart that will best display the data. Click the **Chart** that you desire from the list; then click the **Chart Subtype** that you want. Preview it to ensure that this chart will indeed show the data as you desire—click on "press and hold to view sample" and hold the mouse button down until you see the sample displayed. If this chart is not what you want, go to some of the others and preview them until you find the desired chart. Once you have selected the chart and chart subtype, click **Next**.

Step 2. Because you have already highlighted the range of data and labels, you should see the chart here and can go on by clicking **Next**.

Step 3. Label the chart by typing **January Expenses** in the box under Chart title. Click the tab labeled **Data labels**. If you choose a pie chart, click **Show percent**, and click **Next**. If you choose a bar or column chart, click **Show value** and click **Next**.

Step 4. Click to show the chart **As a new sheet**. Click **Finish**.

d. Print the chart by clicking the printer icon.

3. Using the steps learned here, create and print a column chart (any subtype) that shows a comparison of all of the expenses for the 3 months.

Assignment 1: Create a Simple Spreadsheet
Directions

1. Create a spreadsheet for any of the following:

a. A unit budget that includes last year's costs, this year's cost to date, and projections for next year if costs increase 5%.

b. A drug worksheet that lists the dose by weight for a class of drugs (e.g., emergency drugs for preemies or for cardiac arrest, a comparison sheet for safe doses of narcotics) and formulas for calculating the drugs for individuals of different weights.

c. A personal budget of the living costs for the past year, current year, and projected for next year if all costs increase by 3%.

d. Special topic approved by faculty.

2. Submit both the printed spreadsheet and electronic file showing what happens with formulas and "what if" questions.

Assignment 2: Create a Grade Sheet
Directions

1. Using a spreadsheet to create a grade sheet that includes headings for first and last name, an ID number (social security number), and the test scores for a midterm, a project, a final exam, and the final grade.

2. Enter the data under the headings as it appears here:

ID	Last Name	First Name	MIDT	PROJ	EXAM	FINAL
123–45–6789	Titmouse	Martha	95	98	87	
125–12–4534	Finch	Jerry	87	75	90	
124–65–9087	Cardinal	Sam	65	70	67	
124–65–9087	Robins	Sally	85	80	90	
125–65–1234	Nuthatch	Jamie	85	90	95	
127.12–1234	Wren	Timothy	90	95	90	

3. The midterm and project are each weighted 30%, and the final exam is weighted 40% of the final grade. Enter formulas to calculate the final grade for each student.

4. Using the appropriate functions, enter formulas to calculate the highest and lowest grade and the average for the midterm, project, and final exam grade.

5. Give each grade a percentage weighting so that all three grades total 100%. Place those percentages in a row you add between the headings and first row of data.

6. Using the percentages and grades, determine the final numerical grade for each student.

7. Adjust columns so that the spreadsheet is visually pleasing.

8. Practice creating a scenario showing how Martha's grade would change if she earned a 95 on the final exam.

9. Sort the spreadsheet according to alphabetical order by the last name of the students

10. Print the spreadsheet. Turn in the spreadsheet and the electronic file.

Assignment 3: Create a Chart
Directions

1. Using the data from Assignment 2, create a chart that compares all five students' grades on each of the three different parts that determine the grade for the course.

2. Print the graph. On the back of the paper, indicate why you selected the chart that you did.

3. Turn in the graph.

Introduction to Databases

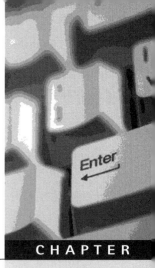

CHAPTER

8

OBJECTIVES

1. Define terms related to database applications.
2. Identify the data types that are best managed through databases.
3. Describe the database design process.
4. Interpret basic directions for operating a database program.

Databases are widely used today. Libraries catalog their collections on databases. Businesses track inventory, manage customer information, and maintain accounting data in databases. Educational institutions track applications and enrollments, drop and add students to courses, and produce class lists using databases. Health care institutions use a variety of database programs to meet their needs as well. These include mainframe and personal computer–level programs. This chapter introduces basic database concepts and terms as well as some introductory keystrokes for completing the exercises. For more detailed information, consult the application program's online help or any related reference book.

Database management systems help to organize, store, and retrieve data. These programs permit the user to create table structures, modify the structures, store data, and retrieve it in a variety of ways. They act as efficient file systems; they are, however, only as effective and efficient as the accuracy and structure of the data.

The main advantages of electronic databases are as follows:

- A reduction in data redundancy (duplicate data in a variety of places)

- A reduction in data inconsistency (data stored differently in the same file, e.g., how to store a person's name—full name, including first and middle, or first, middle initials, and last name)

- Increased data access

Some people treat data security as an advantage. They believe that with centralized data, control over access is much easier. Others believe that data security is a disadvantage because increased access to data results in increased security concerns. To counter this disadvantage, decisions about who has access to what data and at what level must be made. Should everyone have the ability to correct and add data? Do some only need access to viewing it but not changing it? In the health care arena, should receptionists have access to the patient's diagnosis and physician's name, or do they need access to only the patient's name and room number fields? Should the supervisor have the ability to chart medications on all patients, or should only the nurses on the unit have that ability? These are the types of issues that a centralized database raises.

▶ 8.1 DATABASE MODELS

There are three main database models. Each model structures, organizes, and uses data differently. Hierarchical and network models are commonly used on mainframes and minicomputers. Most personal computer database programs use a relational model. The model underlining the design of the database program influences or limits the searching permitted. It also influences the maintenance of the database.

Hierarchical	This model is like a tree or organizational chart. During searching, the program searches sequentially each root and branch and checks for a match. This is commonly called traversing the tree. Some common terms associated with this model are root, parent, and siblings. When designing the database, each child in the hierarchical model can have only one parent.
Network	The network model was developed to solve problems caused by the hierarchical model's inability to store certain types of data easily. The network model permits more than one parent per child. However, it requires multiple links to the various fields, making it much more difficult to revise or edit.
Relational	A relational model relies on so-called flat tables for its structure. Designers use only one data element per field. This means that tables must be reduced to their simplest form. The term used for this process of reduction is normalizing the table. For example, a parent with two children would become two tables that link on a common field.

An alternative database model seen on the Internet or on intranets is the hypertext design. This design relies on objects linked to other related objects. The object may be text, pictures, data files, or sound files. This structure is particularly useful for organizing large amounts of diversified data. The disadvantage to this setup is that it is not possible to perform numerical analysis on the data nor can it be certain how people will access each part of the database.

▶ 8.2 COMMON DATABASE TERMS

These terms describe the structure of a database from smallest unit to largest:

Data	Raw facts consisting of numbers, letters, characters, and dates are data. They are the contents of fields. Other names for data are data items or elements. Some examples of data are Jones, 200–23–1234, and Chicago.

Data Types

Data types refer to the description of what data to expect in a field. They are software dependent; each program defines them. Most programs include alphanumeric (characters and numbers), numeric (numbers), short numeric (short, whole numbers), currency (money), character (letters), date and time, logical (equal to, greater than, or less than), memo (comment), and object (pictures or objects) data types.

Field

A field is a space within a file with a predefined location and length. Another name that describes a field is attribute. Only one data item is placed in each field. For example, place temperature, pulse, and respiration in separate fields; do not place them together in one field such as a vital sign field. Examples of field names are last name, first name, city, state, diagnosis, systolic blood pressure, pulse, and height. Use a field name that reflects the data to be stored.

Record

A collection of fields related or associated with a focal point is a record. For example, a patient is a focal point around whom certain data are collected and stored. A patient chart is a record. A college transcript is a record. Each row of a table, in most programs, is a record.

File

Files are collections of related records. For example, all of the patients in St. Luke's Hospital make a file. Many people compare a file with the file drawer in a filing cabinet. Related data are kept in the same drawer.

Database

A database is a collection of files and is like a file cabinet; it holds related drawers of records. It is organized in such a way that a computer program called a database management system can quickly retrieve the data desired.

Database Management System

Database management systems (DBMS) are the programs that enable users to work with electronic databases. They permit data to be stored, modified, and retrieved from the database.

The following are descriptions of additional database concepts:

Key Field   One or more fields with a unique identifier are key fields. Having key fields ensures that there are no duplicate records in this database because a key field accepts only one record with that combination of text and/or numbers. One of the most commonly used key fields is a social security number.

Link   A link is a logical association between tables based on the values in corresponding fields. This is a connection between two tables in a relational database program. This is what permits a user to query or ask questions of multiple tables and extract only the data desired from these tables. The linked field must be of the same data type.

Table   The table is the structure that is used to store the data. It consists of fields and records. The vertical columns are fields, and the horizontal ones are records.

► 8.3 COMMON DATABASE FUNCTIONS

Common database functions allow users to create table structures, edit data or records, search tables, sort records, and generate reports.

Creating the Database

There are two steps to creating the database: designing the structure (sometimes called the schema) and entering the data.

Designing the structure

Designing the structure of the table requires identifying the field names, field types, and field widths. This structure design is generally stored in a data dictionary, which is a file that defines the basic organization of a database. It lists all of the tables associated with the database as well as the names and types of each field. Many times it also includes comments about the range of acceptable data.

Entering data

Enter data using the designed structure. Sometimes this involves redesigning the structure to facilitate entry of all data. Most databases provide options for verifying accuracy of the data entered. These utilities or tools permit users to set data ranges and data images to help ensure the accuracy of the data entered.

Editing Data or Records

Editing data or records involves adding records, deleting old records, or changing data in active records.

Add	The add function permits placement of additional records into the database.
Delete	Delete permits the user to remove records from the database.
Change	Change permits the user to alter the contents of a record.

Searching the Database

Searching is the process of creating data subsets or locating specific records in the database. Some terms used to describe this process are search, query, find, and ask. The power of the database lies in the search function and the ability to extract data. Described here are additional terms related to searching.

Answer table

In some databases, the answer table is a temporary table in which the program stores search results. It is overwritten when a user conducts a new search or is deleted when a user exits the program. In other databases, the answer tables or results are automatically saved in the Queries object.

Boolean searching

This is using specific strategies to expand or limit a search. Three of the most often used Boolean operators are AND, OR, and NOT. Boolean searching is one of the most commonly used features for searching any database and provides the ability to narrow or expand a search as well as eliminate some records. Although more on searching is described in Chapter 11, "Information: Access, Evaluation, and Use," some basic uses are described here.

AND	This strategy provides records that include both terms on either side of the AND. For example,

computer and health elicits only records that include both terms. If one term is missing, that record does not show in the search results. The match must be exact. If a record has computers and health, it does not show in the search results. Computer is not the same term as computers.

OR This strategy provides records that have either term. For example, computer OR computing finds records that include either the term computer or the term computing.

NOT This strategy provides records that exclude the term following NOT. For example, computer NOT bedside elicits records containing the word computer and eliminates records that have the word bedside.

There are some additional operations such as NEAR and ADJACENT to use, but they are not as common as these three. What is important is that the search strategy is refined to be the most efficient for eliciting the information desired.

Exact Match This search finds only entries that are an exact match for a specified word. Any minor difference results in exclusion of that entry from the results. For example, when searching for child, it finds only child and not children, infants, or teenagers.

Pattern This type of search permits the use of wild cards in place of a character. For example, nur* would match the string nur and any word with nur as the beginning string. Thus, it would find nurse, nurses, nursing, nursery, nurture, and nurturing.

Range These are operators such as greater than, less than, equal to, or some combination of them. They are called logical operators, and they return records that fit the operator, such as all patients with pulses greater than 110.

Select Fields This refers to selecting the fields for displaying in the search results. This involves using some mark to identify the fields to display in the results. All of the fields or selected ones may be chosen. For example, a health care worker may choose to display only the patient name and room number in the results or may choose to display additional fields such as diagnosis, doctor, primary nurse, and laboratory test results.

Sorting the Database

This function permits the user to arrange records in a variety of ways and to work with some subset of them. Many times it is desirable to see the list of names in alphabetic order or all of the zip codes together in numeric order. This feature allows arranging the data in the order that makes sense for the result desired. Two terms used when sorting are ascending and descending. The ascending function sorts in alphabetic or numeric order from A or 1 to Z or NN. Descending is the reverse going from the highest value to the lowest.

Generating Reports

Another powerful feature of databases is the ability to generate multiple reports from the same database or data subset. Most programs permit multiple report formats on the same data.

▶ 8.4 A FEW DATABASE DESIGN TIPS

The most difficult task in developing databases is creating the database structure. This is a time-consuming task and requires the designer to pay attention to detail. Here are some questions to answer before creating table structures.

1. What output is desired?
2. What search questions will be asked?
3. What fields are needed to produce the desired output and to answer the search questions?
4. What is needed to define the record accurately?
5. What field names are desired?
6. What data type will be placed in each field?
7. What serves as the unique identifier for each record?
8. How will this table or file relate to other tables or files? What are the relationships?
9. Is there any redundant (duplicate) data in this table? Should it be normalized?

▶ 8.5 COMMON USES IN HEALTH CARE

Databases have many uses in health care. Administrative use includes databases such as staffing, scheduling, personnel records, quality assurance (improvement), and inventory control. Clinical databases are used for patient records and drug files. Educators use databases for test banks, student experiences, and student records. Research-related databases include literature access, data collection, data storage, and data retrieval. Additional databases are discussed in Chapter 11, "Information: Access, Evaluation, and Use." The National Library of Medicine has a variety of databases that are useful in health care. Selected ones can be seen in Figure 8.1.

▶ 8.6 ADDITIONAL TERMINOLOGY

As things change in the computer world, new terminology develops. Discussed here are three terms related to database concepts.

Data Mining   This concept refers to database applications that look for patterns in already created databases. Do not confuse it with software that presents data in new ways. Data mining software actually discovers new relationships between the data items that were not previously known. This class of database

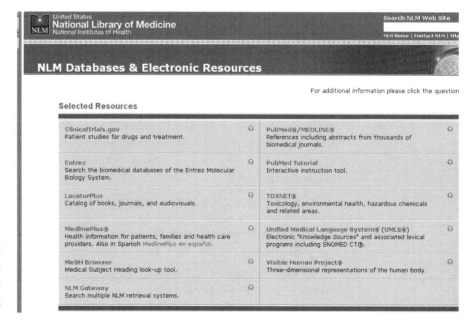

Figure 8.1

Selected National Library of Medicine Databases at http://www.nlm.nih. gov/databases/

	software has great potential for discovering new patterns of patient responses, who responds to what type of treatment, and who is at greater risk for developing certain conditions or side effects.
Data Warehouse	This concept refers to a collection of data designed to support decision making. The purpose of a data warehouse is to present a picture of the general conditions of the entity at a particular time. Software extracts data from other systems and places it in a warehouse database system. This means that many different databases from the institution are collectively scanned for the data relative to or data to support decision making. Generally, a warehouse supports summary data, not detail data. It does not deal with the day-to-day operations of an institution. These data support analysis of trends over time.
Data Mart	A subset or smaller focus database designed to help managers make strategic decisions is a data mart. Sometimes it is a subset of a data warehouse. Like data warehouses, it combines aspects of many databases within the institution, but with a focus on a particular subject, department, or unit.

▶ 8.7 INTRODUCTION TO ACCESS

The remaining part of this chapter describes a relational database program called Access. Basic information to begin using Access is presented here. To learn additional functions, remember to use the help system or refer to the many Access books that are available at most bookstores.

Starting Access
There are many ways to start this program. Some of them are listed here.

Double click on the **Microsoft Access** 🔑 icon if present.
Click the **Start** button, **All Programs**, **Microsoft Office**, **Microsoft Access**.
Double click an **MS Access** file.
Click the **MS Access icon** on the Quick Launch area of the taskbar.

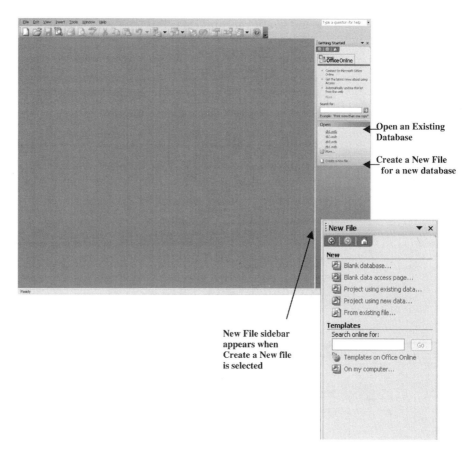

Open an Existing
Database

Create a New File
for a new database

New File sidebar
appears when
Create a New file
is selected

Figure 8.2

Typical Access Screen

In the Getting Started Task Pane, users have the choice to open an existing
database or to create a new blank database. Users will also be asked to name
the database if creating a new one (see Figure 8.2 for the look of the opening screen in Access).

Closing and Exiting the Database

Once a database has been created and used, the database as well as the
Access program needs to be closed. Make sure that the prompts to save data
and the related forms and reports that occur as part of the exiting process
are heeded and acted on. There are two close buttons—one for the database
and the other for the application.

▶ **To close the database:**

Click the **Database close** ✕ button. Be sure to click the close button for
this database and not the application one.

Respond to any prompts regarding saving any unsaved data, forms, and reports.

▶ **To close the application:**

Click the **Application close** ☒ button. Again be sure to respond to any prompts. When the file is maximized, the Close button will be a black X, and not the white X in a red box.

Opening an Existing Database and Creating a New Database

Each database created is stored as a separate file with an extension of .mdb and contains the structure (tables), data, reports, forms, macros, and queries. Once the database is opened, buttons in the database window represent each separate component in the database—tables, queries, reports, pages, and so on. This can be seen in Figure 8.3. In this figure, there are two different close buttons— one for the application and the other for the database. In this view, they appear the same. When the database is maximized, the database button will appear under the Access Program Close button and will be a black X.

▶ **To open a database:**

Start **Access** (mentioned previously here).

▶ **To open an existing database:**

Make sure Access is opened.

On the Getting Started task pane, select an existing database file, and click on it. *If necessary, click the More link to see additional database files that are stored at other locations.* (See Figure 8.2.)

Select location and name of the database to open.

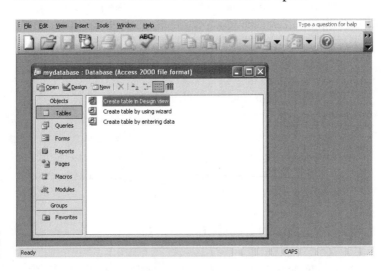

Figure 8.3
Access Database
Screen

▶ **To open a new database:**

Make sure **Access** is open.

Click on the **Blank page** 🗋 icon to create a new file.

When the New File task pane appears, click **Blank database**. *A prompt provides a default name, but it is helpful to give the new database a meaningful name.*

Highlight **Dbl.mdb** in the name text box, and type **Database Name**.

Select the **location** for the file. Be sure to indicate the correct storage device.

Press **Enter**.

Either selecting an existing database or opening a new one will provide the screen shown in Figure 8.3 with the database name in the top left of the dialog box. The following directions provide the steps to create a database table.

▶ **Create the table:**

Click the **Tables** ☐ Tables object if not already selected.

Click the **New** button.

Select **Design View**. Click **OK**, or select Create Table in Design View and Double Click on it.

Type **Field names**, and press **Tab**.

If not a text field, click the **Down arrow** button. Select the **Data type** for this field.

If a text field, press **F6**. Type **Length of field**, and press **F6**. *Pressing F6 toggles to the screen at the bottom so that the length of the field can be entered. By default, the text length is 50 characters.*

Press **Tab**, and type **Description of the field**.

If this is a key field, click the **Key** 🔑 button on the toolbar, or go to the **Edit** menu. Select **Primary Key**, and then press **Tab**.

Continue typing the field names, sizes, and descriptions until the structure is complete.

▶ **Close the table:**

Click the **Table close** ✕ button. Make sure to click the close button on the table window to close this table but not the application.

▶ **Save the table:**

Click **Yes** to save the table. Type **Table Name**, and click **OK**. *The database window now appears.*

▶ **Name the file:**

When naming files it is helpful to label them as:

Table:Name

Query:Name

Form:Name

Report:Name

Here "Name" is the specific identifying name that you give that object. The prefix specifying the type of database file serves as a reminder regarding the nature of the file.

Moving Around the Database

There are two main views for working with a database: datasheet and form views. When opening an existing database, the data are displayed in Datasheet view. That is, they are in rows and columns just like a spreadsheet. To view the data one record at a time, switch to Form view.

▶ **To switch from one view to the other:**

Click the **New Object** ⊞▾ button down arrow for the change view menu. Select **Autoform**. *This presents a view that shows all the fields for one record at a time.*

▶ **To switch back to Datasheet view:**

Click the **View** ✎▾ button, and select **Datasheet view**.

Use the following keys or buttons to move through tables in **Datasheet and Form views**. Figure 8.4 shows the record movement toolbar.

Tab	to go to the next field in the record
Shift Tab	to go to the previous field in that record
Click Next Record	to go to the next record in the database
Click Previous Record	to go to the previous record in the database

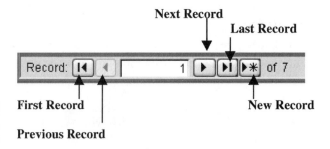

Figure 8.4
Moving Between
Records in Access

Last Record	to go to the last record in the database
First Record	to go to the first record in the database
Double Click Specific Record, Type Record Number	to go to a specific record in the database

Entering and Editing the Data

Once the structure has been created, data may be entered. Entering data is straightforward. Type the data in the appropriate field, and press the tab key to go to the next field.

▶ **To enter data:**

Click **Table Name** in the main Access screen, and click **Open**.

Type the **Data** in each of the appropriate fields.

Press the **Tab** key to go to the next field.

If a mistake is made while entering the data, use the backspace key to erase it and then retype it. Another way to edit the mistake is to place the cursor in the field. Click the field. Use the cursor keys to go to the place of the mistake. Type the correction, and delete the extra letters with the delete key. Use the tab key to move to the next field.

▶ **To add another record to a table:**

Double click the **Table Name**.

Click the **New Object** [icon] down arrow for the change view button.

Select **Autoform**.

Click the **New Record** [icon] button.

Type the **New Data** in the appropriate fields.

Click the **Close** button. Click **Yes**, and click **OK**.

▶ **To change the contents of a field:**

Highlight **Data to replace**.

Type **New Data**, and click the **Close** button. *The change is automatically saved.*

▶ **To delete a record from a table:**

Click the **Record selector** for the record to be deleted (Figure 8.5).

Press the **Delete** key. Click **Yes** to confirm deletion of this record.

Click the **Close** button to close the table.

Another approach is to click the **Delete Record** [icon] button on the toolbar.

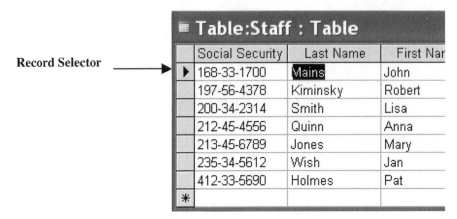

Record Selector ———→

Table:Staff : Table		
Social Security	Last Name	First Nar
168-33-1700	Mains	John
197-56-4378	Kiminsky	Robert
200-34-2314	Smith	Lisa
212-45-4556	Quinn	Anna
213-45-6789	Jones	Mary
235-34-5612	Wish	Jan
412-33-5690	Holmes	Pat

Figure 8.5

Record Selector

Sorting and Finding Records

When using a database and opening a table, the records may not be in the order that is desired for viewing. For example, it may be desirable to review the records by job positions or patient diagnosis or date. It is easier to sort the records than it is to scroll through them to find the ones for which you are looking. Records can be rearranged or sorted by using a sort button on the toolbar. There are two types of sort—ascending and descending. Ascending sort arranges the records in order from the lowest value to the highest value or alphabetically in the field selected. Descending reverses the order going from highest to lowest value or reverse alpha order.

▶ **To sort records in a table:**

Open the **Database** and **Table** to be sorted.

Click the right mouse button anywhere in the column of the field on which the sort will be based. Click the **Sort Ascending** ![icon] or **Sort Descending** ![icon] button.

Sometimes it does not matter what the order is because the goal is to find a specific record to either verify some information or update the record. The find feature searches only the field selected. It does not have the same power that the query feature does.

▶ **To find records:**

Open the **Database** and **Table**.

Click in the **Field** that has the data for the search. The field column does not need to be highlighted.

Click the **Find and Replace** 🔍 button.
Type a value in the **Find What** Box.
Select a **Search** option, and select a **Match** option.
Click **Find Next**.

When the first record to be changed has been found, click back to the table on that record field, and make the change. Then return to the Find dialog box, and click Find Next; repeat the process until all records are found and updated. When all changes are made, click the close button. If there are multiple changes involving the replacement of all or one value with the same different value, the replace feature accessible from the same button works similarly to the find feature but allows multiple changes at one time. Heed the warning that when the replace feature is used it is not possible to undo the operation.

Searching or Querying the Database

Databases allow searching for specific information or records. Searching, however, is an exacting process and requires some knowledge of the database and data. The power of any relational database is the ability to also link multiple tables together and pull only the data needed from each table. Described later here are directions for searching a single table and for linking two tables for a search. Save the query only if it is one that is repeated often. Do not save queries if they are one-time searches.

Several types of searches are possible. One allows users to search all records but to display only selected fields from one or more tables. Another lets users combine two or more tables and display selected fields from them.

▶ **To start the search:**

Start **Access** and open the **Database**.
Click **Queries** 🔲 Queries . Click the **New** button. Select **Design View**, and click **OK**.
Select **Table** to query. Click the **Add** button, and click the **Close** button.
   The query design screen appears.
Adjust windows so that all fields in the **Query Table** are displayed. Refer to Chapter 3 to review how to size windows.
Double click **Each field** listed in the table at the top that is desired for display in the query table (Figure 8.6).

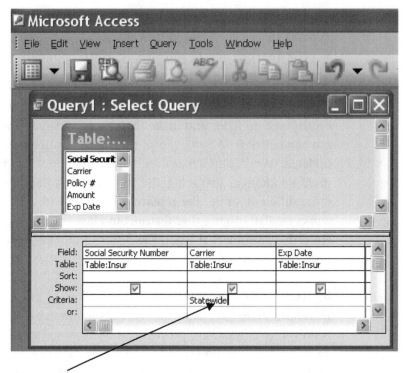

Figure 8.6

Query Design Screen

Criteria Specified in this Example is an Insurance Carrier

▶ **To search one table with selected fields:**

Perform the steps mentioned previously here.

Double click the **Selected fields** to display.

Click the **Run** 🔊 button.

▶ **To search two tables with selected fields:**

Start **Access** and open the **Database**.

Click **Queries**   🗐 Queries . Click the **New** button. Select **Design View**, and click **OK**.

Select **Table** to query, and click the **Add** button.

Select **Second table**. Click the **Add** button, and click the **Close** button.

Adjust windows so that all fields in the table are displayed.

Double click **Selected Fields**—those fields to display in your query re-sults—from both tables.

Click the **Run** button.

Another database feature allows creating a subset of records meeting specific criteria. It is possible to use a single criterion, such as city, or multiple criteria, such as city and state. The criterion is set by typing the condition in the Criteria cell for the field to which the criterion applies (see the example in Figure 8.6). To limit a search to a specific group of records, comparison operators can be used. These include equal to (=), less than (<), greater than (>), less than or equal to (<=), greater than or equal to (>=), and not equal to (<>). It is also possible to use wild-card characters such as the asterisk (*) to substitute for any number of characters and a question mark (?) to substitute for one character. Search operators AND and OR may also be used. Using search criteria is further described later.

Heart*	To find any number of characters after heart, such as heartburn, heart attack, and heart condition.
*Heart	To find any number of characters before the word heart, such as ace of hearts and coronary heart.
??art	To find two characters in that location ending with art, such as chart and heart.
AND	The AND search means that both conditions in both fields must be true to return the record. To search using the AND, type the criteria on the same criteria line for each field to which it applies.
OR	The OR condition means that one or the other has to be true to return the record. To search using the OR condition, type in the related OR row.

▶ **Using specific search criteria:**

Start **Access**, and open the **Database**.

Click **Queries**. Click the **New** button. Select **Design View**, and click **OK**.

Select **Table**, and click the **Add** button.

Adjust windows so that all fields in the table display.

Double click the **Selected Fields** to be in the query results display.

Type the **Criteria** on the Criteria line in the related Field name column.

If using an OR search, type the Criteria on the OR line.

Click the **Run** button.

Generating a Report

One of the primary reasons for creating and maintaining a database is the reporting feature. It is possible to report the total contents of a table or to generate multiple reports for each table with each report providing a different view of the data. Creating a report of the results of queries allows them to be displayed in formats pleasing to read. Access has both an AutoReport and Report Wizard feature to help create reports.

Because this is an introductory chapter, forms are not covered in this book. The major difference between forms and reports is that reports are intended for printing and not for display in a window. Forms are for displaying in a window on the screen. Reports are designed to report some result. Forms are used for entering or changing values of fields.

There are six basic types of Access reports: single column, tabular, multi-column, grouped, mailing labels, and unbound reports. Which report type selected depends on the data and how they are to be displayed. Here are guidelines for creating simple column and grouped reports.

▶ **Creating a simple report:**

Select the **Table or Query** tab.

Highlight the **Table or Query**.

Click the **New Object** ![icon] ▾ button down arrow.

Select **AutoReport**.

Click the **View** ![icon] ▾ button down arrow. Select **Design View**.

Make whatever changes to the report needed by dragging the objects to their new location. To move a field name or field separately, click the top left corner of the field box, and move it to its new location. To move all of the fields on the same horizontal row, click on the ruler; then place the curser, now in the shape of a hand, and drag all of the fields to the new location.

Once the design is complete, toggle to the Preview ![icon] button. Use properties to change fonts, add colors, and so on. It is possible to toggle between the two views until the report is as desired.

▶ **Creating a grouped report:**

Grouped reports allow organization of data in a particular fashion by grouping like records together. For example, a health care worker might group records by department or diagnosis or health care provider. The example here uses the Report Wizard to help design and layout a report.

Select the **Table or Query** for the report.

Click the **New Object** ![icon] ▾ down arrow button. Choose **Report**.

Select **Report Wizard**, and click **OK**.

Add the **Fields** wanted in the report, and click **Next**.

Select the fields to **Group** the report by, and click **Next**.

Set the **Sort** order. Click the **Next Button**.

Select a **Layout** and **Orientation**. Click **Next**.

Select a **Style** for the report. Click **Next**.
Click **Finish**.
Click **File**, **Save As**, type **Report: Name**.

▶ **Modifying and formatting a report:**

Reports can be modified using some of the design tools available with the program. Remember reports contain fields and field labels that can be rearranged. Adding descriptive text to the data as well as headers and footers is also a feature of the report. Use the steps given here to modify and format a report.

Select the **Report to modify**.
Click the **Design** button.
Make the Modifications.

▶ 8.8 USING DATABASES WITH OTHER OFFICE APPLICATIONS

Just as there are functions within other Office products that allow interaction among them, data from Access can be exported for use in Word and in Excel. For example, databases with information about customers and their addresses can be used in mail-merged letters and address labels. The specifics of this are beyond this basic text, but help is available within the applications or in other books about their use.

SUMMARY

This chapter presented basic database concepts necessary to understanding the world of databases. The database structure and related terms are discussed. Specific directions for using Access as an example of one database then followed. Learning how to use databases increases the ability to retrieve and use information in them and helps greatly in making decisions.

Exercise 1: Create Table and Enter Data
Objectives
1. Create two tables with a linked field.
2. Enter and save the data.
3. Edit fields and add records.

Activity

1. Start the program.

   Insert a diskette into Drive A or into whatever removable storage device being used. Tables will be created on the removable storage device.

   Double click the **Access icon.** You may need to access the program by selecting Start, All Programs, and Microsoft Office, Microsoft Access OR by using the Microsoft Office desktop shortcut or the Access icon on the Quick Launch area of the taskbar.

2. Create the table structure.

   Click **Create New File, Blank Database** to open a new blank database (see Figure 8.2 for the dialog screen).

   Click the **Down arrow** button in the Save in text area, and click **the appropriate storage device** icon to switch to it.

   Highlight **dbl.mdb** in the file name box. Type **Staff Insurance**, and press **Enter.**

   Click the **Tables button** ☐ Tables if not already selected, and click the **New**

   ☐New button on the menu bar.

   Select **Design View**, and click **OK.**

   Type **Social Security Number.** Press **Tab.** Press **F6.** Type **11.** Press **F6.** Press **Tab.** Type **Unique Identifier, Separate numbers by dashes.** Pressing F6 toggles you to the screen at the bottom so that you can type in the length of the field. By default, the length is 50 characters.

   Click the **Key** button on the toolbar to make this a key field, and press **Tab.**

   Continue typing the field names, sizes, and descriptions as outlined here.

Last_Name	Text	10	Staff person's last name with first letter capitalized
First_Name	Text	10	First_name
Street_Name	Text	20	Street Address
City	Text	15	City
State	Text	2	State, use the two-letter all-cap abbreviation
Zip_code	Text	5	Five-digit zip code
Phone	Text	12	Phone number, including area code
Dept	Text	2	Department two-letter code

   When finished your screen should look like Figure 8.7.

   Click the **Table close** button. Make sure that you click the second one down to close this table, not the application.

   Click **Yes** to save the table, and type **Table:Staff.** Press **Enter.**

   What type of data does the program accept in the field Zip_code?

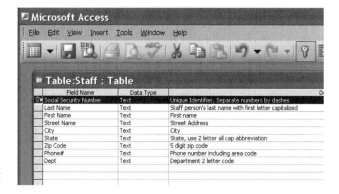

Figure 8.7

Staff Table Structure

What other data types can you use in Access?

Where can you find this information?

3. Create a second table.

Use the directions mentioned previously to do this. Call this one **Table:Insur**. Enter the following field names and data types:

Field Name	Data Type	Value	Description
Social Security Number	text	11 key	Unique identifier, separate numbers by dashes
Carrier	text	30	Insurance carrier
Policy_#	text	11	Individual's policy number
Amount	currency		Policy value amount
Exp_Date	date		Expiration date of policy

Make sure to save this structure.

4. Enter data.

Enter data into both of the tables created previously. If you make a mistake while entering the data, use the backspace key to erase it, and then retype it. Another way to edit the mistake is to place the cursor in the field. Click on the field. Use the cursor keys to go to the place of the mistake. Type the correction, and delete the extra letters with the delete key. Use the tab key to move to the next field.

Click **Staff** table in the main Access screen, and click **Open**.

Type the following data in each of the appropriate fields.

Table: Staff

200-34-2314	213-45-6789	197-56-4378
Lisa Smith	Mary Jones	Robert Kiminsky
34 Terry Blvd.	5997 Irish Place	99 Moonlight Lane
Pittsburgh	Bethel Park	Forest Hills

PA 15267	PA 15102	PA 15343
412-675-3333	412-833-7659	412-635-3557
PT	4W	6S
412-33-5690	235-34-5612	212-45-4556
Pat Holmes	Jan Wish	Anna Quinn
45 White St.	7886 Center Ave.	912 Modern St.
Carnegie	Greentree	Moon City
PA 15106	PA 15106	PA 15111
412-276-1122	412-355-5195	412-567-3227
4W	OR	ER

Click the **Printer** 🖶 button on the toolbar to print a copy of this data.

After entering the data, click the **Close** ✖ button for that dialog window.

Select **Table:Insur**, and repeat the process to enter the data for the Insurance Table. Remember to provide a print of this data too, and close this window.

Table: Insur

200-34-2314	213-45-6789	197-56-4378
Allstate	Statewide	Mutual Care Provider
A20034231	2345612	M197564378
1,000,000	500,000	2,000,000
2/12/06	6/20/06	4/10/06
412-33-5690	235-34-5612	212-45-4556
Statewide	Fireman's	Statewide
4562340	F345612	8976002
1,000,000	500,000	1,000,000
10/1/05	12/5/05	11/18/05

5. Edit records.

   Add another record to the Staff table.

   Double click on **Staff** table to open it.

   Click on the down arrow of the **New Object: Autoform** 🗗▾ button. Select **Autoform**.

   Click the **New Record** ▶✱ button.

   Type the following data: 168.33-1700, Mains, John, 123 Irish Place, Whitefish, PA, 15261, 724-333-1234, ER.

   Click the **Close** button. Click **Yes**. Click **OK**. Close the **Staff** table.

   Change the contents of one record.

   Open the **Staff** table.

Highlight **333-1234** in the phone number field of the John Mains record.

Type **345-1234**, and click the **Close** button. The change is automatically saved.

Delete a record.

If necessary, open **Table:Staff**.

Click the **Record selector** for Mains record (Figure 8.4).

Press the **Delete** key, and click **Yes** to confirm the deletion of this record.

Click the **Close** button to close the table. You should now have six records in the table.

6. Close Access.

Click the **Close** button to close the application.

Remember to remove your disk.

Exercise 2: Create Search, Sort, and Generate Report
Objectives

1. Search (Query) the database using one table, two tables, all fields, and selected fields.
2. Sort the database.
3. Prepare and print a report.

Activity

1. Preliminaries.

Start **Access**. Place your **Diskette into Drive A**.

Open the **Staff Insurance** database. Make sure that you change the Look in to the A drive.

2. Search.

You are now ready to search. First we want to know the answer to the question, "Do any of the staff have an insurance policy with Statewide?" If yes, how many?

Basic Search.

Click **Queries**. Click the **New** button. Select **Design View**, and click **OK**.

Select **Table:Insur**. Click the **Add** button, and click the **Close** button.

The query design screen appears (Figure 8.6).

Adjust windows so all fields in the Insur table display. Refer to Chapter 3 if you do not remember how to size windows.

Double click **each field** listed in the Table:Insur to display the field in the query table.

Type **Statewide** in the cell that is the intersection for carrier and criteria.

Click the **Run** ⚡ button.

Click the **Printer** 🖨 button on the toolbar to print a copy of this query.

Do any of the staff use Statewide as their insurance carrier? _____ If so, how many staff use Statewide as their insurance carrier? _____ Hint: You should have three records. If you do not, check your query table to make sure that it is correct. Then check your data in the tables to make sure your data are correct. This was an example of a simple search displaying all of the fields from a single table.

Click the **Close** button for the query window.

Click **No** to not save this query.

Search all records but selected fields.

Click **Queries**. Click the **New** button. Select **Design View**, and click **OK.**

Select **Table:Staff**. Click the **Add** button, and click the **Close** button.

Adjust windows so all fields in the Staff table display.

Double click **Social Security Number, Last_Name, First_Name, and Dept** fields listed in the Table:Staff to display the field in the query table.

Click the **Run** button.

Click the **Printer** button on the toolbar to print a copy of this query.

Click the **Close** button for the query window.

Click **No** to not save this query.

Do a more complex search on two tables.

This query is "What staff have liability policies due to expire in October, November, or December, 2005?" Based on the query results, a reminder to renew and provide current information on their policies can be sent.

Click **Queries**. Click the **New** button. Select **Design View**, and click **OK.**

Select **Table:Insur**. click the **Add** button.

Select **Table:Staff**. Click the **Add** button, and click the **Close** button.

Adjust windows so that all fields in the **Staff** table are displayed.

Double click **Social Security Number, Last_Name, First_Name, and Dept** fields listed in the **Staff** table to display the field in the query table.

Double click the **Exp_Date** field of the Insur Table.

Type **>=10/1/05 AND <1/1/06** in the cell of the intersection of Criteria and Exp_Date field.

Click the **Run** button.

Click the **Printer** button on the toolbar to print a copy of this query.

How many have insurance policies that are about to expire? (You should have three.)

What departments are they in?

Click the **Close** button for the query window.

Click **Yes** to save this query. Type **Query:expdate**. Press **Enter**, or click **OK.**

3. Sort the data.

Sometimes you want to place the records in a different order from that in which they are displayed.

Open the **Table:Staff**.

Click the **Last_Name column** heading. That is, click over the words Last-Name. The total column is now highlighted.

Click the **Sort Ascending** ![Sort Ascending icon] button.

Click the **Printer** button on the toolbar to print a copy of the data in this order.

Click the **Close** button of the table window.

Click **No** to not save the sort changes.

4. Find a specific record.

To find a specific record for the purpose of checking some information in it.
Open the **Table:Staff**.

Click in the City field. The field column does not need to be highlighted.

Click the **Find** ![Find icon] button.

Type **Carnegie** in the Find What box.

Select **All** in Search option, and select a **Whole Field** in the Match option.

Click **Find Next** twice, and click **OK** to the prompt for no more records found.

Click the **Close** button in the Find window.

To find a record to update it.
Click in the **Last_Name** field. The field column does not need to be highlighted.

Click the **Find** ![Find icon] button.

Type **Smith** in the Find What box.

Select **All** in Search option, and select a **Whole Field** in the Match option.

Click **Find Next**, and click the **Close** button to close the find window.

Press the **Tab** key until you are at the phone number field.

Highlight the **3333**, and type **1234**. Click the **Close** button.

5. Generate reports.

Select **Queries**.

Highlight the **Query:expdate**.

Click the the **New Object** ![New Object icon] button down arrow.

Select **AutoReport**.

What is wrong with this report? Hint: Look at the location of the date.

Click the **View** ![View icon] button down arrow. Select **Design View**.

Click the **Date place holder** (the second box labeled exp date), and then click the **Left** justify button. Click the **Label** ![Label icon] button on the toolbox bar. Click in the

Prepared by Nancy Nurse

Social Security Number	412-33-5690
Last Name	Holmes
First Name	Pat
Dept	4W
Exp Date	10/1/2004
Social Security Number	235-34-5612
Last Name	Wish
First Name	Jan
Dept	OR
Exp Date	12/5/2004
Social Security Number	212-45-4556
Last Name	Quinn
First Name	Anna
Dept	ER
Exp Date	11/18/2004

Figure 8.8

Completed Staff
Report

Page Header band, and type **Prepared by Your Name**. If the toolbox bar is not displayed, you may either click the toolbox button or select View from the menu and click **Toolbox**. Figure 8.8 shows you what the report should look like when you have added your heading.

Click the **Close** button and **Yes** to save it. Type **Query:expdate**, and click **OK**. If prompted to replace the Query:expdate report, click Yes.

Click the **Report** tab. Highlight **Query:expdate**, and click the **Preview** button.

Close the **Report Preview** window.

6. Using the Table Wizard.

Click **Tables**.

Select the **Table:Staff** table.

Click the **New Object** down arrow button. Choose **Report**.

Select **Report Wizard**, and click **OK**.

Click the >> button to place all of the fields in the Report window.

Click **Next**. Select **Dept field**. Click >, and click **Next**, **Next**.

Select **Block** and **Landscape**. Make sure to adjust the field width to fit.

Click **Next**. Select **Corporate**. Click **Next**.

Type **Staff Report**, and click **Finish**.

Click the **Printer** button. Click the **Close** button, and click window **Close** button. Exit **Access**.

Exercise 3: Design a Small Clinical Database
Objectives
1. Design a record structure to use in generating a reminder or work list for caring for a group of patients.
2. Enter data for 10 patients.
3. Print a report.

Activity
1. Complete the table designed in #2 below by adding at least five additional rows with appropriate data for a patient record to provide the information that you would need to provide patient care. Consult a reminder sheet, worksheets, and patient plans or progress notes from your clinical facility for ideas of data to include.
2.

Field Name	Field Type	Field Size	Description Data
Last Name	Text	20	Patient last name
First Name	Text	15	Patient first name
Room Number	Number	4	Four-digit room number
Gender	Text	1	F or M for female or male
Primary Dx	Text	25	Main reason for hospitalization
Secondary Dx	Text	25	Secondary reason for hospitalization, if any

3. Enter the data for eight patients.
4. What problems did you encounter?
5. Save the data.
6. Search for an individual patient.
7. Search for all patients with a specific diagnosis.
8. Add two more records.
9. Generate a work list or reminder sheet for a group of patients.

Assignment 1: Clinical Experience Database
Directions
1. Construct a table structure(s) to use for monitoring your clinical experiences. Use a table similar to the one in the previous exercise that identifies the fields, data type, and field size.

2. At the bottom of your table(s) (or on the back), explain the rationale behind the table(s). What questions were you trying to answer? What experiences were you trying to monitor?

3. Open Access, and create the table(s). Then enter records for 10 of your experiences. Provide a printout of the table structure as created and the data in the table.

4. Conduct a search to answer one of your questions. Print the results.

Assignment 2: Data Classification, Taxonomy, and Data Sets
Directions

1. Read two references on the Nursing Minimum Data Set or any other Clinical Minimum Data Set.

2. Answer these questions.

Questions

1. Define classification systems, taxonomies, and data sets. Review an article or two about one of these listed here. You can use the following:

International Classification of Diseases, 10th Clinical Modification (ICD-10 CM)

The Physicians' Current Procedural Terminology (CPT-4)

Diagnostic and Statistical Manual of Mental Disorders (DSM-IV)

Systematized Nomenclature of Pathology (SNOP)

Systematized Nomenclature of Medicine (SNOMED)

Nursing Intervention Classifications (NIC) (McCloskey and Bulechek)

International Classification of Nursing Practice (ICNP) (working paper on international classification)

Home Health Care Classification (HHCC) (Saba)

North American Nursing Diagnosis Association (NANDA)

Omaha Visiting Nurses Association System

Nursing Minimum Data Set (NMDS) (Werley)

Nursing Lexicon (Grobe)

2. What are the major advantages/disadvantages of doing this type of work?

3. What are the database and automation implications of this work?

4. Design the table structure(s) using elements from any of these.

Using the World Wide Web

OBJECTIVES

1. Describe the Internet and the World Wide Web.
2. Define related Internet terms.
3. Describe the meaning of the components of World Wide Web addressing.
4. Identify the hardware and software that are needed to connect to the Internet.
5. Use browsers to explore the World Wide Web.
6. Download various files from the Internet.
7. Evaluate and create web pages.

This chapter focuses on the fastest growing use for a computer—accessing the Internet. Computer users access the Internet for the purpose of communicating with others, obtaining information and files, and purchasing products. A brief definition and description of the Internet and a discussion of the World Wide Web begin this chapter. This is followed by a discussion of the services that are available on the Internet, connecting to the Internet, browsing for and locating information, using search engines, and downloading files. A brief discussion of creating web pages is also included. Additional information on Internet communication (e-mail, newsgroups, list services, etc.) and informational resources (searching and search strategies) is included in Chapters 10 and 11, respectively.

► 9.1 THE INTERNET

The Internet, sometimes referred to as the information or global superhighway, is a loose association of thousands of networks and millions of computers around the world that all work together to share information. It is a true global network providing people with quick access to information from all over the world.

No one source foots the bill for the Internet. Everyone pays for his or her part. For example, colleges and universities pay for their connection to some regional network. This regional network in turn pays a national provider for access. Many institutions and companies donate their computer resources in the form of servers and computer technicians to hold up some part of the Internet. Other companies own and operate components of the Internet in the form of communication lines and related switching equipment. The main lines that carry the bulk of the traffic are collectively known as the Internet backbone. In the United States, these were called network access points (NAPs), each owned by a different company, and metropolitan access exchanges (MAEs). These designations are changing and in many parts of the world are now referred to as Internet Exchange Points or IXPs. Some of the major players are MCI, Sprint, and WorldCom. These companies sell access to Internet service providers (ISPs), organizations, and other large businesses.

By connecting to each other, these networks create high-speed communication lines that crisscross the United States. These high-speed communication lines also extend to Europe, Great Britain, Australia, Japan, Asia, and the rest of the world. However, all points along the route may not be as well developed as the network in the United States and some other countries. In the United States, the backbone has many intersecting points. If one point fails or slows, data are quickly rerouted over another part. This redundancy was one of the key points in its development. In some parts of the world, the network may have less redundancy, making it more vulnerable to slowdowns or breakdowns.

Although no one entity owns or controls the Internet, a handful of organizations are influential in its development and maintenance. Here are a few of them.

- The Internet Society (ISOC) is a supervisory organization that is made up of individuals, corporations, nonprofit organizations, and government agencies from the Internet community. It holds the ultimate authority for the direction of the Internet and provides a home for several organizations that deal with Internet issues and standards (http://www.isoc. org).

- The Internet Architecture Board (IAB) is responsible for defining the overall architecture of the Internet (the backbone) and all of the networks attached to it. It approves standards and the allocation of resources like Internet addresses (http://iab.org).

- The Internet Engineering Task Force (IETF) focuses on operational and technical issues related to keeping the Internet running smoothly as a whole (http://www.ietf.org).

- The World Wide Web Consortium (W3C) works with the standards for HyperText Mark-up Language (HTML), other related web standards for SHTML, SML, and CSS, and other specifics as they relate to the web part of the Internet. They promote interoperability for the web (http://www.w3.org).

- Backbone ISPs, cable and satellite companies, regional and long-distance phone companies, and various agencies of the United States and other countries' governments contribute to the Internet telecommunications infrastructure.

- The Internet Assignment Numbers Authority (IANA) and the Internet Network Information Center (InterNIC) are the two organizations responsible for assigning IP addresses and domain names, respectively (http://www.iana.org and http://www.internic.org).

A network communications protocol called Transmission Control Protocol/Internet Protocol (TCP/IP) is what makes all of this work. This is a communications protocol that is the basis for computers talking to each other over the Internet. Every computer on the Internet must use and understand this protocol for sending and receiving data. This protocol uses what is called a packet-switched network that minimizes the chance of losing data sent over the transmission medium. The TCP part of the protocol breaks every piece of data into small chunks called packets. Each packet is wrapped in an electronic envelope that contains the web addresses for both the sender and the recipient. Once the packets are created, the IP protocol determines the best route for getting the packet from one point to another point. Each packet may arrive at its destination by a different route. Routers examine the destination address and then send the packet to another router until it finally reaches its destination. The router sends the packet by the best route available at that time. When the packet arrives at its destination, TCP takes over. Its function is to identify each packet, to make sure that it is intact, and to reassemble the packets into the original data.

▶ 9.2 SERVICES ON THE INTERNET

Many services are available on the Internet. Most people, when using the term Internet, use it to mean the World Wide Web. The web is just one part of the Internet, albeit the fastest growing one. Basically, the services available can be placed into three categories: electronic communications, information services, and information retrieval.

Electronic Communications	These services permit the users to communicate with other people on the Internet via electronic mail, bulletin boards, chat rooms, instant messages, list services (listservs), and news groups. These are discussed in Chapter 10.
Information Services	Information services are commonly referred to as remote login, or information access. These services permit users to log in to other computers from their computers for the purpose of obtaining information. The two main services in this area are telnet (used by many librarians) and the web (used by all).
Information Retrieval	These services permit users to obtain files from other sites and bring them to their computers. This is commonly referred to as file transfer. File transfer protocol (ftp) is the most commonly used protocol for transferring files from one computer to another. Since the development of the web, the interface for transferring files has become more user friendly and not command driven.

One thing that is happening regarding services on the Internet is that all of them are becoming easier to use. For example, when transferring a file, the user does not need to know all of the earlier commands for downloading files or for activating ftp. Most of the time, it is a matter of clicking on a download hyperlink and responding to prompts. Graphics may even be downloaded by right clicking on the graphic and selecting save target as from the shortcut menu. The user is isolated from the background commands necessary to use these services.

Another trend regarding services on the Internet is the closing of some sites that use other protocols such as telnet and gopher as the web part continues to grow. Telnet sites permitted the user to log in to a computer at another site for the purpose of accessing its information. Many of these sites permitted anyone to use them. Librarians continue to use telenet services, but most of the general public does not. Gopher sites were hierarchically based menus for accessing information available on the Internet. The user selected from the menu and a submenu until the information was found. Now the web and search sites make it easier to find and access this information by using search engines, directories, and hyperlinks. The services, once provided by telnet and gopher sites, are now being replaced by websites and searching facilities.

► 9.3 WORLD WIDE WEB

Some consider the World Wide Web (WWW) the easiest of the Internet services to use. This part of the Internet is the graphical portion that stores electronic files, called web pages, on servers that are accessed from a computer. Keywords in a document are highlighted. Selecting a keyword takes the reader to another part of that document related to that word, to another document at that site, or to another site. In addition, some graphics and buttons are also hyperlinked, permitting the user to go to different sites or to obtain more information at this site.

Presented here are some of the terms related to the World Wide Web.

Client-server   The client is the web browser software that knows how to communicate with a web server. A personal computer is the client. The server is the remote computer that stores the web page files and communicates with the client. The user's computer communicates with the server.

Hyperlinks   Hyperlinks are text or graphics linked to other parts of a file or to other files at the same site or other sites. When over a hyperlink, the pointer turns to a hand (🖑).

HTML   HyperText Markup Language is the tagging that is used to code the web page files so that they display on a variety of computers. Included in these tags are commands for linking text and graphics.

HTTP   HyperText Transfer Protocol is the communications protocol that is used for accessing and working with the World Wide Web. Do not confuse it with HTML.

Web Browser Software   This software is used to access web pages on the Internet and to interpret HTML code into readable form. Two of the major browsers are Internet Explorer and Netscape Navigator. Safari is the browser of choice for the Mac OS.

► 9.4 UNDERSTANDING ADDRESSING

When connecting to the Internet, the computer is identified by a unique address. This address allows the computer to access information from a web server and in turn have other computers send information to it. Although humans like words and graphics to communicate, computers prefer using numbers.

This section discusses the IP address, Domain Name, and uniform resource locator (URL), which are all terms used to locate and differentiate one computer and its files from all other computers and files on the Internet.

IP Address

The IP or Internet Protocol number is a unique identification number for each computer on the Internet. To communicate effectively, no two computers can have the same number at the same time. A computer may be assigned a fixed or static address or a dynamic address that changes each time the user accesses the Internet.

The IP address uses a number from 0 to 255 for each part of its four-part number. This number may be something like 208.34.242.17. Because the number of computers is fast approaching the 4.2 billion possible addresses for the IP system, work is proceeding on finding alternative numbering systems that do not require major hardware or software changes.

Domain Name

A domain name is an address, similar to that used by the postal service, that points to a computer with a specific IP address. It is a description of a computer's location on the Internet. Domain names create a single identity for a series of computers used by a company. A special Domain Naming System (DNS) computer looks up the name and matches it with its assigned number. One needs to remember that computers like numbers, whereas people prefer names. Examples of domain names are www.adobe.com or intranet.school.edu.

The domain name contains a few components, separated by a period (Figure 9.1). On the left is the more specific name for the computer; to the right is the category that describes the nature of the organization. The first item is the name of the host itself (www or intranet). The next item is the second level domain name (adobe or school). An organization or entity like INTERnet Network Information Center (InterNIC) registration services registers the domain name. This is the part of the domain name that is registered. The last item (com and edu) is the top-level domain name and describes the purpose of the organization or entity that owns the second-level name.

Here are a few of the common top-level domain names. For a more complete listing and description, consult http://www.iana.org/gtld/gtld.htm. Additional top-level domain names are always being proposed.

aero   Air transportation industry
com   Business or other commercial enterprises
edu   Postsecondary institutions

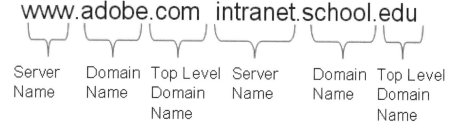

Figure 9.1
Domain Name
Scheme

gov   Government agency or departments

mil   Military

net   Network service provider or resource

org   Organizations, usually nonprofit or charitable

pro   Professionals or other licensed people

These are all United States top-level domain names. There are also country top-level domain names such as .ca for Canada and .nz for New Zealand.

A domain may also contain other components between the host (web server) and second-level domain; these are called subdomains. Subdomain names are used by large organizations that support many Internet servers. For example, the US government and its many agencies differentiate one agency from another through use of the subdomains. An educational institution may have subdomains for each school or department. For example, there might be one like this www.nursing.school.edu where nursing represents the nursing school or department's web server (www). Also, other countries sometimes do this: Virginia.co.uk where co is the equivalent of .com and uk represents the United Kingdom.

Anyone can register with the InterNIC for a second-level domain name. However, there is a fee for having one's own second-level domain name. To see who owns specific domain names, go to http://www.internic.net/whois. html. Some enterprising people have registered a variety of names of big corporations and now make money selling the rights to these second level domain names to those organizations.

Understanding the domain names will help to identify the type of information likely to be obtained from a certain site. Knowing that the site is a government agency, such as the IRS (http://www.irs.gov), means that the forms and their instructions provided there are legitimate. Obtaining health information from the National Library of Medicine (http://www.nlm.nih. gov) or Centers for Disease Control and Prevention (http://www.cdc.gov) means that the site is probably providing accurate and reliable information. However, information from someone's personal home page may or may not be accurate or reliable.

URLs

URLs help a computer locate a web page's exact location on the web server. Although IP addresses and domain names locate the computer, they do not

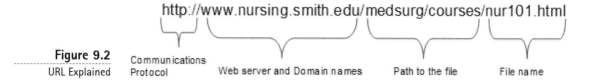

Figure 9.2
URL Explained

locate the web documents on the server. The URL helps the computer find the actual web pages (see Figure 9.2 for an example).

In this example, http://www.nursing.smith.edu/medsurg/courses/nur101.html, the first part, http://, identifies the communications protocol that the computers are using to communicate with each other. Other examples are ftp and telnet.

The second part, www.nursing.smith.edu, is the web server or host computer where the page is located. Remember that the first part of this address describes the local host site, and the second part describes the domain name that is registered to that institution. The institution can decide how it wants to set up its local host. For example, the local host might be www or www.healthschools or www.dept.

The third part, /medsurg/courses/, tells the server where the file is found. The slashes represent folders, just like those on a user's computer. This provides the computer with the information about the location of a web page file.

The last part, nur101.html, is the actual filename for the browser to display. Most of the time it will be an HTML or HTM file. HTML files are static web pages in which the content is created at the time the page is created. With increasing frequency, a web page may be dynamic, meaning that it is interactive. It can accept and retrieve information from and for a user. These web pages generally require some form of HTML and either a program or script. Programs and scripts are instructions that tell the computer how to perform a task. Examples of these programs and scripts include CGI (common gateway interface), ASP (active server pages), and Java applets.

Most of the URLs start with http:// because most users are accessing the World Wide Web. Remember that when typing these URLs in the location or address box, there are no spaces between the parts; they always use forward slashes, and they must be typed exactly as given. If a one (1) is typed for a lower case L (1), the computer will not be able to find the site and will return an error message. If the URL is in an electronic form, highlight the

URL, and use the copy and paste feature to place it in the Address or Location text box to avoid typing errors.

▶ 9.5 CONNECTING TO THE INTERNET

This section provides a brief outline of the equipment and software that are needed to access the Internet. What determines the equipment needed to access the Internet depends on what services are desired. For example, using the web and accessing multimedia files require a higher level computer than accessing a text-based e-mail program on a Unix computer. In addition, software is needed for each type of service accessed. To make things easier software-wise, most ISPs and browser programs now come with many features bundled into one easy-to-install program.

As discussed previously, the computer will need an IP address and a host domain name. The university or service provider assigns these to the computer. The IP address might be fixed, meaning that it needs to be configured with the software; if it is dynamic, the IP address is assigned by the ISP each time the computer connects to the Internet. This IP address is only good for the current Internet session. Most places require the user to obtain a user ID and password for signing onto the Internet. The user ID and password may be chosen by the user or assigned by the institution using their user naming standards. For example, some institutions use the user's last name, first letter of first name, and middle initial; others use last name, first letter of first name, and a number. Thus, a user name might be joosir or joosil. Many ISPs let the user choose his or her own ID as long as someone else on the system does not have that ID. The ID could then be ngtcrawler, nurseJane, or hojo. What is important is that each user on that system must be uniquely identified in the system. No two users can have the same user ID. Some ISPs and institutions handle this by assigning numbers to the end, and thus, ngtcrawler becomes ngtcrawler2, and nurseJane becomes nurseJane2.

Although the user ID is public knowledge, the password is private. Passwords should be safeguarded like a PIN from an ATM account. They should not be given to anyone or written where others can see them. In addition, each system has criteria for what are acceptable passwords. For example, many systems require a minimum number of characters and a combination of letters and numbers. Thus, the password might be bri8ll. Dictionary words and common knowledge words such as a spouses name or pet's name should not be used. These are too easy for someone to break. Use nonsense combinations that make sense to you. An example might be gcle95 where g = green, cle = camry le, and 95 = year of the car.

Computer

Although the computer requirements are not very demanding for accessing the Internet, the computer must have sufficient RAM, a fast processor, and free hard drive space. To use the web and take advantage of its graphics capabilities, use a computer that has been manufactured in the last 3 years. At the least, it needs to run Windows 98 or Macintosh OS 8. The operating system then dictates some of the hardware specifications. Today, Windows 98 is the minimum to consider for accessing the Internet, whereas Windows XP and its variations are desired. For the MacOS, 10.3 is the desired operating system. For the processor, a Pentium level with 500 MHz speed is minimal, whereas computers running in the gigahertz range are ideal. Remember that hardware requirements change rapidly as expectations and demands grow, and thus, chances are great that most users will own several computers in their lifetime. The level of the computer really depends on what the user wants to do on the Internet. If one expects full multimedia information to appear on the computer instantly, he or she will need a higher level computer with higher speed connections and full multimedia capabilities—sound cards, speakers, and good graphics. If the expectation is to use primarily e-mail, a basic computer will do.

Network Connection

From home, the computer needs to have a connection to the host computer. This is generally accomplished through a phone line, a DSL (Digital Subscriber Line) line, or a TV cable connection. When connecting on campus through a dorm or office, the connection is done through the campus network connections.

Modem
A modem is used to provide an interface between the computer and the transmission channel for converting the data into a form that can be transmitted via the selected transmission line. At home, this can be a dial-up modem, a DSL modem, or a cable modem. Dial-up modems are still in high use in many parts of the country because of the costs and unavailability of other

types of connectivity. They are the slowest means of connecting, and they tie up the phone line; however, they are readily available and are relatively inexpensive.

DSL modems provide connectivity by using the digital portion of the regular copper telephone line. This is faster than a dial-up connection, does not tie up the phone line, is a little more expensive, and is always "on." The downside is the lack of availability in many areas, and security issues exist because the computer is always connected.

The cable modem is designed to work with a cable TV line and is specified by the cable provider. It provides faster access to the Internet than traditional phone modems and DSL. A cable modem typically has two connections, one to the cable wall outlet and the other to the computer via an Ethernet card. Costs vary greatly depending on location and cable provider; speed fluctuates based on how many people are sharing the bandwidth at the same time. Security issues exist with cable as well.

Wireless Card

A wireless card is used to provide connectivity via mobile computers. It converts the data into radio signals. It can be very fast and may be available in areas not serviced by cable or DSL. The downside is that the device must be within a 10- to 20-mile radius of an access point. The number of wireless access points is increasing daily.

Network Card

This is a card installed into a computer that enables a direct connection to the network. This is the typical connection from college dormitories, laboratories, and offices. This type of connection does not need a modem but requires a special cable and an active network port.

In any case, the user needs to use one of these devices to move the data from the computer to the access provider.

Access Providers

Access providers are organizations that provide access to an Internet host computer. These access providers often supply the software needed to connect to the Internet. There are several different types of access providers, as outlined later. Users need to choose the type of access that is appropriate for them.

ISPs

Two types of ISPs are (1) online providers who provide access to a variety of special services and databases as well as the Internet and e-mail and (2) ISPs who provide access to the Internet and e-mail but no other special services or databases. Two examples of this first group are America Online and Microsoft Network. Two examples of the second group are EarthLink (merged with MindSpring) and AT&T Worldnet. In addition, Comcast (cable) and Verizon (DSL) also serve as ISP providers.

When selecting an ISP, consider the following points:

- Is there a flat rate that covers all connecting time, or is the price per hour? Is there a setup fee?
- What is used to connect to the Internet—T1 or T3 lines?
- Is the connectivity fast and reliable at ALL times of the day? In other words, what is the ratio of subscribers to bandwidth?
- Is there reliable and responsive technical support?
- Is there space on the server for personal home pages?
- Do they provide all of the desirable services such as e-mail, instant messaging, web and related multimedia files, ftp, newsreader, and telnet?
- What is the maximum size for file attachments and for the e-mail account?
- What is available for privacy and security? Do they offer a firewall? Parental controls? Free virus protection?
- For dial-up connections, are there local access phone numbers or 1-800 numbers with national access?
- Do they offer only dial-up, or do they also include broadband connectivity?
- Do they provide backup services to store personal data?

Free-net access

These can be community-based computer networks designed to help the local citizens access and share information and resources, or they can be free ISPs that make their money from paid sponsors or advertisers. Funding to support community-based access is generally done through local libraries, government funds, and interested local businesses. Some areas offer free net access through the local libraries and other types of organizations; others charge a small fee for access. This type of service is generally restricted to people who live in the community or meet specific criteria. Many of these networks rely on a group of volunteers to assist in developing and maintaining the system.

The free ISPs such as United Online (formerly NetZero and Juno) provide 10 hours of free access per month (most of them no longer provide unlimited access). If the user wants more, he or she can sign up for a fee. The tradeoff here is advertising and a lack of privacy. Some of these services require the completion of lengthy forms that are then used to market products to the user or to sell the information to marketing companies.

Company or Institutional Access

This type of access is provided to an employee or student in an institution. Access is then provided through the organization's computer and connection facilities. A user installs and uses the software provided by the company for dialing into the computer at the company or institution. Once connected to the company's computer, the user now has access to all of the capabilities provided by the company, including Internet access. An advantage to this type of access is that the user generally makes a local phone call with no monthly Internet access fees. Disadvantages are that the user must remain an employee or student, and he or she is subjected to the policies of that organization or institution (acceptable user policies).

Software

The software needed to access the Internet depends on how it is being accessed and who provides the connection service. Communication protocols that coordinate data transfer to and from the local computer and the Internet (like TCP/IP) and protocols for the various services (such as e-mail, web, and ftp) are needed. If access comes through a university or corporate network, often special software is needed. This software is generally obtained from the company and works behind the scenes once installed. Most Information Technology (IT) departments provide easy-to-use instructions for installing the program.

The Internet front-end software is the software with which the user interacts. This might be a comprehensive program, such as Netscape or

Internet Explorer, or one provided by the service provider. Most of the time this software is provided free of charge when becoming a subscriber (AOL), is available for free downloading (Netscape), or is available as part of the operating system (Internet Explorer).

► 9.6 USING WEB BROWSERS

Once connected, the user can start using the web. A web browser is the software program that is used to display web pages on the World Wide Web. Although many different browsers are available, the two most commonly used are Microsoft Internet Explorer and Netscape Navigator. Both are based on an earlier browser called Mosaic, which was the first browser that accessed the graphical portion of the Internet. Both browsers are available for Windows and Macintosh systems. However, slight differences exist in the two versions of each browser. Learning the basics of using a browser should not take long.

Although much competition exists between these two browsers, they are very similar in how the user interacts with them. Both are available for free from each company's website (Internet Explorer from http://www.microsoft.com/windows/ie and Netscape Navigator from http://www.netscape.com). Safari is bundled with any Apple computer. The main elements of web browsers follow the conventions for all windows programs. For example, they both have a title bar, a menu bar, a toolbar, scroll bars, and status bars. Discussed next are the toolbars for both Internet Explorer and Netscape Navigator.

Because browsers, like most software, are constantly being revised, occasionally check the version of the browser, and update it as needed. To check for the current version, open the **browser**. Select **Help** from the menu bar, and select **About browser name**. The version number is displayed. To update the version, the user can go to each website and select the update. Sometimes there are options to set the browser settings to check for updates automatically. For example, Internet Explorer will automatically check for updates if this setting is turned on (**Tools**, **Internet Options**, **Advanced tab**, and click to **Automatically check for updates**). With each new version, more capabilities are built into the browser for using the web. The basic functions, however, remain constant: the ability to use the back, forward, stop, search, print, and home buttons.

Orientation to Internet Explorer and Netscape Navigator

Because the toolbars for both are more similar than dissimilar, this discussion presents both.

The Toolbar

Figures 9.3 and 9.4 show the basic layout of the screen for Internet Explorer and Netscape Navigator, respectively.

Internet Explorer	Netscape Navigator	Function of the Toolbar Buttons
		The Back button retrieves the last page viewed this session. It permits retracing steps backward one web page at a time.
		The Forward button retrieves the previous page viewed this session. It allows retracing steps forward one web page at a time. It is only active once the Back button is used.

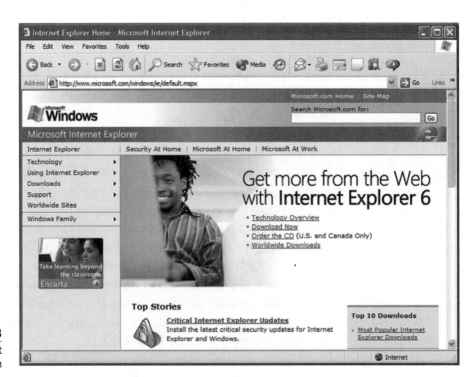

Figure 9.3
Microsoft Internet Explorer Main Screen

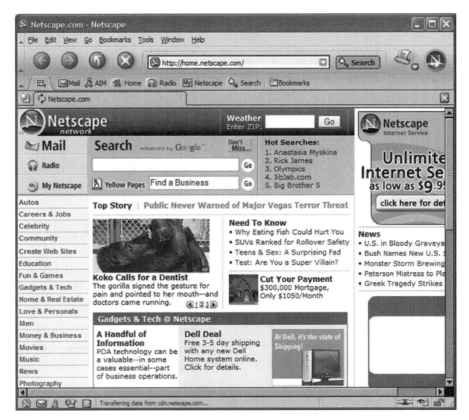

Figure 9.4
Netscape Navigator
Main Screen

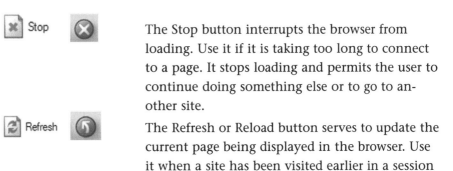

The Stop button interrupts the browser from loading. Use it if it is taking too long to connect to a page. It stops loading and permits the user to continue doing something else or to go to another site.

The Refresh or Reload button serves to update the current page being displayed in the browser. Use it when a site has been visited earlier in a session and the contents change frequently. For example, a stock or sports page needs to be refreshed often.

The Home button retrieves the page displayed when the browser opens. This is called your home page. Use it to return to that page. Do not confuse it with the term *home page*, that is, the main page of a host's site.

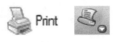 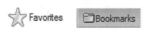

The Print button prints the current web page or frame. In Explorer, one copy of the current page is sent to the default printer. In Netscape, the print dialog window appears. Select the appropriate printer settings from the printer dialog box, and press OK.

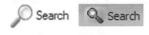

The Search button accesses a search engine to permit searching for information on web sites.

The Favorites and Bookmarks buttons (located below the standard toolbar) allow one to mark favorite places so that they can be accessed quickly and easily later. The URL does not even need to be remembered; just select the favorite site or bookmark from the menu and click.

The History button permits revisiting sites from previous sessions. These sites stay in the history folder for a set number of days. To access this in Netscape, choose **Go**, **History**, or **Ctrl + H**. There is no button for it on the standard toolbar, although it can be added to the My Sidebar area.

Starting the browser

Remember from Chapter 4 that there are several ways to start programs. To start the browser, double click the **Browser** icon. If the browser is not on the desktop, click the **Internet Explorer** or **Netscape Navigator** option on the Quick Launch area of the taskbar. If that option is not available, use the **Start** button and **All programs** to find the browser. When the browser starts, a specific home page opens. This page might be the institution's or the browser's. The user has the ability to change this home page by using the Set Preferences feature that is found in both browsers.

▶ **To change the home page in Internet Explorer:**

Select **Tools**, **Internet Options** from the menu bar.

Make sure that the **General Tab** is selected.

If it is not selected, select the text in the **Address** text box of the home page options section of the window.

Type the new **URL**, and press **Enter**.

Click **OK** to close the Internet Options dialog box.

▶ **To change the home page in Netscape Navigator:**

Select **Edit**, **Preferences**.

Select the text in the **Location** text box of the home page section of the window.

Type the new **URL**, and click **OK**.

Now when the browser starts, it will point to the new home page. This is also the process that is used to change how long sites stay in the history folder (the Internet Options or Preferences dialog boxes).

Surfing the Net

Surfing the Net refers to clicking hyperlinks to go to another part of a document, to a different document, or to another site. To use a hyperlink, click it. Most web pages identify text hyperlinks by placing them in a different color and often by underlining them. Hyperlinks can also be identified by the changing look of the pointer. It changes to a hand (🖑) when placed over a link. Be patient because it sometimes takes time to load the web pages. Intensive graphic pages come in faster through an Ethernet connection than over a modem. Heavy traffic on the Internet also slows the loading time.

If the user has the URL for the site, the user can simply type the URL in the locator or address text box located under the standard toolbar. Most current browsers do not require typing the http:// part of the address. They automatically insert that part. The computer requires the user to be exact; thus, make sure that the address is correct.

▶ **Go to a site by typing the URL:**

Click the **Text** in the **Locator** or **Address** text box to select the text.

Type the **URL** and press **Enter**.

Click any **Hyperlink** objects or text to surf.

Using the history list

The history list keeps track of sites that have been visited over the past several days and offers a convenient means of redisplaying those pages. Unlike favorites or bookmark lists, which store page locations that the user designated, history items are saved automatically when visiting a site. Most browsers store all sites visited in this folder regardless of how the user arrived at the site. Some locator or address drop-down lists only store sites where the URL was typed.

▶ **To use the history list in Internet Explorer:**
Click the **History** (History) button.
Click the **Day of the Week** that the site was visited.
Click the **Site** and/or related **Actual pages** at the site.

▶ **To use the history list in Netscape:**
Choose **Go**, **History**. There is no button for it on the standard toolbar.
Click the **Day** that the site was visited.
Click the **Site**.

Printing a web page

Note the subtle difference between the two browsers in printing. Internet Explorer sends one copy of the current document to the default printer, but Netscape brings up the print dialog window for the user to choose a printer, select pages, and select the number of copies. When the computer prints a web page as a result of the print command, it will print both the graphics and the text.

▶ **To print a web page from Internet Explorer:**
Go to the **Web** page to be printed.
Click the **Printer** button.

▶ **To print a web page from Netscape Navigator:**
Go to the **Web** page to be printed.
Click the **Printer** button.
Make the appropriate selections in the printer dialog box, and press **Enter**.

If printing from a website with frames (the screen is divided into several sections, each with its own scroll bar), make sure that the correct frame is selected before issuing the print command; otherwise, it will print the active frame.

Saving a web page

Sometimes, users might want to save a web page because of the content or the tagging. When saving a web page, several options are available:

- **Web Page**, **Complete** saves all of the files that are needed to display the page in its original format. This includes graphics, frames, and style sheets.
- **Web Archive** saves a snapshot of the current page in a single MIME-encoded file. This option is not available in earlier versions and in some browsers.
- **Web Page**, **HTML only** saves only the code and text on the web page, not the graphics, sounds, or any other files displayed on the page but not embedded in the page.
- **Text Only** saves just the text from the current web page in straight text format, permitting it to be imported into any word processor.

▶ **To save a web page:**

Select **File**, **Save as**.

Select the **Location** and **File name**.

Select one of the options for **File type**.

Click the **Save** button.

The graphic objects are separate files. They are not embedded in the HTML file; the file points to the graphic file, which contains the image.

▶ **To save just a graphic from a web page:**

Right click the **Graphic**.

Select **Save Picture** or **Image** or **Target as**.

Select the **Location** in which to download the graphic.

Type a **File name**.

Under Save as type, select gif or jpg.

Click the **Save** button.

▶ **To copy information from a web page into a document:**

Select the information to be copied.

From the **Edit** menu, select **Copy**.

Go to the document, and click **Paste** when the cursor is at the appropriate spot.

Be very careful of copyright rules and plagiarism.

▶ **To create a desktop shortcut to a web page accessed frequently (option not available in Netscape):**

Right click somewhere in the web page (not on a graphic).

Select **Create Shortcut** from the shortcut menu, and click **OK**.

Two other saving features can be used with web pages. One is to save the file as a desktop background, and the other is to send a web page through e-mail. These features can be found on the shortcut menu.

Creating a bookmark or favorite

This is the feature that permits saving frequently visited sites. Use this feature to help organize a list of web pages so that they can be found easily later. There are basic functions needed to use this feature in all versions of both browsers. Although the exact procedure will vary, the basic function will exist in all versions of both browsers.

The basic functions are as follows:

- Adding and removing Bookmarks or Favorites from your list.
- Organizing the list of URLs into categories or folders.
- Editing and arranging the bookmarks or favorites.

A number of factors make it difficult to create bookmarks. Many laboratories provide a prescribed set of bookmarks or favorites designated by the library or the laboratory. There may be limitations to what may be changed or added to this set. In addition, users may not have access to the bookmarks and favorites when using a different computer. For these reasons, it is recommended that users create a folder on a removable storage device and not on the hard drive. The procedure for doing this is described in Exercises 1 and 2 at the end of this chapter. If using a personal computer, creating and managing bookmarks and favorites is similar to the procedure discussed in Chapter 3, "The Computer and Its Operating System Environment."

Managing Internet Files

When surfing the Internet, visited sites send temporary files to the computer. These files are stored in one of two folders located on the hard drive under Documents and Settings, User, cookies and temporary Internet folders.

Cookies

The cookie files are designed to enhance the online experience by recognizing the visitor when the visitor returns to a website and recording what was done at that site. It can remember what reservations were made the last time the visitor accessed hotels.com or a credit card number that was used to order something from LLBean.com. Although this should be harmless when one is using a personal computer, it may pose a problem when using laboratory or work computers. Cookie files usually have the name cookies.txt associated with them. Sites can only read cookie files it placed on the hard disk; they cannot read files placed by other sites.

Temporary internet files

These files are sent to the computer for the purpose of speeding the loading of graphics files when the site is visited again. The problem with these files (both cookie and temporary) is that they take up space on the hard drive and are not deleted automatically. Therefore, users must periodically delete these files. How often this needs to be done depends on how many sites have been visited. Failure to purge these files periodically could lead to a full hard drive. These files are also a record of places visited on the Internet. The user can manage these files through the browser interface or directly from the hard drive.

History files

A history file keeps track of where the user has been on the web. (Look in the user's Documents and Settings folder, Local Settings for a subfolder called History.) If anyone else uses that computer, it may be wise to delete the history folder contents. Some laboratories have the setting set to automatically delete the content of this folder when the user logs off.

▶ **To delete the cookie, temporary files, and history files through Internet Explorer:**

Open **Internet Explorer**.

Select **Tools**, **Internet Options**.

In the Temporary Internet files section, click the **Delete Cookies** and **Delete Files** buttons.

Click the **Clear History** button.

▶ **To delete cookies and history files through Netscape:**

Open **Netscape Navigator**.

Select **Tools**, **Cookie Manager**.

Click the **Remove all cookies button**.

Close that dialog box.

At the main Netscape Navigator window, select **Edit**, **Preferences**.

Click the **History** folder in the left Category area.

Click the **Clear history** and **Location bar** buttons.

▶ **To clear these files manually (which computer users do):**

Double click **My Computer** and the **Local disk (C:)** icons.

Double click the **Documents and Settings** and the correct **User** folder.

Double click the **Cookies** folder.

Highlight **All the files**.

Press the **Delete** key.

Respond **Yes** to any prompts about deleting these cookie files.

Repeat the process with the **Temporary Internet Files** and **History** folders located at documents and settings/user/local settings.

This section of the chapter presented some basic functions for working with a browser. Both Netscape Navigator and Internet Explorer were presented to demonstrate how similar the browser functions are. The next section focuses on some basics regarding evaluating quality of design and creating simple web pages.

► 9.7 SEARCH SITES (ENGINES)

The Internet contains a vast amount of information. There is no single source to index the Internet like there is for the Library of Congress, which indexes books. One should design a search of the Internet to find relevant information in an effective and efficient manner (more on this in Chapter 11). Search sites are places on the Internet where users go to find information. Search engines are software that are used to find and index information. Several hundred different search sites and engines are on the Internet. Generally, they are divided into three main categories, but differences between them are disappearing as each increases its functionality.

Directory

A directory is a hierarchical grouping of WWW links by subject and related concepts. These are created by people who searched the web and then grouped the links by subject. Therefore, they preselect the information appearing in the directory. The amount of irrelevant returns in directories is far less than in either of the other two groups. Not all search sites include directories.

These sites are great for finding information quickly when one knows little about the topic and the topic is broad or common. They are not good for obscure facts. Links to outdated or moved web pages is another problem. Yahoo and About are two popular directory sites.

Keyword Search Site

This is a server or a collection of servers dedicated to indexing Internet web pages, storing the results, and returning lists of links that match particular queries. They provide access to the largest portion of information on the Internet but many times return a lot of irrelevant information. The indexes are normally generated using spiders or bots. Sometimes the word search site and search engine are confused, but they are two different terms.

Most of these have advanced search features for narrowing the search, but still the results are large. Google and AllTheWeb are two popular keyword search sites.

Meta Search Engines

Meta search engines are not really search engines. These work by taking the user's query and searching the web using several different keyword search sites at one time. These are gaining in popularity because they permit one stop searching.

Metasearch engine sites provide a good picture of what is available because they use several different search engine sites and the information is not preselected like in directory sites. They may restrict some of the advanced search features. A few examples are Ixquick, Vivisimo, DogPile, ProFusion, and Turbio10.

Each one has a different interface or appearance, but they all have several common features. Understanding how to use search sites begins by understanding a few relevant terms.

Hits

Hits are a list of links that are returned as search results when a search engine is used.

Query

Query refers to the combination of terms that the user enters into a search engine in order to conduct a search.

Ranking

This is a process of indicating how relevant a hit may be. Many times a search engine will organize the search results by their ranking. However, the methods used by search engines to rank pages varies; thus, ranks may not always be useful.

Robot

Robots are used to create a database of links that are accessed when a user conducts a search. These are special kinds of computer programs that can search the web, locate links, and then index the links to create the database. Indexing is usually done by using the words in the URL and title of the HTML file and counting the frequency of words used at the Internet site. Some robots search the full text, whereas others review a portion of the site. Robots are also called spiders and crawlers.

Search Site Issues and the Invisible Web

Information on the Internet is being published faster than search sites can index it. They cannot keep pace with the sheer volume of information. Adding to the problem is the issue of who is publishing to the Internet. Early web pages were published by government agencies, nonprofit institutions, and educational institutions. Now more and more websites are being published by commercial companies that are trying to market or sell their products and services.

In addition, the current search engines are limited in what they can index. This is creating an area of the web now referred to as the Invisible Web (Bergman). The most comprehensive search site indexes less than 20% of the information on the Internet. In addition to the shear volume of information, other factors influence what a search site can index, such as editorial policies like family-friendly sites and news sites, databases that require typing in search strings like the CDC databases, sites that require the visitor to log in like certain parts of the Chronicle of Higher Education, pages with nothing but images, certain file types like pdf and exe, dynamically generated pages, and documents behind firewalls.

Accessing Search Sites

Using a search engine begins by accessing the search engine site on the Internet. Search engine sites can be located by clicking on the search icon in both Netscape and Internet Explorer or typing in the URL for a search site. In addition, there are portal type directory structures like the **Librarians' Index to the Internet** and clearinghouses or reference sites like **Search Enginewatch** and **Reference Desk** that provide links to the most popular search sites. Many ISPs and college/university libraries also provide links on their main pages for accessing search sites.

▶ 9.8 CREATING AND EVALUATING WEB PAGES

This section of the chapter covers some basics of web page creation as well as evaluating the design of a web page. This is not intended to make readers into web designers but to provide some pointers with which to start as well as some help on evaluating design. Material on evaluating the quality of the content of a website is covered in Chapter 11, "Information: Access, Evaluation, and Use." After visiting various websites, most users begin to appreciate a site that is well designed and develop criteria for what they find most appealing in a site's design.

Creating Web Pages

Although the first thing that most web page creators want to do is start tagging the documents, there is in fact a process for designing web pages. This process is outlined here and serves as a guide for things to consider when creating web pages. Paying attention to these items at the start saves time and energy in the long term.

- Decide what is to be accomplished with this site. Answer these questions: What is the intent of this site? What do I want to accomplish with this site? What are the purposes and goals of this site? Create a statement that reflects the answers to these questions to serve as a guide during the development and maintenance of the website.

- Identify the target audience to help focus the design and content. Many websites are created without identifying the Who. A design for teenagers may not be appropriate for professional audiences.

- Develop a site map showing the relationship between the parts. What pages will be there? How will they link or relate to others? Keep in mind that users may access these pages in varying ways and may not always start at the beginning.

- Develop criteria for inclusion of content. How will decisions be made about what content to include? What is the criterion for inclusion? Keep in mind the intent of the site and the target audience.

- Decide who will be responsible for maintaining each part of the site. Consider how often the data may need to be updated, and then determine a schedule for reviewing and updating the parts.

- Decide on a design that best presents the content. A consistent look to the site helps keep the user oriented as to place. Some things to consider are placing navigational aids consistently in the same place on each page identifying the who, what, when, and where of the content. Make these navigational aids, such as buttons, easy and clear to follow. Set these standards at the start, and then use them.

Once these guidelines are addressed, some specific things should be considered regarding design and layout. Although these points serve as a guide, good design is a matter of a person's own personal taste and style, not someone else's. Good design also keeps in mind the intent of the site and the target audience.

- Use common sense. Remember that many people access the Internet through dial-up modems and not the faster Ethernet, cable, or DSL connections. Graphics take longer to load than text, and the audience will be lost if they have to wait too long for the graphics. Use the 10-second rule; that is, the page should load from many different types of connections in 10 seconds. Also, consider that not everyone will be using the latest technology, and thus, many may not have the latest version of a browser or the same size of monitor used during the design. When in doubt about design, keep it simple.

- Design a template or layout to use with most of the pages. This means to make sure that each page has a descriptive title located in the same place on all pages, buttons and navigational aids to take the user back to the original site home page and to other pages at this site, and identifying information such as who created the page, when it was created or last revised, and how to contact the webmaster with questions. Many pages also include information about copyright.

- Use graphics and sound as appropriate. The graphics and sounds should add something to the content, not detract from it. Just because it is possible to place many graphics on the page, do not do so unless the graphics help convey the message of the page. Keep in mind the rules "simple is better" and "white space is good." Consider that many users find graphics and sound distracting. Other users may access the page in settings where sound is distracting to others. Pay attention to copyright requirements, especially when using graphics created by others.

- Keep graphics reasonable in size. Try to maintain a balance between size, resolution, color, and look. That means to try and keep the size between

25K and 30K with a resolution of 72 dpi. Use the appropriate graphic file format—gif files for images and jpg for photos. Use thumbnail graphics (small postage-sized pictures), and give the user the option to look at the graphic in a larger version. Keep in mind that what most users see when the page loads is the first 4 inches of a printed page.

• Select colors carefully. Make sure that the colors work together and are easy to read or are pleasing on the eyes. If the designer lacks color sense, have someone else design the color scheme or use an already developed color scheme. Be especially careful of colors if users will be printing the web pages.

HTML Files

Once the documents are designed in terms of layout and content, the documents need to be coded or tagged. The concept of HTML exists to provide a mechanism for displaying text and graphics based documents in web browsers. It describes the contents of a web page by specifying fonts and font-related attributes as well as location or layout of the text and graphics. HTML is a series of tags embedded in the web document that tell the browser how to display the page. The tags look like the example here.

```
<HTML>
<HEAD>
<TITLE>Document Title</TITLE>
</HEAD>
<BODY>This is my first attempt at a web page.</BODY>
</HTML>
```

The first and last tags (<HTML>) tell the browser that this is an HTML file. Tags between the HEAD tag are for informational purposes and do not display in the browser window. The TITLE tag displays the web page title in the title bar of the web browser. All text between the BODY tags displays in the browser window.

When a browser locates a web document by using the URL or by being sent there through a link, it interprets these tags regardless of the platform the user is using. This means that the web pages can be displayed on Windows, Unix, and Macintosh computers and that basically they will look the same.

Many tools are available for creating HTML documents. They are divided into three groups.

- ASCII Editors require the creator to type the tags and text directly into the document. NotePad, which comes with the Windows operating system, is an example of an ASCII editor.
- HTML converter programs take a document created in another program and convert it to an HTML file by adding the tags. The Microsoft Office suite is an example of this type of program. The user saves the file created as a web page.
- HTML editors are software programs with a graphical user interface that helps the developer create HTML files without having to type the tags. FrontPage and Dreamweaver are two popular HTML editors.

Each of these tools has advantages and disadvantages. For example, using a converter program such as Word results in documents appearing differently than they do in the word processor. The program has to interpret the formatting and convert it into HTML tags. This is not always done cleanly, and thus, the creator may still need to play with the tags to have the document display as designed. ASCII editors are tedious to use but provide excellent control over the web page. HTML editors are more powerful than converters, but the creator gives up some control over the web page design. Exercises 4 and 5 provide experience with creating a simple web page.

▶ 9.9 TRANSFERRING FILES

One of the functions that most Internet users want is the ability to transfer files from a server on the Internet to their computers. Before the advent of the web, using ftp was the only way to transfer files from one computer to another over the Internet. Ftp is the communications protocol and program that is used to transfer data from one location to another. To do this, the user had to access ftp and then type commands such as fetch and put to tell the computer what to do. Now with web browsers, transferring files is as simple as following directions on the screen.

If the need is to save the current web page in HTML format or capture a graphic, follow the directions given earlier in this chapter. The browser is great for transferring these files. If, however, the need is to transfer a variety of other types of files like compressed (Zip), program (exe), and preformatted files (pdf), use the file transfer protocol (ftp). The use of ftp is becoming easier as many web documents that facilitate file transfer embed the ftp commands in the HTML code. That means the user clicks something like a download button and follows the directions on the screen.

▶ **To use ftp, the following items are needed:**

- A local computer that is capable of running ftp with an Internet connection.
- A remote computer running ftp with an Internet connection.
- The Internet address for the remote server. This is usually ftp.same-second-domain.same-high-level-domain.
- An account on the remote server might be needed. Many ftp sites are run as anonymous, which means a login is not needed, or if a login is needed, it is something like anonymous for the login and the user's e-mail address or nothing for the password.

▶ **To start the ftp protocol:**

Click the **Start** button, and then **Run**.

Type **ftp ftp.irs.gov** where ftp starts the protocol, and rest is the ftp address for the Internal Revenue Service.

Follow the directions to log in.

Remember that this is a command-driven system, and thus, it requires the user to type the commands followed by pressing the enter key.

▶ **To access ftp through a web browser:**

Start the **Web** browser.

In the location or **Address** text box, type **ftp://ftp.domain.domain**.

Select the **File** to transfer, or click the **Download** button.

Click **OK** to save the file to disk.

Select a location in which to place the file and filename if needed, and click **OK**. The file is now being transferred.

Two commonly used terms regarding transferring files are download and upload. Download is moving a file from one computer (generally a server) to another (generally a local PC). It is a generic term that does not specify how it is done, just that the files were transferred. Uploading is transferring a file from a local computer to a remote server. This is the reverse direction and is used when moving local HTML files to the web server for publishing on the Net. Although a communications protocol called telnet can be used to run TCP/IP and remotely log in, the discussion here focuses on implementing ftp through web browser facilities.

Here are some points to consider when retrieving files from the Internet.

- Know what to download. Some ftp sites are cryptic and assume that the user knows the filename and how the site is organized. When at an ftp site, look for a file that describes the site and how it is organized. This is usually a text file titled index, read.me or files.lst. Select it, and read how things work at that site.

- Keep security in mind. Downloading files from the Internet can introduce a virus into your system. Most sites take precautions to prevent viruses in their files, and thus, the chances are good that the files will be clean. However, to be on the safe side, it does not hurt to check the downloaded files (especially exe and com files) with an antivirus program before installing them on the computer. Many people believe that there is a greater chance of getting a virus from e-mail files than from ftp sites.

- Know the system requirements for the file. Many sites also assume the user knows the operating system—Windows 98, NT, 2000, XP—as there are different versions of files for the different systems. Many sites will also tell the downloader how large the file is, how much space is needed on the hard drive to run the program, and how much memory the program requires. Make sure that the file is the correct one for the system in use.

- Obey copyright laws. Several different types of files are available for download. Freeware files are available without cost. Many free graphics files are available for use in creating web pages. Although some are totally free for use, others have restrictions such as free for use at nonprofit websites. If the file is used, some sites require acknowledgment of the developer or site on the website. Shareware files can be tried for free, and if users like the program, they pay a small fee to register the program. Many times the registered version is a later, better version than the shareware one. The last types of files are program files; these require payment for them. Some of these programs provide a trial version before the users actually pay for it; others require the user to buy the program before it can be downloaded. The trial versions usually last 30 days and then become unusable.

SUMMARY

This chapter covered some basics of using the Internet, specifically, some terminology and concepts such as web, URL, ftp, and HyperText. An introduction to connecting to the Internet and the related requirements followed. A brief orientation to the two most commonly used browsers was presented to show how similar they are. Because the web is composed of web pages, the chapter concluded with a brief discussion of the creation of web pages and the evaluation of web page design.

References

Bergman, M. (2001). The deep web: Surfacing hidden value. *The Journal of Electronic Publishing*, University of Michigan Press. Retrieved June 2, 2004, from http://www.press.umich.edu/jep/07-01/bergman.html

Additional Resources

Bare bones (http://www.sc.edu/beaufort/library/pages/bones/bones.shtml): This site is a great tutorial site for learning about searching and search sites.

InvisibleWeb.com (http://invisibleweb.com): This is an interesting catalog of deep web resources.

Librarians' Index to the Internet (http://www.lii.org): This site is a searchable annotated collection of resources selected by librarians. Although sites are selected primarily for the general public, many are of use to those in higher education as well.

Search Engine Showdown (http://searchengineshowdown.com): This site has some interesting statistics about search engines. It also includes some tutorials.

Search Engine Watch (http://searchenginewatch.com/): This site has excellent descriptions of searching and search engines. It tries to keep up to date with what is happening in the world of Internet searching. It is a good reference source.

Exercise 1: Introduction to Microsoft Internet Explorer and Browsing

Objectives

1. Define selected words related to a website.
2. Identify different types of web addressing.
3. Use Internet Explorer to access the World Wide Web and to connect to different sites.
4. Create and edit a Favorites Folder.
5. Print a document from the World Wide Web.
6. Transfer both a home page and a graphic file from the web.

Activity

1. Define the following words and answer the related questions.

   Home page. Hint: there are two different meanings.

   What home page is opened when connecting to the college computer laboratory or your workplace computer?

   What is a link or hyperlink?

2. Understand web page addresses.

What is the difference between an e-mail address and a web address or URL? Here are some addresses. Decide what type of address each is.

43.134.020.12

cdc.gov

Nancy_Drew

Frogger@microsoft.com

What might be the host name for a computer at the National Library of Medicine?

Nancy works in the Nursing Department at the University of Pennsylvania. What might be the full Internet address of that department?

Do you want to find out who owns a particular domain name?

Double click the **Internet Explorer** icon.

Click the **Address** text box to highlight the text.

Type **http://www.networksolutions.com/** in the address text box, and press **Enter**.

Click **WHOIS** hyperlinked words at the top of the screen.

Type **upmc.com** in the search text box, and press **Enter**.

Who owns this domain name, and what is the primary IP address?

Click the **Back** ⬅ Back button on the standard browser toolbar. Highlight the text in the search box.

Type **nbc.com** in the query text box, and press **Enter**.

Who owns this domain name, and what is the primary IP address?

Click the **Back** ⬅ Back button on the standard browser toolbar. Highlight the text in the search box.

Type **nursing.com** in the query box, and press **Enter**.

Who owns this domain name, and what is the primary IP address?

Click the **Back** ⬅ Back button on the standard browser toolbar. Highlight the text in the search box.

Type **healthcare.com** in the query text box, and press **Enter**.

Who owns this domain name, and what is the primary IP address?

3. Use Internet Explorer to connect to sites.

Click the **Text** in the **Address** text box in Internet Explorer to highlight it.

Type **http://www.mapquest.com**, and press **Enter**.

Click the **MAPS** 🌐 button, and type your **Address, City, State**, and **Zip code** in the correct text boxes.

Click the **Get Map** [Get Map] button. How accurate is your map?

Click the **Text** in the address text box in Internet Explorer to highlight it.

Why might this be helpful to a home care nurse?

Now type **weather.com**, and press **Enter**.

Type **Your Zip code** (your actual zip code, not the words) in the zip text box, and click **Go**.

What is the forecast for the next 5 days in your city?

Click the **Back** Back button until you are back at mapquest.

Click the hypertext word **Print** at the top of the screen.

Click the hypertext **Send to printer** to print a copy of the map.

4. Create and work with **Favorites**.

Click the **Favorite** Favorites button and then the **Organize Favorites**
Organize... text on the side task bar. *The organize favorites dialog box appears* (Figure 9.5).

Click **Create Folder** in the organize favorites dialog box, and type **Learning Folder**. Press **Enter**, and click the **Close** button.

Click the **Drop-down Address** button on the Internet Explorer address bar, and click the **weather.com** site.

Click the **Add** Add... button on the Internet Explorer task pane.

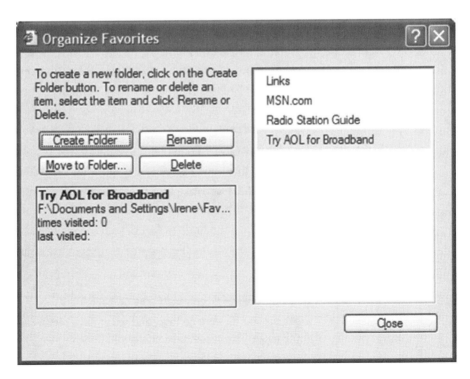

Figure 9.5

Organize Favorites
Dialog Box

Click the **Create in** button. Click the **Learning Folder**, and click **OK**. *The weather site is now added to the favorites folder.*

Type **pacprod.com/card.htm** in the address text box, and press **Enter**.

Click the **Learning Folder**, and select **weather.com**. *This leads to the weather site.*

Click the **Favorites** task pane close button to remove the folder list from the task pane.

Because users may not be able to keep a favorites folder on the hard drive in the laboratory, they will want to keep their folders on a diskette. They can do this one of two ways—create the favorites, and at the end of each session, copy them to a diskette OR create a word file and paste the URLs of favorite sites into it. If using this approach, write a short description of the site so that in a few months it will be easy to remember the essence of that site.

Click the **Favorites** ⭐ Favorites button to open the favorites task pane.

Right click the **Learning Folder**, and select **Send to**.

Select the **3$^1/_2$" floppy drive icon** or your removable storage device. *The folder is now copied to the storage device.*

To access this folder in the future from a browser, select **File**, **Open** and the **Browse** button. Make sure that the list of file types is set to **All Files***. Select the correct storage device. Highlight a **Site** or **Folder**, and click **Open**.

To access the Word file, open **Word** and the correct **Folder**. Click the correct **URL**. If not in a laboratory with a direct connection, make sure that the browser is running in the background. This means that you access your ISP service or the link will not work.

5. Save web pages.

Type **www.cdc.gov** in the Address Text box, and press **Enter**.

Click the **Emergency Preparedness and Response** option.

Select **Fact sheet and overview** and **Anthrax: What You Need to Know**.

Select **File**, **Save as**. Make sure to select the correct location and save it as HTML Only. Click the **Save** button.

Open **Word** and the **Anthrax** file. What do you notice about this file? Close **Word**.

Now open the **Anthrax** file in a web browser. What is missing?

To save a graphic file:

Go to the college or university's home page.

Right click on the **college logo**, and select **Save picture as**. Select the location and file name (if it needs to be changed).

Close any open windows and exit the browser.

Check the file on the storage medium. There may be limitations regarding using a
company or school's logo!

Exercise 2: Introduction to Netscape Navigator and Browsing
Objectives
1. Define selected words related to a website.
2. Identify different types of web addressing.
3. Use Netscape Navigator to access the World Wide Web and connect to different sites.
4. Create and edit a Bookmarks Folder.
5. Print a document from the World Wide Web.
6. Transfer both a home page and a graphic file from the web.

Activity
1. Define the following words and answer the related questions.

   Home page. Hint: There are two different meanings.

   What home page is opened when connecting to the college computer laboratory?

   What is a link or hyperlink?
2. Understand web page addresses.

   What is the difference between an e-mail address and a web address or URL?

   Here are some addresses. Decide what type of address each is.

   43.134.020.12

   Firstgov.gov

   Martha_Rodgers

   Joos@laroche.edu

   What might be the host name for a computer at the US Government's Veteran's
   Administration Hospital?

   Martha works in the Nursing Department at Pennsylvania State University. What
   might be the full Internet address of that department?

   Do you want to find out who owns a particular domain name?

   Double click the **Netscape Navigator** icon.

   Click the **Location** text box to highlight the text.

   Type **http://www.networksolutions.com/** in the location text box, and press **Enter**.

   Click **WHOIS** hyperlinked words at the top of the screen.

   Type **disney.com** in the search text box, and press **Enter**.

   Who owns this domain name and what is the primary IP address?

Click the **Back** button on the standard browser toolbar. Highlight the text in the search box.

Type **mercyhospital.com** in the query text box, and press **Enter**.

Who owns this domain name, and what is the primary IP address? What is this person trying to do?

Click the **Back** button on the standard browser toolbar. Highlight the text in the search box.

Type **nursing.com** in the query box, and press **Enter**.

Who owns this domain name, and what is the primary IP address?

Click the **Back** button on the standard browser toolbar. Highlight the text in the search box.

Type **healthcare.com** in the query text box, and press **Enter**.

Who owns this domain name, and what is the primary IP address?

3. Use Netscape Navigator to connect to sites.

Click the **Text** in the **Location** text box in Netscape Navigator to highlight it.

Type **http://www.mapquest.com**, and press **Enter**.

Click the **MAPS** button, and type your **Address**, **City**, **State**, and **Zip code** in the correct text boxes.

Click the **Get Map** Get Map button. How accurate is your map?

Click the **Text** in the location text box in Netscape Navigator to highlight it.

Now type **weather.com**, and press **Enter**.

Type **Your Zip code** (your actual zip code, not the words) in the zip text box, and click **Go**.

What is the forecast for the next 5 days in your city?

Click the **Back** button until back at MapQuest.

Click the hypertext word **Print** at the top of the screen.

Click the hypertext **Send to printer** to print a copy of the map.

4. Create and work with **Bookmarks**.

Click the **Bookmarks** Bookmarks button on the toolbar and then the **Manage Bookmarks** text from the drop-down menu. *The Bookmark Manager dialog box appears* (Figure 9.6).

Click the **New Folder** in the manage bookmarks dialog box, and type **Learning Folder**. Click **OK**, and then click the **Close** button to close the dialog box.

Click the **Drop-down Address** button on the Netscape Navigator location bar and click the **weather.com** site.

Select **Bookmarks** from the menu bar, and then **File bookmark**. Click the **Learning Folder**, and click the **OK** button. *The weather site is added to the Learning Folder.*

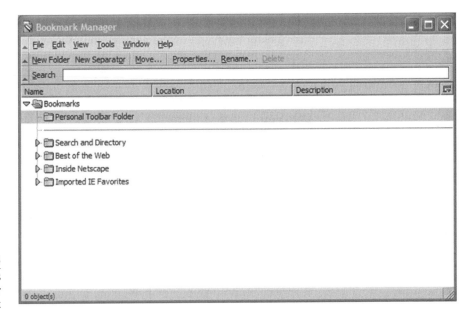

Figure 9.6

Netscape Navigator's
Bookmark Manager
Dialog Box

Type **pacprod.com/card.htm** in the location text box, and press **Enter**.

Click the **Learning Folder** and select **weather.com**. This leads to the weather site.

Because users may not be able to keep a bookmarks folder on the hard drive in the laboratory, they will want to keep their folders on a removable storage medium. This can be done in one of two ways—create the bookmarks and at the end of each session copy them to a disk, OR create a word file and paste the URLs of favorite sites into it. If using this approach, write a short description of the site so that in a few months, it will be easy to remember the essence of that site.

Click the **Bookmarks**   Bookmarks   button and **Manage Bookmarks** from the drop-down menu.

Select **Tools**, **Export** from the menu in the Bookmark Manager dialog box.

Select the **storage device**, and click **Save**. *The whole bookmarks file is saved; there is no option to save just part of it.*

To access this folder in the future from a browser, select **File**, **Open**. Select the correct storage device. Click the **bookmarks.html** file and **Open**.

To access the Word file, open **Word** and the correct **Folder** and **File**. Click the correct **URL**. If not in a laboratory with a direct connection, make sure to access the ISP service or the URL will not display in the browser.

5. Save web pages.

Type **www.cdc.gov** in the Location Text box, and press **Enter**.

Click **Emergency Preparedness and Response** option.

Select **Fact sheet and overview** and **Anthrax: What You Need to Know**.

Select **File, Save as**. Make sure to select the correct location and save it as HTML Only. Click the **Save** button.

Open **Word** and the **Anthrax** file. What do you notice about this file? Close **Word**.

Now open the **Anthrax** file in a web browser. What is missing?

To save a graphic file:

Go to the college or university's home page.

Right click on the **college logo**, and select **Save image as**. Select the location and file name (if it needs to be changed).

Close any open windows, and exit the browser.

Check the file on the storage medium. There may be limitations regarding using a company's logo or a school's logo!

Exercise 3: Downloading Files from the Web
Objectives

1. Download a variety of file types.
2. Identify the differences between downloading, file save, and save target or image as.

Activity

1. If necessary, start a **Browser**.
2. Obtain a file through a browser from a website.

    In the **Location** or **Address** text box, type **www.download.com**, and press **Enter**.

    Click **Utilities** from the directory structure.

    Click **File Compression**, and scroll to **WinZip for Windows 98/NT/2000/XP**.

    Click the **WinZip** file. What is the version, date, and size of this file?

    Will it fit on a floppy diskette?

    Click the **Download** button. Click **Save** to save this program to a disk.

    Select a location, and click **Save**.

    Note the address toward the top of the window in Figure 9.7. *The file is now downloading.*

3. Obtain a file through a browser from an ftp site.

    In the **Location or Address** text box, type **ftp://ftp.pkware.com**, and press **Enter**.

    What do you need to know to obtain the correct file? How different is this site from the one in number 2?

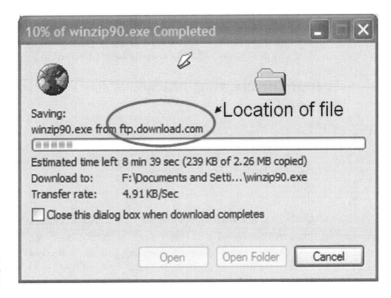

Figure 9.7

Download Screen

Click **files.1st**. What is the filename and size of the file that will run in Windows XP or 2000?

Click the **Browser's back** button.

Click **the correct file**. At this point, the process is the same as that in number 2; thus, click **Cancel**.

Now, go to **www.pkware.com**. This is the website for the same file.

What is the difference in the user interface?

Click **Windows platform** and then **Free Downloads**.

Click the **Correct file**. At this point, the process is the same as that in number 2; thus, click **Cancel**.

Files in numbers 2 and 3 are compressed files. Before you can use them, you need to unzip or execute them. To do this, double click the file, and follow the on-screen directions.

4. Obtain another file through a browser from an ftp site using the right click technique.

Type **ftp://ftp.irs.ustreas.gov** in the location or address text box.

Double click **Pub** directory, **Irs-pdf** directory.

Right click **f1040ez.pdf**, and select **Copy this item**.

Select the **correct storage device**, and click the **Copy** button. *The file is now downloading.*

Close the **browser**.

Double click the **f1040cz.pdf** file that was just downloaded.

What happened?

To display pdf files, the system must have Acrobat Reader installed. Some files require special programs to read and display them. Most sites that use pdf files have a link to a free copy of the Acrobat Reader software.

Exercise 4: Creating a Simple Web Page with HTML

Objectives

1. Design a simple HTML file.
2. Use a text editor to enter HTML tags.
3. Add a graphic and links.

Activity

1. Obtain a quick reference guide for HTML tags. Use the methods for searching outlined in Chapter 11 and search for a reference on HTML tagging. Why do you feel that this is a good site for beginners? Justify your answer.

   Include the URL here:

   Select two of the following sites to provide reference sources about HTML tagging. Either save them to a disk or print them for reference when doing your home page design.

   http://www.mcli.dist.maricopa.edu/tut/tags/tag1.html

   http://archive.ncsa.uiuc.edu/General/Internet/WWW/

   http://www.w3schools.com/default.asp

2. Find the following images needed for your HTML document. Download them to a disk.

   Graphic: Filename: URL:

   An icon or button to use on your home page

   A line to separate some of your content

   A background image or color for your home page

   A picture that represents something for your home page

   Try to find at least one site that has medical clip art (hint: Search in Google for "medical clip art").

3. Create HTML pages with an ASCII editor.

   Go to **Start, Programs, Accessories**, and click **Notepad**.

   Type **<HTML>**. Press **Enter**. Type **<HEAD>**, and press **Enter**.

   Type **<TITLE>Your Name Homepage</TITLE>**, and press **Enter** (that means to type your name and not the capitalized words **YOUR NAME HOMEPAGE**), for example, Irene's Homepage.

   Type **</HEAD>**, and press **Enter**.

   Type **<BODY>**, and press **Enter**.

Type **<H1>Home Page of Irene Joos</H1>**, and press **Enter**.

Type **Welcome to my website. <P>** and press **Enter**.

Type **This is my first attempt at tagging HTML files. <P>** and press **Enter**.

Type **Here is a picture that represents who I am . . . <P>** and press **Enter**.

Type **<IMG SRC="images/file name and extension"> <P>** Use one of the images that you downloaded previously, and type its filename and extension. Make sure that it is in the same folder as your html file and in the images folder. For example, **<IMG SRC="images/angry_bear.gif">**.

Type **<A HREF="http://www.yahoo.com">Click here for Yahoo! </A>**, and press **Enter**.

Type **</BODY>**, and press **Enter**.

Type **</HTML>**.

Save the file on a disk as **index.html**. Make sure that you type the extension.

Open **Netscape Navigator** or **Internet Explorer**. Choose **File**, **Open file**.

Select **index.html**, and click **OK**.

Print it and **attach** it to this exercise.

It should look similar to the one in Figure 9.8. If you are having trouble with this, make sure that the coding is exact (all tags must be correct, and no extraneous marks can be present). Check to make sure that the location and name of the graphic are correct. Check to make sure that the tags are opened and closed (/). Make sure it is saved as an HTML text file.

Click on the **Click Here for Yahoo!** Did your link work? If not, make sure that you are connected to the Internet.

Using the guides from the earlier part of this exercise, learn one new tag, and add it to the file created during this exercise.

Did it work? Did you have any problems with it? How did you solve them?

That is all there is to it. Most people who do not tag all of the time refer to references when looking for the appropriate tags or use the source code from other sites when they find something they like. However, in order to do that, you have to have some basic understanding of the codes. When creating your page, refer to the quick guides mentioned previously.

Exercise 5: Creating a Simple Web Page Using Microsoft Word
Objectives

1. Design a simple home page using Microsoft Word.
2. Edit the page.
3. Add a graphic and links.

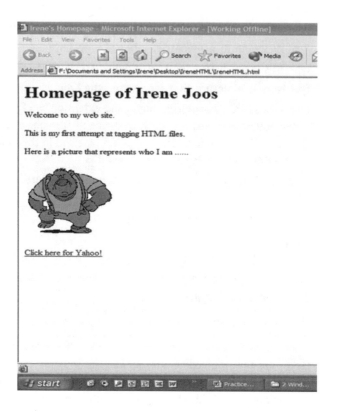

Figure 9.8

Sample HTML File

Activity

1. Plan. First, you are to create two web pages—one will be the index page or home page, and the other one will be the Favorites page that will teach you how to link to and from the home page. Create a folder to hold all of the HTML files created for this exercise. Call it WordHTML. In that folder, place a subfolder called graphics. Load the graphic images into that folder.

2. Create an HTML file.

    Start **Word**.

    Select **File**, **New**, and click the **Web Page** option from the New Documents task pane on the right side of the window.

    Select **Format**, **Theme** from the menu bar and pick **Blends**.

    Type **Welcome to My Website!**

    Select the text. Format it as **Heading 1**, and **center** it.

    Press the **Enter** key two times.

    Type **This site is my first one created using a converter program—Word.** Press **Enter**.

    Type **I'm starting to get the hang of this!** Press the **Enter** key twice.

Type **Here are some things I want you to know about who I am:** and press the **Enter** key twice.

Click the bullet button on the formatting toolbar and type

Where I go to school and press **Enter**

Where I work and press **Enter**

Something about my family and friends and press **Enter**

A few of my favorite sites and press **Enter** three times.

Type **School**. Press **Tab**. Type **Work**. Press **Tab**. Type **Family & Friends**. Press **Tab**. Type **Favorites**.

Select the previous line of text, and set left tabs at **1.5**, **2.5**, and **4.5** inches.

Save the document on the storage medium in the WordHTML folder as **Index.html**. Make sure that it is saved as an HTML file.

3. Edit the document created in number 2, and insert a graphic.

Select the **Heading**, and format it as **Comic Sans** or some other related font.

Place the pointer to the left of the W in welcome.

Select the **Insert**, **Picture**, and **Clip art** options from the drop-down menu.

Type **school** in the search text box, and click **Go**.

Insert the **book and apple** clip art (or some other related one).

Change the size to about **2" square**.

Editing the document is just like editing other Word documents.

Click the **Save** button to update the file.

4. Insert another graphic.

Use the clip art **Search for** feature to search for a **graphic line**.

Insert it into the space above the words at the bottom of the file.

5. Create a second HTML file.

Follow the previously mentioned directions, and **create** a **second file**. Use the same theme and formatting as the previous file.

Call the file **Favorites** and include the following text:

Heading   **Favorite Things.**

Text   **I love to travel with my family throughout the US and abroad.**

Pictures   Two either **scanned** or from the **Internet** of a place you like.

Create a 2 × 2 table, and place one picture in each cell with text explaining the pictures in the other two cells. Remove the lines around the table. Align the text appropriately in the cell.

Type **Home**. Press **Tab**. Type **School**. Press **Tab**. Type **Work**. Press **Tab**. Type **Family & Friends**.

Select the previous line of text, and set left tabs at **1.5**, **3**, and **4.5** inches.

Save the file.

6. Create links to each other.

Select the text **Home** at the bottom of the page of the favorites file.

Select **Insert, Hyperlink**.

Click **From existing file or web page** button on the left side of the dialog box.

Make sure to look in the **WordHTML** folder. Select **index.html**.

Open the **Index.html** file in Word—not the browser.

Select the text **Favorites** at the bottom of the page.

Select **Insert, Hyperlink**.

Make sure that **the Existing file or web page** option button is selected and that the location is the WordHTML folder.

Click the **Favorites** file and **OK**. *You have now created a link from the file to the favorites file.*

Save the file.

7. Show the documents.

Start a **Browser**.

Select **File, Open**, and click **Browse**.

Select the **Index.html** file on the removable storage medium.

Click the linked text, **Favorites**, to open the favorites file.

Click the **Home** linked text in the index file to go back to it.

Print each document. They should resemble Figure 9.9.

8. Now make two more files (school, work, or family and friends).

Add appropriate content and graphics.

Link all of the files together.

Save the files. Print the files.

Figure 9.9

Sample Word
HTML Files

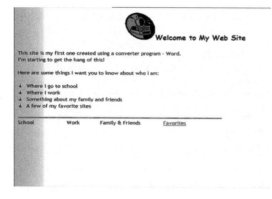

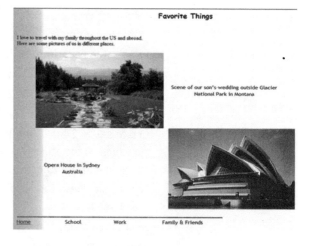

Assignment 1: Evaluating Web Design Quality
Directions

1. Use the methods for searching outlined in Chapter 11, and search for a reference on evaluating quality design for web pages. Why do you feel that this is a good site?

2. Write the URL of the site you visited here.

3. Go to **http://www.cyberbee.com/guides.html**. Select the design guide links. What are the indicators of quality design discussed at this site?

4. Go to **http://www.webstyleguide.com/index.html?/index.html**. Look around this site. What are the indicators for quality design discussed at this site?

5. Go to **http://www.colin.mackenzie.org/webdesign/**. What are some of the criteria discussed at this site?

6. What do you think constitutes quality in design? Are there other things you might add to these lists that are not there?

7. Select a website to critique using selected design criteria. List five design criteria and compare this site against those criteria.

8. Type your responses to these questions using your word processor.

Assignment 2: Creating a Personal Home Page
Directions

1. For this assignment, you will create a personal home page. You may use whatever software you prefer to create it (anything from an ASCII editor to HTML converter to HTML editor).

2. The following is expected for this home page:
   - Follows the guidelines given in class and in the references for good design.
   - Include at least one of each of the following:
     - One button
     - One graphic or image found on the web
     - Colored background
     - One picture (make sure that you are not violating copyright; it is easier if you use a picture that you have and scan it)
   - A link to your biosketch
   - A link to a web page at another site
   - A link to your college or university home page
   - Uses only graphics that are appropriate for the content.
   - Has at least four HTML files linked together

3. Part of your grade will be a presentation of your home page to your classmates. Be prepared to show your home page and talk about its development. This means that

you need to make sure that all of your graphic and HTML files are on your diskette in the proper places.

Assignment 3: Creating an E-Portfolio
Directions

1. Complete a search on e-portfolios. What are they? Why are they important?

2. Read the article that appeared in the 12/1/2002 issue of *Syllabus* (also available at http://www.syllabus.com/article.asp?id=6984). What is the essence of the article?

3. Think about projects completed and courses/seminars/workshops/experiences that you have had since coming to college. The idea here is to demonstrate the experiences, knowledge, and skills that you have acquired while in school. Assemble an example of what you learned and experienced in each of these areas:

    Communication skills (written and oral)

    Computer literacy skills

    Information literacy skills

    Knowledge of and experience in the global arena

    One or two skills required to demonstrate competency in your major

4. Create a front page to access these materials (call it index.html). Now design some web pages that highlight your experiences, knowledge, and skills. Obtain web space on the school server to publish these pages.

5. Present your pages during a class presentation, and talk about what you were trying to highlight and why.

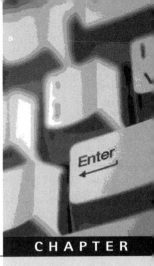

Computer–Assisted Communication

OBJECTIVES

1. Identify the components needed to establish computer-assisted communication.
2. Describe computer communication modalities: e-mail, listservs, bulletin boards, chat rooms, Internet conferencing, and threaded discussions.
3. Identify security threats when using e-mail.
4. Send e-mail messages and attachments.
5. Join a listserv and participate in the discussion.
6. Access newsgroups, bulletin boards, and chat rooms.
7. Identify criteria for selecting the World Wide Web for online learning.

Communication is the process and structure of sending and receiving messages by a variety of means. In computer-assisted communication, the computer enhances the communication process by either structuring the message or providing a channel to send and receive messages. This chapter focuses on using a computer system as a channel for communicating messages over both short and long distances. Messages sent by a computer system take many forms. For example, they may take the form of a short e-mail note, an article published online, a database, a downloaded computer software program, or an online course.

► 10.1 TERMS RELATED TO COMPUTER–ASSISTED COMMUNICATION

The following terms are important to understand when examining different computer-assisted communication modalities. They are introduced here, and more specific information about some of them appears later in the chapter.

Asynchronous	This term was first used in data transmission, referring to sending and receiving data a byte at a time with a start and stop bit delimiting each byte. Now it is also used to reference a communication exchange when the people involved are communicating at different times. For example, e-mail is asynchronous because communicants do not need to be on the computer at the same time.
Bulletin Board	Similar to their counterparts hanging on a wall, these are public areas for messages. They are typically organized around specific topics and may be part of an online service and accessed through Internet search engines. Bulletin boards may be open to everyone or may be restricted to members of certain groups and accessed through passwords (see Figure 10.1 for examples of bulletin boards accessible from http://www.healthboards. com/).
Chat	Chat is real-time communication between two or more users via a computer. Most Internet service providers have built-in chat features.
Chat Room	A designated area or "room" where individuals gather simultaneously and can "talk" to one another by typing messages. Everyone who is online usually sees the messages (see Figure 10.2 for an example of a website to access chat rooms related to health at http://www.chatmag.com/topics/ health/).

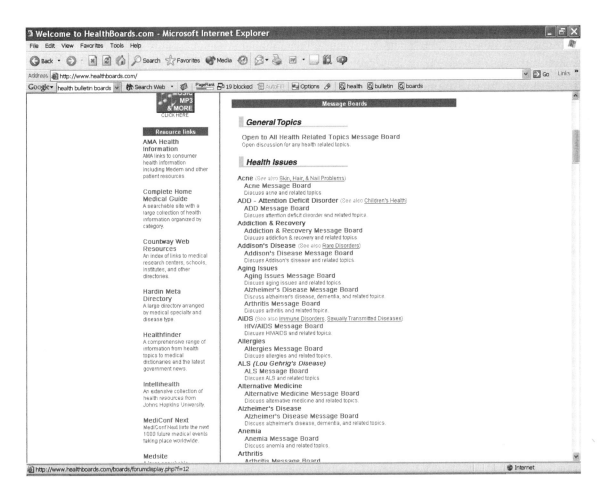

Figure 10.1
- - - - - - - - - - - - - - - - - - -
Accessing Bulletin
Boards about Health

E-mail

Electronic mail is a message that is composed and sent over a computer network to a person or group of people who have an electronic mail address. E-mail can be sent over a local area network or over the Internet.

Emoticon

Emoticons are a way to show an emotion via text on the computer to help make up for the inability to read body language or to hear the inflection in the voice.

Instant Messaging

Abbreviated IM, this communication service permits the user to send real-time messages via a private chat room to other individuals who are

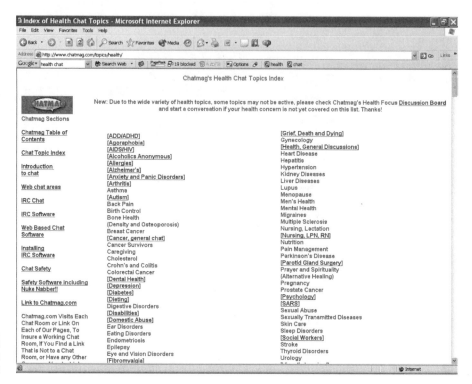

Figure 10.2

Accessing Chat
Rooms about Health

online. Because systems are not standard, individuals communicating with one another must use the same system and must be registered through the system to get an IM address.

Internet Conferencing

This occurs when two or more persons interact over the Internet in real time, receiving more or less immediate replies. This can involve interaction via text, audio, or video.

Listserv

Listserv is the name for a software program that manages automated mailing lists; however, it is commonly used to refer to all mailing lists. When someone posts a message to a listserv, everyone on the mailing list receives the message via e-mail. Figure 10.3 shows some listservs that might be of interest to nurses.

Organization	What's There	Web Address
American Nurses Association	Links to a Variety of Listservs	http://nursingworld.org/listserv/
National Institute of Health		http://list.nih.gov/cgi-bin/show_list_archives
Maternal and Child Health Bureau		http://www.mchb.hrsa.gov/training/listserv.htm
American Mental Health APH	Listserv Information	http://serendip.brynmawr.edu/sci_cult/mentalhealth/list.html
AHRQ Child and Adolescent Health	Listserv Information	http://www.ahrq.gov/child/flyrlist.htm
CDC Environmental Health	Listserv Information	http://www.cdc.gov/nceh/ehs/Listserv/listserv.htm
*GLOBAL*RN (Focus on culture and health)	Listserv Information	http://nurseweb.ucsf.edu/www/globalin.htm
Health Education AIDS Liaison (HEAL)	Listserv Information	http://thorup.com/HEAL/listserv.html
National Association of Neonatal Nurses	Listserv Rules	http://www.nann.org/i4a/pages/index.cfm?pageid=839
School Health	Listserv Information	https://secure.serve.com/jcooper/school_listserv_reg.html

Figure 10.3

Partial List of Listservs of Interest to Nurses Accessed from http://nursingworld.org/listserv/

Newsgroup

A group of information and articles organized around a particular topic, such as Alzheimer's Disease or Child Abuse, is a newsgroup. News-readers can post a message to the newsgroup for all to read and respond.

Online Course

This refers to educational experiences and/or materials on the Internet. The actual amount of "online" experience in a course varies. Course materials may be online; other learning experiences may take place through traditional methods, or all learning experiences may be initiated and conducted through websites, e-mail, and other online computer experiences.

Phishing

This is sending fraudulent e-mail that solicits private information such as passwords or credit card numbers. This can result in identify theft.

Spam   This is electronic junk mail. This type of e-mail is unsolicited and/or not from an identifiable source. As well as being irritating, it may be deceptive.

Spim   This is the spam of instant messaging—part spam and part instant messaging, being used by an increasing number of advertisers.

Synchronous   This term was originally used in data transmission to mean moving streams of data at the same time and rate. When applied to communication among people on the computer, it refers to individuals communicating in the same time set. Chat rooms or NetMeetings are examples of synchronous communication as individuals involved are all on the computer at the same time.

Threaded Discussion This online information exchange is similar to a bulletin board, except that topics within each interest area are identified and organized together so that users can access and read just those discussions rather than all items posted.

Video Conferencing This is a conference involving a computer, video camera, microphone, and speakers. Along with hearing audio, whatever images appear in front of the video camera are delivered to the participant's monitor. Video conferencing can involve just two participants or multiple ones in a "virtual" conference.

► 10.2 COMPONENTS NEEDED FOR COMPUTER-ASSISTED COMMUNICATION

Both the sender of the communication and the receiver of that message must have the appropriate hardware, software, and a connection to the network in order to communicate. The basics of computer-assisted communication require a sender, channel, medium, and receiver. In computer-assisted communication the sender includes not only the person creating the message, but also the computer. The communications medium and channel refer to the "how" of the communications—how the message is being transferred from one place to the other. The medium may include such devices as telephone wires, twisted pair, fiber optic cables, radio waves, or satellites. The computer must be connected to the communications medium by either a modem or connection card (network card or wireless card in the computer). It is essential that both computers use software that supports the same communications protocol so that they can "talk" to each other. Chapter 9 provides more detail on computer hardware and the basic communication software needed.

Most computer laboratories and hospitals are networked. The network consists of all of the computers and related devices that are connected together for the purpose of sharing devices, programs, and data. Other terms related to these connections include the following:

Server

The computers in the network act as a manager for the network. The server runs user and computer software programs, stores data, and controls network traffic.

Local Area Network (LAN)

A network that exists within one or more buildings. Networks vary in size and have a variety of organizational structures. There may be several small LANs connected together within one institution.

Wide Area Network (WAN)

Several LANs that are separated by distance and connected by a backbone are referred to as a WAN.

Backbone

The backbone is a high-speed network connecting several powerful computers or LANS.

Internet

The Internet is a worldwide system for linking computer networks using Transmission Control Protocol/Internet Protocol (TCP/IP) communication standards.

TCP/IP Standards

TCP/IP is the basic communications standard for using the Internet.

▶ 10.3 ELECTRONIC MAIL

E-mail or electronic mail is a way to send messages to others in electronic form. Users write e-mail just like they would write a letter with the word processor. However, instead of printing the message and sending it via the postal system, e-mail users typically click a "Send" button on the e-mail program and the mail arrives at its destination within a matter of seconds or minutes, depending on where it is going. Just as there are many different word processing, graphics, and spreadsheet programs, there are different mail programs. Often one comes with the computer. Outlook, Eudora, and Pegasus are popular mailers. Mailers are also included with both Netscape and Internet Explorer and from the Internet service provider. Many search sites, as well as other service providers, provide free mail services. All of these programs typically involve a point-and-click approach to accessing and sending mail. Some institutions, however, use a mail system that is dependent on typing commands rather than selecting them from a menu. Although this chapter provides general information about using e-mail, it does not provide step-by-step procedures for using a specific program. Check the help information online or the documentation for the system in the institution for assistance using a specific e-mail system.

E-mail messages consist of two parts: the header and the body. The body is the actual message. The header has at least four sections that provide useful information.

Date   This includes the date and time that the message was sent.
From   This identifies the sender and the sender's e-mail address.
To   This identifies the receiver and the receiver's e-mail address.
CC   This is an option in some e-mail systems to send a copy of the message to a recipient. Some programs also provide an optional BCC (blind carbon copy).
Subject This is the topic discussed in the e-mail.

E-mail users are given a certain amount of space for e-mail messages on the server of their institution or by the Internet service provider or e-mail provider. If e-mail messages are not read and deleted, eventually the space allotted will become filled and other messages will be returned to the senders. Thus, people with e-mail accounts should read the mail often and delete messages that are no longer needed. Most programs also allow users to store systematically the messages that they wish to keep in folders located off the mail server either on the local drive or another network server. By moving previously read messages to folders, the Inbox of the mail system is kept uncluttered and new messages are more readily visible when the mail program is started.

E-mail Addresses

All e-mail systems provide users with individual addresses. On a local area network, an e-mail address operates much like interoffice mail. A user's local e-mail address usually consists of the user's ID only. Mail sent over a WAN is like mail sent via the postal service in that a full Internet address is needed. Web page and e-mail addresses are different, however. In an e-mail address, there is always an @ symbol that separates the user ID from the rest of the address. A URL never has an @ symbol in the address and always starts with http://. Chapter 9 provides more information about URLs.

There are three parts to an Internet e-mail address. For example, the address might be whitman_n@mail.lynchburg.edu.

User ID or **Distribution ID**	The first component, the *user ID*, is the e-mail name of the individual on the computer system where he or she receives mail. No one else on that system has the same user ID. The user's ID in the previous example is whitman_n. One of the e-mail functions that is especially useful when sending e-mail to a group of people is the creation of a distribution list. It is also called an **alias** or **mailing list**. The *distribution ID* is the name assigned to the list. Each time the sender addresses an e-mail message using the distribution ID, each person whose e-mail address is on the list receives the message. For example, there might be a list called classN402 to identify the students in a certain nursing class. When addressing a message, selecting the distribution list provides a list of all of the members' user IDs.
@	The "at" sign is always between the user's ID and the user's mail system address.
User's domain or mail system address	This is the location address for everyone who uses that local computer mail system. This part of the address functions like the home address. Everyone in the family uses the same apartment or house address. In the previous example, the location address is mail.lynchburg.edu.

E-mail Netiquette

Just as there are rules governing what is acceptable to say and do during social interactions, guidelines exist for acceptable ways of communicating using e-mail. Netiquette is the name given to electronic communication conventions. Some of the main rules of netiquette include the following:

1. Start the message with a greeting, just like with any communication, and make it specific to the recipient(s): "Hi Kurt," "Mary," or "Greetings Colleagues."
2. Include in the message only what is appropriate for others to read. Never assume the message is private.
3. Be clear and concise. E-mail messages include only the words. When people communicate face to face, they use intonation and body language as well as words to send the message. With e-mail, no observation of the recipient is possible, and thus, no immediate feedback or the ability to adjust the message midway occurs. "Emoticons," like the smiley, have been developed to signify feelings. Standard emoticons include the following:

:-)	Basic smiley
;-)	Winking smiley—means "just kidding"
:-(	Sad face
8-)	Smiley with sunglasses
-o :	Surprised face

   For other emoticons, visit http://www.windweaver.com/emoticon.htm or http://www.computeruser.com/resources/dictionary/emoticons. html.
4. Keep it short. Do not quote huge amounts of material or include the entire original message in a reply unless it is pertinent to the reply. When replying, put the reply early in the message body so that readers do not have to wade through material to get to the response.
5. Limit formatting. Some programs do not read underlining, bold, etc.
6. Use the underscore symbol before and after words to represent underlining when needed, for example, for a journal title.
   a. Keep the line length to 60–70 characters.
   b. Use *asterisks* around a word to make a point.
7. Always specify the content of the message in the subject line so that readers know what to expect. This can also help readers discriminate between what might be a legitimate message from someone known and what might be a message with a virus.

8. Never type in all caps. THIS IS CONSIDERED SHOUTING.

9. Make the message one that is well presented. Check the spelling and grammar.

10. Respect copyright. Always give credit to others for their work and follow copyright rules for using material (see Chapter 12 for guidelines related to copyright).

11. Avoid flaming, which is voicing very strong antagonistic opinions or attacking someone.

12. Sign the message. The signature should include at least the name and e-mail address. It can also include the postal mail address, telephone number, title, and professional affiliation but should be no longer than four lines. It is possible to create a "signature" file ahead of time and use it as a standard on all the mail.

13. Never send chain letters. They are forbidden on the Internet.

E-mail Attachments

A file sent along with an e-mail message is called an attachment. Any type of file can be sent via e-mail—text files, graphics, spreadsheets, and even video. E-mail systems are set up to handle text, not the binary files associated with graphics and color images often included in attachments. Therefore, attachments are encoded by the sender's system to a text file that can be sent via e-mail; on arrival, they are decoded by the receiver's system. Attaching files to e-mail messages is no longer difficult; few programs involve having to know the commands for encoding and decoding that were once necessary. When sending attachments, find out what the computer receiving the message can decode. Also, be certain that the recipient of the file has the software to run the file being sent and can handle the file size. Some e-mail systems limit attachment sizes. For example, if sending an Excel document, the recipient will need to have Excel software.

E-mail has been growing in popularity as a rapid method of communication. However, along with its advantages has come the irritating problem of unsolicited messages, or spam. Spam has grown so great in its impact that a federal law regulating junk mail went into effect January 1, 2004. The Controlling the Assault of Non-Solicited Pornography and Marketing (Can Spam) Act, although resulting in a few prosecutions, has not greatly reduced spam. Many Internet providers offer spam-blocking products for their customers, and some e-mail programs have filters that may be set to block spam related to specified subjects or from specified addresses. It is wise never to open messages from anyone or any company not known and never to provide personal information in response to an e-mail message. Some e-mails fraudulently represent commercial companies and request such information; this phishing scam can lead to identity theft. In an attempt to prevent advertising spam from coming into e-mail accounts, some individuals set up a separate account for any ordering that they do so advertisements come to that e-mail account rather than their standard account. Viruses attached to e-mailed files are also an increasing problem. These are discussed more under Reading Attachments.

A few commonalties related to sending and receiving attachments are discussed here. Review the documentation or online help to learn more of the specifics for handling attachments on the system.

Inserting attachments

Most mail packages have a menu command or a tab that starts a separate dialog screen to insert an attachment. Once on the dialog screen, users can browse the computer and point and click the file to be added. Some mail programs provide the ability to send multiple attachments at once; others will zip (compact them into one file) multiple files before sending them.

Reading attachments

Most programs use an icon on the e-mail message list screen that indicates an attachment is present. For example, Microsoft Outlook uses a paper clip image to indicate an attachment. In order to open and view it, the receiver must have the same software or something that will interpret the original file and allow it to be read. Typically, clicking on the attachment indicator either opens the file or opens a dialog box that allows the viewer to save the attachment to a file or to open the attachment. To protect the computer, it is wise not to open attachments without checking them for a virus unless certain of the sender. Malicious computer hackers have now developed systems that enable them to access a user's address file and send messages to everyone in the list, making it appear as if the message is from that user. Thus, it is prudent not to open attachments, even from known individuals, unless they are expected. Executable (.exe) attachments may contain viruses, and once opened, they will create a variety of problems on the computer. Save the attachment to a file—just be sure to note in what folder the file is being saved—and then check it with an antivirus program such as Norton Utilities or McAfee Antivirus software before opening. If a file with a virus is found, delete the file from both e-mail and the computer's delete folder without opening it. Some systems routinely check all attachments before permitting the user to open them.

Listservs

People with common interests frequently join to form an organization. The type of interests and the structures of organization have wide variations. The joining of people with common interests also occurs in the virtual world of the Internet. The term listserv comes from one of the software programs used to support this process. Individuals subscribe to a group with a specific focus and send e-mail, called "posts," to the listserv. The post is automatically sent to all members of the list. Some examples of listservs of interest to nurses are found in Figure 10.3.

Listserv Program

This software program maintains the mailing list for a group of people with common interests. To join the group, or to subscribe, individuals send an e-mail message to the listserv's e-mail address. Because this message will be read and answered by a computer program, the message must follow the specific format required by the listserv software. Several different listserv software programs exist. Some examples of common listserv programs include Listproc, ListServ, and Majordomo.

The List

The membership list includes the group of people who have joined together by subscribing to the same list. The list will have a computer name that reflects the interest of the group. For example, snurs-1 is the name of a list for undergraduate nursing students. To communicate with other people on the list, participants send a message to the list's e-mail address. The message will then be sent as an individual e-mail message to each person on the list. When the message is distributed to each member on the list, it is referred to as "posted to the group."

Types of Lists

There are two types of lists. On a moderated list, each e-mail message to the list is reviewed and approved by a person before it is posted. On an unmoderated list, no one reviews posts before they are sent to members. Most lists are unmoderated. The list relies on the integrity of its members to abide by the list rules.

Joining a List

Most lists have directions that can be accessed either through e-mail or on the website that introduces the listserv. Be sure to save the directions for later use after subscribing to a listserv. Procedures for joining listservs are similar. The following steps represent the typical approach to joining a list.

1. Address the e-mail message to the listserv's e-mail address, not the list's e-mail address. For example, **listserv@listserve.arizona.edu** is the address of a listserv.
2. Put no other information in the header. Leave the subject line blank.
3. In the body of the message, type the following:

   Subscribe <list name> <firstname lastname>. For example: **subscribe nursenet Nancy Smith**

   Some listserv software programs accept the word sub in place of the word subscribe, whereas others require the word join. Some listserv software programs require the e-mail address in place of the first and last name.
4. Put no other information in the body of the e-mail message. Do not sign your name or thank the listserv. Remember this is NOT a communication with a person but is rather a set of commands being sent to a computer.
5. If unsuccessful, an error message from the computer will be e-mailed back. This message will try to indicate what mistake was made. If the message is not meaningful, get help at the local site.
6. If successful, a welcome message from the listserv will arrive. It may contain a great deal of information that is not entirely meaningful initially, but save this message!
7. If there is a time when participation in the listserv will be decreased and e-mail not read, send a message to the listserv suspending the mail service. To stop receiving mail from the list, send an unsubscribe message to the listserv's address. The specific directions for stopping mail or for unsubscribing are included in the Welcome Message from the list. Failing to stop listserv mail results in a full mailbox, and messages are bounced back to the listserv. This is very poor list etiquette. Some lists permit archiving messages while on vacation.

Posting an E-Mail Message to a List

It is wise to read several postings on a list before posting a message. Each list has its own culture. It is helpful to know the list and the nature of the list before posting.

1. Send the appropriate message to the list's address. NURSENET is a global forum on nursing issues. Note the difference in the list's address **(nursenet@listserv.arizona.edu)** and the listserv's address **(listserv@listserv.arizona.edu)**. In both cases, the domain part of the address is the same, but the user ID part of the address is different. When posting a message to the list, users are communicating with people and not a computer. Many lists require users to type an ID and password before the messages can be posted.

2. Put the topic of the message in the subject line. This is very helpful to receivers reading their e-mail directory. If the posting is a response to another person's e-mail, use the same words to identify the subject topic as the previous sender used. Many mail programs will insert the subject and address if the reply function is selected. If selecting the reply function with an e-mail message from a listserv, check to be sure that the mail program inserted the correct list address.

3. When typing the message, use appropriate netiquette.

4. Because some mail programs clip off the header on incoming messages, always sign the message with the name and e-mail address at the end of the message.

Newsgroups

Usenet is an informal group of computer systems that exchanges news. The news exchanged is organized into newsgroups. These newsgroups can be conceptualized as a cross between a listserv and a bulletin board. People with a common area of interest subscribe to a listserv. The same is true for a newsgroup. Once a user subscribes to a listserv, each message that is posted to the list is sent to the user individually. This does not happen with a newsgroup. With a newsgroup, the messages are posted to a central location in the local system. To read these messages and interact with the group, users must use a software program called a newsreader. Today, most web browsers have newsreaders built into them, and thus, more people are involved in newsgroups.

Newsgroups are organized by topics in a hierarchical tree structure. The first part of the topic identification is general. Each successive part becomes more specific. For example, the newsgroup related to nursing has the following name: sci.med.nursing. The newsgroup for nurse practitioners is named alt.npractitioners.

Individuals may read a newsgroup by linking on "Groups" from Google at http://www.google.com/. Google provides a service that maintains a list of newsgroups and allows web access. Figure 10.4 shows general Usenet names and the opening screen that allows searching for the desired group. To select a group, use the name, for example, sci.med.nursing, or search a specific topic to see what newsgroups are of interest. After finding a newsgroup on the desired topic, current postings can be accessed by clicking on the articles from this newsgroup.

Internet Conferencing

Internet conferencing involves two or more people interacting with one another over the Internet, engaging in a real-time conversation and receiving more or less immediate replies, depending on the speed of their connections. Chat, or text-based interactions, was the original and main initial form of this conferencing. Now audio and video conferencing via the Internet is common. Rather than calling a meeting or phoning colleagues, Internet conferencing uses a software program and the appropriate audio

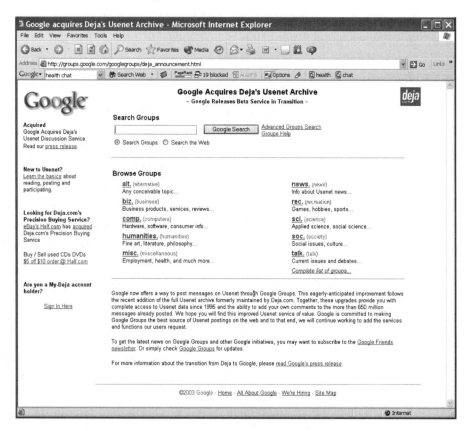

Figure 10.4

Accessing
Newsgroups

and video accessories to allow participants to speak to and see colleagues over the Internet. Currently, programs such as Microsoft's NetMeeting allow audio and/or video conferencing, sharing of a whiteboard (writing space like a blackboard that everyone in the meeting can see), and sharing applications. Sharing applications means that users can open and show a colleague a spreadsheet of quality assurance data, for example, and the colleague does not need to have the spreadsheet software to see this application. NetMeeting comes with Internet Explorer and can be downloaded free from the Microsoft site on the Internet if not already included with the computer software bundle.

Chat

Although some chat rooms support graphics and voice, the basic chat interface is text. Text chat involves two or more people communicating by typing messages that appear in a text window, visible to the other people in the same chat room. People use chat to communicate about specific topics and to meet new people online and because it offers a more rapid response than e-mail. In fact, chat rooms are one of the most used resources on the Internet. However, like chatting in a crowded room, often many simultaneous conversations are taking place. In text chat, the participant will see all of the messages that are part of those different conversations in the order that they were entered into the system. Thus, following the sequence of a particular line of the conversation may be confusing at first.

Most chat systems allow participants to send private messages to individuals in the chat room as well as to participate with the group. Some chat programs, such as ICQ and ichat Pager, allow users to compile a "buddy list" of friends on the Internet. Using these programs, users can set up personal chat rooms and chat privately with friends. The same "instant message" is available to AOL subscribers; their buddies do not need to subscribe to AOL but can simply download the software. Instant messaging, or private chat, is becoming increasingly common. The process for participating in chat rooms is similar in most programs:

- Log in.
- Choose a username, the name that everyone else in the chat room will see. Register as required by the chat room. Some people use a real name, but others use a nickname for better privacy—that is a personal choice. As with other user IDs, each name must be unique.

- Read messages in the current chat session. Messages from those participating in the chat session as well as system messages and information about people entering and leaving the room appear in a box on the screen. Each message is preceded by the username of the person submitting the message so that each can tell who said what.

- Type the message into the text entry box, and press Enter.

Using one of the many search engines on the Internet, it is possible to find a chat room of interest. Most search engines support chat rooms. There are also topic-specific chat rooms located on many other websites; for example, the Chatmags page shown in Figure 10.2 lists some health-related chat rooms. Chat rooms are usually organized around topics of interest, age, or other categories. Chatiquette is similar to netiquette in terms of the words and behavior acceptable while participating in a chat room. For more information about chatiquette, visit http://www.ker95.com/chat101/html/chatiquette.html.

Online Learning

With advances in technology, educators are commonly putting educational materials online. Software such as Blackboard and WebCT support the use of the Internet for class activities such as posting syllabi, assignments, grades, testing, and discussion groups. In some instances, entire courses are being taught via the web with no regularly scheduled classroom sessions and no in-person contact among students or teacher. Web-based systems are asynchronous; thus, students are able to use Internet-based materials from wherever they are, whenever they want, and as often as they want. Traveling to an educational site is no longer necessary, as students can access materials from any computer that has Internet access. However, there is more to facilitating learning than merely having course materials on the web. When exploring an online course, examine it to determine how well it includes the following:

- A list of goals or outcomes that describes what can be achieved from the course and how this will be useful.

- Clearly outlined expectations for the projects/homework expected and how the grade is achieved.

- A variety of learning experiences guided through online information and resources.

- Modules that organize topics into manageable units for learning.

- Opportunity for interaction between the students and teacher.
- A way to ask questions and receive answers.
- Control, to some extent, of the learning environment to set the pace and progression through course modules.
- Examples to facilitate understanding of material being studied. The opportunity to practice using material and to apply material to problems or cases.
- Feedback on practice and the use of the material.
- Tools to help reflect on what is being learned and to guide setting the next steps in the learning process.
- Resources in the form of hyperlinks, tables, charts, summaries, and references.

Students who are looking for an online learning experience should also consider their own motivation as well as the structure of the course. When examining whether an online course is appropriate, ask the following questions:

- Am I self-directed so that I can identify what I want from the course and use the course materials to do so?
- Am I disciplined so that I will keep up with the work without the structure of a regular class session?
- Can I feel satisfied from interaction online versus in person?

Learners who are goal directed, disciplined, and comfortable interacting on the computer might find online learning of interest.

SUMMARY

This chapter introduced terminology and procedures for using common methods of computer communication. Using e-mail, subscribing to listservs and newsgroups, and accessing chat rooms are all useful methods of exchanging ideas and information about health and health care delivery. Trends toward using the computer for Internet conferencing and educational experiences are expanding. Criteria for evaluating online learning were provided as a basis for making personal decisions about this method of learning.

Additional Resources

Chat guide. (n.d.). Retrieved August 13, 2004, from http://www.best-of-web.com/entertainment/chat.shtml

Computer User High-Tech Dictionary. (n.d.). Retrieved August 13, 2004, from http://www.computeruser.com/resources/dictionary/noframes/

Email privacy. (n.d.). Retrieved April 5, 2004, from http://lookoff.com/privacy/privacy_email.php3

Gumbrecht, J. (2004, August 15). Spim mixes with spam with online chats. *Dallas Morning News.* Retrieved August 15, 2004, from http://www.indystar.com/articles/4/170299-2224-223.html

Metz, C. (2003, April 22). Spyware: It's lurking on the machine. *PC Magazine Online.* Retrieved July 25, 2004, from http://www.pcmag.com/article2/0,4149,977889,00.asp

Michael Lerner Productions. (2004). *Master the basics: Netiquette.* Retrieved August 13, 2004, from http://www.learnthenet.com/english/html/09netiqt.htm

Online netiquette.com. (2004). Retrieved August 13, 2004, from http://www.onlinenetiquette.com/

Protect the PC. (n.d.). Retrieved August 13, 2004, from http://support.microsoft.com/default.aspx?scid=%2fdirectory%2fworldwide%2fen-gb%2fprotect.asp

Protect thyself online. (2004, September). *Consumer Reports, 69*(9), 12–19.

Spies lurking in the PC? The basics of spyware (adware). Retrieved July 25, 2004, from http://www.webtechgeek.com/center_Frame_Spyware.htm

Swartz, J. (2004, July 27). Poll shows some look forward to reading spam. *USA Today*, p. 4B.

The core rules of netiquette. Retrieved July 13, 2004, from http://www.albion.com/netiquette/corerules.html

Webopedia: Online electronic dictionary. Retrieved August 13, 2004, from http://www.webopedia.com/

What you should know about spyware. (April 16, 2004). Retrieved July 25, 2004, from http://www.microsoft.com/athome/security/spyware/devious-software.mspx

Self-evaluation for potential online students. Retrieved August 14, 2004, from http://www.webct.com/oriented/ViewContent?contentID=876625

What you should know about spyware. (2004, April 16). Retrieved July 25, 2004, from http://www.microsoft.com/athome/security/spyware/devious-software.mspx.

Exercise 1: Using e-mail
Objectives
1. Access an e-mail system.
2. Change the password.
3. Read, save, and delete the mail.

Activity

1. Obtain an account from the computer center.

   An account gives the user permission to use the system. This permission comes in the form of a user ID and a unique password. If the instructor or school has not provided you with an account, a computer account needs to be set up before doing this exercise. If you have a user ID and password, you are ready to begin this exercise.

2. Find the documentation.

   Most institutions have documentation for computer programs available to users. Short handouts are usually available free either in print or at the institution's website. More detailed documentation may be sold through the computer center and/or bookstore. Find out where and how you can obtain documentation in the institution. Obtain a copy of the documentation for signing on to the system and for using e-mail. With an account, you may also be able to access online help.

3. Sign on.

   Follow the directions for signing on to the computer system. Generally, this means type the **User ID**, and press the **Tab** key to go to the next text field. Type the **Password**, and press **Enter** or click **OK**.

   Remember that the password will not appear on the screen. In most mail programs it appears as ****** in the **Password** text box.

   If a message appears on the screen saying **invalid password**, **login incorrect**, or something similar, try typing the user ID and password again. Some systems are case sensitive; thus, you need to note whether you should or should not use capitals in either the user ID or password. However, most systems give you three tries to get in and then the account is locked out; you will then need to see the account administrator to have it unlocked.

4. Change the password.

   When signing on for the first time, some computer systems require you to change the password before proceeding. If the system does not require you to change the password, this should be the first action after signing on. Check the documentation for the specific process for changing a password.

   In newer mail programs:
   Click the password **Icon**, OR Select an option on a **Menu**, OR Click a **Hypertext** link.

   In older or mainframe based systems:
   Type a command such as **Set password** or **Passwd**, and press **Enter**.
   When prompted for the current password, type the **Current password**, and press **Enter** or click **OK**.
   When prompted, type the **New Password**, and press **Enter** or click **OK**.
   When prompted, type the **New Password** a second time, and then press **Enter** or click **OK**.

When typing passwords throughout this procedure, the passwords do not show on the screen. Processing the change is usually instant, although on some systems, there may be a time lag before the new password takes effect. Check the system documentation.

5. Access and read the mail.

Start the **Mail** program.

Click the **Icon**, or type the **Command** to open the Inbox containing the mail.

6. Open and read each message.

Double click or highlight the **Mail message**, and press **Enter**.

If this approach does not work, look at the screen for directions, and read the written documentation for the system. After you read each e-mail message, look at how the mail directory changed.

7. Exit the mail program.

In windows-based e-mail programs,

Click the **Close** button in the upper right corner or

Click **File**, **Exit** from the menu bar.

In command based programs,

Type **exit**, **quit**, **eoj**, **logoff**, or **logout** or some such command, and press **Enter**.

8. Send a message.

Find the **E-mail address** of a friend. Asking the friend for his or her address is the easiest way to do this. In college settings, there may be a faculty, staff, and student directory online that contains listings of addresses.

Start the **E-mail** program.

Type the **E-mail address** of the friend in the To: text box. Many programs permit you to select the address from the e-mail address book by double clicking it.

Press the **Tab** key twice, or click in the Subject text box. You do not need to CC yourself, and pressing the tab key twice passes the CC textbox. Most newer mail programs place a copy of all e-mail sent out in your sent folder.

Type in the **Subject**, and press **Tab** or click in the **Message** text box.

Type and format the **Message**.

Click the **Send** icon.

The procedure for composing an e-mail message varies greatly from one system to another. The previous information is the general process for many of today's e-mail programs. If this does not work, read the local documentation for the following information:

1. How do you initiate the function to compose a message?

2. How do you enter the address of the person who will receive this message?

3. How do you enter the e-mail message?

4. When the e-mail message is ready, how do you give the send command?

One way to test the understanding of the correct procedure at the location is to practice by sending yourself a message. Once you master the procedure, practice sending messages to a friend.

9. Reply to a message.

Open a **Mail Message** (double click it).

Click the **Reply to Sender** button. *The program inserts the sender's address and subject in those textboxes. The Subject text box uses the same subject and adds a RE: to it.*

Compose the **Response**, and click the **Send** button.

In some mail programs you will need to type the **Reply** command. If you have received a message as part of a distribution list, find out how to reply to the author and how to reply to everyone on the list.

10. Save or delete each message.

Highlight the **Message**.

Press the **Delete** key or button.

In some web-based mail programs, you delete messages by clicking in the square box next to the message, and then click the delete button.

Read the local documentation for the save and delete procedures. If you do not delete messages, the mailbox will become full and eventually new messages will be bounced back to the sender. Some mail programs leave the undeleted messages in the inbox, whereas others move them to an older message folder. You will know the message is in the inbox if the message is listed in the message list each time you start the mail program. Most systems permit you to move messages into online folders. Read the documentation for a procedure for saving messages in folders.

11. Exit the e-mail program.

In Windows e-mail programs:

Click the **Close** button in the upper right corner, or select **File**, **Exit** from the menu bar.

In command based programs:

Type the **Command**, as indicated in the system documentation (**exit**, **quit**, **eoj**, **log-off**, **logout**), and press **Enter**.

It is important to exit the e-mail system with the computer still running. If you turn the computer off or just walk away without exiting e-mail, someone else may be able to access the account without signing on. Once you exit the e-mail program, complete the computer sequence for shutting down the computer as specified by the laboratory, library, or other locale.

Assignment 1: Set Up an Online E-mail Account
Directions

1. Type this address into the Internet address box: **http://www.msn.com/** to access MSN, and click on the **hotmail** tab.

2. Click the **new user sign in**, and follow the instructions given. Be sure that you read all privacy information. When given the choice, be sure that you select the free e-mail. How much storage space do you get for the mail in this system?

3. Once you have registered, read the welcome message from MSN Hotmail. How often do you need to use this system for it to remain active?

4. Print this message to hand in, and answer the previous questions on the printout.

Assignment 2: Accessing a Newsgroup
Directions

1. Access Google's newslist from the Web browser (**www.google.com**).
   Click **Groups**. Click **Misc**. Click **Misc.Health** or **Misc Fitness**.

2. Look at the groups listed across the page. Note how active they have been by the amount of shading in the activity line. Select a group of interest. Print the web page that contains the subject threads.

3. Select a subject thread that has at least eight articles, and follow that thread. In the frame on the left of the page, select the discussion thread by clicking on the first message; read that post, and then click on the next in the list and so on.

4. Use the word processing package to answer the following questions:
   - What discussion topic did you select?
   - What was the general theme of messages to this topic?
   - What were the reactions to reading about this topic?
   - Would you like to participate in a newsgroup? If so what topics might be of interest? If not, what are the reasons?

5. Submit the responses to these questions and the web page printout.

Assignment 3: Compare and Contrast Listserv and Literature Search
Directions

1. Subscribe to a health-related listserv. Review the messages each week for the next 4 weeks. Make an annotated list of the topics discussed during those 4 weeks. At the end of 3 weeks, send a post to the listserv. At the end of 4 weeks, send a message to the listserv to unsubscribe. Turn in a copy of messages that you have posted as well as the list of the five top topics discussed.

2. Use an automated literature database to do a literature search. Limit the search to the last 2 years. Search for articles related to the focus of the listserv. For exam-

ple, if the listserv relates to home health nursing then use the words home health nursing as keywords when doing the literature search.

3. Turn in an annotated list of the five most common topics discussed in the literature. Write a brief paper comparing and contrasting the two lists of topics.

Assignment 4: Internet Resource Document
Directions

1. In this assignment, you will create an Internet resource document that can be used by other students. The document should include only those resources that can be accessed from the site. Resources on the Internet change frequently; thus, check each resource before adding it to the document. This means to make sure the address is correct and the site is still available.

2. Work in small groups (three to five people) to create the resource document. The resource document should include each of the following related to specific topics of interest to the discipline:

   a. A list of chat rooms with information on how to access them

   b. A list of listservs with directions for subscribing

   c. A list of newsgroups with directions for how to access them

3. After each small group completes its document, the class will create a master document identifying all resources found by the class.

Assignment 5: Evaluating Online Courses
Directions

1. Use a search engine (see Chapter 11) to search for online courses. You might try the terms "distance learning" and "online courses." When you find one that is not password protected and that you can explore, compare it to the criteria for examining online courses at the end of this chapter.

2. Using the word processor, make a flyer listing each criterion. Beside or under each of these, identify how well the course you examined meets these criteria. Give enough information to lure someone to a good course or steer them clear of one that you think has not yet been well developed. Be sure that the course title and web address are on the flyer. Be creative with the design, and include graphics if you wish.

3. Submit the flyer.

Information: Access, Evaluation, and Use

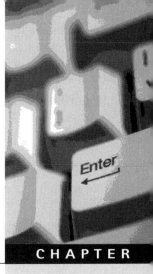

CHAPTER

11

OBJECTIVES

1. Define an information need, including concepts and terms, that can be used to search for information.
2. Develop a variety of search strategies to access information from library and Internet resources.
3. Use a systematic approach to evaluate the quality of information from a variety of sources.
4. Identify appropriate and inappropriate uses of information.
5. Explain general principles for documenting information resources.

Starting in the late 1980s, a growing body of literature called for all nurses to be information literate. Examples of these are presented in Table 11.1. Note the concepts that are reflected in these titles. Critical thinking, evidence-based practice, and life-long learning all require information literacy. In 2001, the American Nurses Association described information

Table 11.1   Early Calls for Information Literacy

Author	Title of Article and Journal	Year Published
Cheek, J. & Doskatsch, I.	Information Literacy: A Resource for Nurses as Life-Long Learners in *Nursing Educator Today*	1998
Weaver, S.M.	Information Literacy: Educating for Life Long Learning in *Nurse Educator Today*	1992
Fox, L. M., Richter, J. M. & White, N.E.	Pathways to Information Literacy in *Journal of Nursing Education*	1989
Fox, L. M.	Teaching the Wise Use of Information — Evaluation Skills for Nursing Students in *Western Journal of Nursing Research*	1989

literacy as a required skill for all beginning nurses. (Staggers et al. 2001). Information literacy is defined by the American Library Association (2000) as the ability to recognize when information is needed as well as the ability to locate, evaluate, and use the needed information effectively. The American Library Association went on to identify five information literacy standards for higher education. An information literate person is able to

- Determine the nature and scope of an information need.

- Effectively and efficiently access that information.

- Critically evaluate the information and its sources and incorporate that information into one's knowledge base.

- Use information effectively for a specific purpose.

- Appreciate the economic, legal, and social issues surrounding the use of information and use that information in an ethical and legal manner.

The five standards, along with an emphasis on information related to health, provide the organizing structure for this chapter. The chapter begins with a discussion of how information can be effectively accessed. More specifically, the emphasis will be on how to access information that has been stored in computer systems. The ability to access information makes it possible to access all kinds of information from a wide variety of sources. That information may be accurate or inaccurate, objective or biased, current or outdated.

Inaccurate and misleading information does not come with a label indicating that there is a problem. In fact, many times the author will try to ensure that the information appears to be high quality. The reader must determine the quality of the information.

Even good information can be misused. For example, the Internet includes many excellent sites with information about the importance of adequate vitamin intake during pregnancy. However, referring a patient to one of these sites with no appreciation of her ability to read and understand the data is a misuse of information.

► 11.1 IDENTIFYING AN INFORMATION NEED

Information needs come from a variety of sources. Some common examples include a classroom assignment, a health problem in the family, or a clinical assignment. In each case, the first step is to write a statement describing the question to be answered. For example, in preparing to write a pamphlet on exercise for an older population, what information would be needed?

- Exercises that are valuable and not valuable for older clients
- Writing materials about the general population and health literacy
- Signs and symptoms appropriate to the older population if one is overexercising or underexercising

Several other information needs can be identified. In addition, it is important to identify other terms that can be used to find the same or related information. How many different terms can be used for "older persons"? Each of the information needs that is identified and the terms that are used to express these needs can be used to access information.

► 11.2 ACCESS

Accessing information begins by understanding how data are stored in the computer. Data are stored in an orderly and systematic structure called a database. As was explained in Chapter 8, a database is built of tables that contain records. Each record refers to a specific entity and includes a set number of fields. Data related to the entity are stored in the fields. For example, if the entity is a journal article, the fields most likely include the author(s), article title, journal source, and an abstract of the article, along with several other fields. The process of searching for data in a database involves matching specific attributes about the entity with the field where the datum is stored. For example, if a search request was looking for a book that was written by the author Joos, the database management system would search in the author field for the name Joos. Each time Joos was found in an author field it would refer to a book written by Joos. However, if a record included Smith in the author field and Joos in the title field, this book would not meet the search criteria. This would not be a book written by Joos, but rather a book about Joos.

A specific type of database designed to store information about articles, books, and other print materials is a bibliographic database. The fields in a bibliographic database include the title, author, abstract, date of publication, along with several other details about the item being indexed in the database. Increasingly, bibliographic databases also include the full text. Table 11.2 lists common bibliographic databases that are used in health care. These are only a few of the many important health-related bibliographic databases. Access to these databases may be provided by the group or organization that produced the database, or access to the database may be provided by an information vendor who has leased the database. Table 11.3 lists examples of the most

Table 11.2   Selected Bibliographical and Full Text Databases in Health Care

Database	Description
AMED	The Allied and Complementary Medicine Database (AMED) is produced by the Health Care Information Service of the British Library. This database covers journals in complementary medicine, palliative care, and several professions allied to medicine.
CINAHL	Recently purchased by Elton B. Stephens Company (EBSCO), the Cumulative Index to Nursing & Allied Health (CINAHL) database provides coverage of the literature related to nursing and allied health. More than 1600 journals are regularly indexed along with publications from the American Nurses Association and the National League for Nursing. This database overlaps MEDLINE; however, there are several citations in CINAHL that are not included in MEDLINE.
ClinicalTrials.gov	ClinicalTrials.gov provides regularly updated information about federally and privately supported clinical research using human volunteers.
Cochrane Database of Systematic Reviews	This database produced by the Cochrane Library includes full text articles that review the effects of healthcare. The reviews are highly structured and systematic, with evidence included or excluded to minimize bias.

Table 11.2 Selected Bibliographical and Full Text Databases in Health Care. (continued)

Database	Description
LexisNexis	This resource is a full-text legal information service covering newspapers, magazines, wire services, federal and state court opinions, federal and state statutes, federal regulations, and SEC filings such as 10-K's, 10-Q's.
MD Consult	This full text database provided by Elsevier Company includes medical texts, articles from clinical journals, peer-reviewed clinical practice guidelines with integrated MEDLINE searches, customizable patient education handouts, and a drug database of more than 30,000 medications.
MEDLINE	MEDLINE® (Medical Literature, Analysis, and Retrieval System Online) produced by the US National Library of Medicine is considered the primary bibliographic database of biomedical literature. It includes citations from over 4,600 journals including nursing, dentistry, veterinary medicine, pharmacy, allied health, and pre-clinical sciences. Increased coverage of life sciences such as aspects of biology, environmental science, marine biology, plant and animal science as well as biophysics and chemistry began in 2000. By the end of 2001, most citations previously included in separate NLM specialty databases have also been added to MEDLINE.
MedlinePlus	Produced by the National Library of Medicine this database of health information is designed for health professionals and consumers alike. It combines references from MEDLINE with extensive information from the National Institutes of Health and other sources on over 650 diseases and conditions.
PsycInfo	Produced by the American Psychological Association this database includes citations and summaries of journal articles, book chapters, books, dissertations, and technical reports in the field of psychology as well as the psychological aspects of related disciplines, such as medicine, psychiatry, and nursing.
SPORTDiscus	Produced by the Sport Information Resource Centre (SIRC) this database covers all aspects of sport, fitness, recreation, and related fields.

Table 11.3 Electronic Information Vendors in Health Care

Company Name	URL
EBSCO Informational Services	http://www.ebsco.com/home/
Elsevier	http://www.elsevier.com/
OVID Technologies	http://www.ovid.com/site/index.jsp
ProQuest Company	http://www.proquest.com/
StatRef	http://www.statref.com/default.htm
The Thomson Corporation	http://www.thomson.com/

common information vendors in health care. Most of these vendors produce their own databases as well as lease access to databases produced by other groups. Table 11.4 provides examples of the databases offered by selected information vendors. Although a large number of databases and several vendors provide electronic access to health care information, some significant gaps

Table 11.4   Examples of Databases offered by Selected Information Vendors

Examples of Health Related Databases Provided by ProQuest®

Database Name	Focus and Content of the Database
CINAHL	more than 1,200 health-related publications: 270 of them are in full text format.
MEDLINE	more than 4,300 publications; over 400 are full text.
ProQuest® Nursing Journals	over 350 full text journals.
ProQuest® Medical Library	more than 400 full text references from the MEDLINE Database.
PsycINFO	over 1,900 psychological, psychiatric, and related publications; over 350 full text.

Examples of Health Related Databases Provided by Thomas Gale

Database Name	Focus and Content of the Database
Health and Wellness Resource Center	over 700 health/medical journals with hundreds of pamphlets; 75% are full text.
Health Reference Center – Academic	over 400 pamphlets and selected health related topics.

Examples of Health Related Databases Provided by EBSCO

Database Name	Focus and Content of the Database
CINAHL	over 1700 nursing and allied health journals.
Clinical Pharmacology	drug monographs on all US prescription drugs, over the counter drugs and hard-to-find herbal and nutritional supplements.
Health Source Consumer Edition	collection of consumer health information resources including nearly 300 full text journals.
Health Source: Nursing/ Academic Edition	more than 550 scholarly full text journals and as well as abstracts and indexing for nearly 850 journals.
MEDLINE	abstracts from over 4,600 current biomedical journals.
PsycINFO	nearly two million citations and summaries of journal articles, book chapters, books and dissertations, all in the field of psychology.
Psychology and Behavioral Sciences Collection	nearly 550 full text journals covering topics such as emotional and behavioral characteristics, psychiatry & psychology, mental processes, anthropology, and observational and experimental methods.

exist. For example, at least two vendors offer access to online full-text medical books but no vendors offer access to a collection of online nursing books.

Whichever company or organization is providing the access will determine the specific database management system and in turn the user interface for searching that database. Many users become confused between the bibliographic database and the bibliographic database management system. PubMed is an example of a bibliographical database management system. PubMed is a World Wide Web retrieval service developed by the National Library of Medicine. It provides access, free of charge, to MEDLINE. It also contains links to the full-text versions of articles at participating publishers' websites. The URL for PubMed is http://www.ncbi.nlm.nih.gov/PubMed/. However, several other bibliographic database management systems can be used to access MEDLINE. Because vendors and information providers use different bibliographic database management systems and user interfaces, this book does not contain specific commands for using them. Each bibliographic database management system does contain a help section. This is where the specific information for searching is found.

General Principles for Searching

Two factors determine how much time and effort one needs to exert when searching for information—one's level of expertise with the topic and one's knowledge of search strategies. An expert in a specific field will find it much easier to do an efficient and focused search. For example, if the searcher is an expert in maternity who is looking for information about a specific complication of pregnancy, the information is usually found very quickly. This is because an expert knows the language and how knowledge is organized within the field.

However, if the searcher is not an expert, the process of searching for information is in many respects recursive. A student usually begins by identifying a topic about which more information is needed. For example, a student may take a course on managed care and may be assigned to report on a controversial issue related to managed care. As the search for information on the topic of managed care begins, often related information that does not really apply to the assignment is found. At the same time, there might be more information about this topic than can be used. In the process of selecting materials that will apply and eliminating materials that do not apply, the search will become more focused. This initial exploration can be frustrating, but it is very important. It is during this initial stage that one becomes familiar with the terminology and the way that the related information is organized. Just looking for a few related articles or Internet sites and then stopping the search means much will be missed.

Indexing, Standard Languages, and Keywords

A record within a database will include several fields. The database management system that interfaces with the database will offer the user the opportunity to search on these fields. Database management programs are usually designed for both experienced and inexperienced users. The experienced user will understand both the concept and the procedure for searching on specific fields. For example, many literature database management systems are designed so that the user can search for a specific author. In these systems, the user would enter a command such as au-Whitman or a-Whitman. The search results from these systems would include all books that were authored by Whitman.

On the other hand, these same literature database management systems can function well for a user who is less familiar with these concepts. With these systems, any term that is entered by the user will be compared with several fields. For example, the user could enter the term Whitman, and if this term occurred in the title, author, or even the abstract, it would be included in the search results. Some database management system offer the opportunity to search on a specific field; some of the more common fields and commands available are included in Table 11.5.

The two fields that are most frequently confused are keywords and subject. Both of these fields identify the topic discussed in the reference being accessed. However, keywords and subject terms are developed very differ-

Table 11.5   Common Searchable Fields in Bibliographical Databases

Abbreviation	Field
Au or A	Author
Ti or T	Title
Yr	Year Published
Pb	Publisher
K	Keyword
Su	Subject

ently. Using the same term as a keyword and then as a subject will often produce overlapping but different search results. Keywords are terms that may have been selected by the author, publisher, or the developer of the literature database management system to identify the topic of the article. Some literature database management systems are designed so that any word that appears in the title, author field, and/or abstract will function as a keyword. However, keyword terms are not standardized in any way. For example, an article about cirrhosis may be indexed on the keyword "liver" or "hepatic disease" or "cirrhosis." The same article in different literature database management systems may have different keywords that are associated with it.

Subject terms, on the other hand, are very standardized. Individuals who are experts in understanding indexing and taxonomy concepts develop these in a systematic process. Standard sets of subject terms are often referred to as a controlled vocabulary. One example of a controlled vocabulary is MeSH (Medical Subject Headings). MeSH is used in indexing MEDLINE. This means that there are people who read each article and then select the specific indexing terms from the controlled vocabulary. If a subject term is used, one can expect to find all of the materials that relate to that term. Because keywords are not standardized, searching on a keyword may lead to incomplete results.

It is also important when planning a search strategy to understand that different databases may be indexed with different subject terms. For example, CINAHL (Cumulative Index of Nursing and Allied Health Literature) has its own controlled vocabulary that is different from MeSH. This means that the same article may be indexed under different terms in CINAHL than it is in MEDLINE.

By understanding how keywords and subject differ, it is possible to maximize the advantages of both of these indexing approaches in developing a search strategy. Using terms and concepts that were developed in clarifying the information needed, one can select a specific database or group of databases. For example, if the information needed is related to the concept nursing diagnosis, CINAHL would be a better database than PsycInfo. Because most library information systems permit the user to search several databases at the same time, the next step is to use the library information system to indicate which databases to include in the search. The identified terms are entered into the library information system as keywords. The resulting hits from the search are reviewed to find references that fit best with the information need. These best-fit citations are then reviewed to determine the subject terms that were used to index these references. There will be several different subject terms. For example, an article describing the types of injuries that occur when children are abused may be indexed on subject terms related to trauma, children, or abuse. Select the subject term that fits best with the identified information need. A new search using the subject term will result in a more comprehensive list of hits. However, that list of hits may include too many or too few references.

Boolean Search Strategies

Several approaches can be used to expand or exclude references from search results. These approaches are built on the concept of Boolean search strategies. Chapter 8 introduced these concepts, and they are explained in more detail here.

And

By searching on two topics using the word **AND** between the two topics, one is able to find materials that are about both topics. For example, if searching for information dealing with computers and nursing diagnosis, the search might look like this: **Computers AND "nursing diagnosis."** In many systems, using the symbol + (plus) in front of both terms will function the same as using the term **AND** between the terms. Each of the citations that was listed in the search results would be about both computers and nursing diagnosis. The term **AND** is used to narrow the search results to a more focused group of hits. There are quotes around the phrase nursing diagnosis. Using quotes usually results in the terms being used as a phrase rather than as two separate terms. If nursing diagnosis is seen as two separate terms, any articles that were indexed with the term nursing and the term diagnosis would be included in the search results. With quotes, the two terms must be next to each other.

Or

Sometimes a concept can be represented by several different but closely related terms. Many of these terms would be identified when analyzing the information need. For example, the concept abuse is related to the terms intimate partner abuse, family abuse, or family violence. If the term **OR** is used between each of these terms, the citations in the search result will include references indexed on any of these terms. **OR** is used to expand a search.

Truncation

Sometimes the topic may have several words with the same base. One example is nurse, nursing, and nurses. In this case, using truncation may be more efficient than **OR**. With truncation, type the beginning of the term, and then use a symbol to indicate that the search includes any citation that has a term beginning with these letters. The specific symbol will depend on the specific database management system in use. Some common symbols include nurs*, nurs?, and nurs$. Remember that when one uses truncation the search results will include every term that begins with the beginning letters. For example, what other terms begin with the letters nurs in addition to the terms nurse, nurses, and nursing?

Not

The term **NOT** is used to eliminate references. For example, one might need information about assistive heart devices but not want citations dealing with pacemakers. In this case, the search would be "assistive heart devices" **NOT** pacemakers.

Near

The term **NEAR** is used when the terms should be located within the next few words. For example, the search may be for information on teaching people about computers. In this case, **teaching NEAR computers** might be useful.

Figure 11.1 is a diagram that demonstrates the concepts of **AND**, **OR**, and **NOT**. Several other operators can be used to expand or limit a search. These strategies are usually explained in the help section of the library information system or the Internet search site.

Figure 11.1

Understanding
Boolean search
strategies

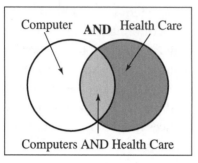

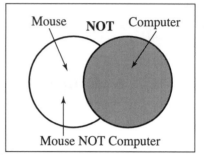

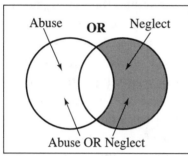

Search Sites and Engines

The Internet contains a vast amount of information. However, important differences exist between information on the Internet and information resources in an academic library. Table 11.6 compares key differences.

Search sites are places on the Internet where one can go to find information. Search engines are software that is used to find and index information. Several hundred different search sites and engines are available on the Internet. Table 11.7 lists the URLs for selected general and health specific search sites. Each has a different interface or appearance, but they all have several common features. Understanding how to use search sites begins by understanding relevant terms.

Refer to Chapter 9 for definitions of directory, keyword search sites, meta search sites, hits, query, ranking, and robot. Listed here are additional search site terms.

Meta-directory   A meta-directory is a directory of links to other directories. These are sometimes called a directory of directories or directories of directories.

Ranking   See Chapter 9 for a definition. The methods used by search engines to rank pages vary. For example, the number of times a site is linked from

Table 11.6 Key Differences Between Library And Internet Resources

Library Resources	Resources on the Internet
Resources go through a review process.	Many resources are posted without a review process.
Resources are purchased by the library and distributed free or at a discount.	A wide variety of financial approaches are used and these may not always be obvious.
There is a professional staff available to assist in finding resources.	The Internet does not usually provide personal assistance.
Library resources are indexed and organized.	There is no organizational plan for the Internet.
Library resources are selected to ensure a comprehensive collection related to key topics.	The Internet provides an eclectic hodgepodge of information.
Information found in a library can usually be accessed at a later date.	Information on the Internet may or may not be available at a later date.

other sites can be used to determine ranking. Some search engines will sell ranking placement; thus, ranks need to be viewed with caution. However, they are very important. On August 31, 2004, the search strategy (nursing AND Computers) on Google (www.google.com) returned 1,990,000 hits. If one spent 10 seconds looking at each hit, it would take a little over 7 months to skim over all of these hits. This conclusion is based on the assumption one was viewing these results 24 hours a day and does not spend more than 10 seconds on any site.

Table 11.7 URLs for General and Health Specific Search Engines.

General Search Sites	Health Specific Search Sites
Google: http://www.google.com	**MedHunt:** http://www.hon.ch/MedHunt/
Yahoo: http://www.yahoo.com	**MedNets:** http://www.mednets.com/
Ask Jeeves: http://www.askjeeves.com	**PubMed:** http://www.ncbi.nlm.nih.gov/entrez/query.fcgi
Teoma: http://www.teoma.com	**Entrez:** http://www.ncbi.nlm.nih.gov/gquery/gquery.fcgi

Stop Word   A stop word is a word that is ignored in a query because the word is so commonly used that it makes no contribution to relevancy. Examples are words such as *and, get, the,* as well as *you.*

One uses a search engine by accessing the search site on the Internet. There are several ways to find sites. For example, most academic libraries provide links to several sites. Search Engine Watch located at http://www. searchenginewatch.com/ provides a directory of several different types of search sites. On the home page of the search site, there will be a field or box where search terms are entered to create a query. Before trying a query, it is often helpful to access the help section. Sometimes this section is referred to as search tips. Because each of the search sites is different, there will be variations on each search site. Think of it like a car. Each model is different, but there are many common functions. The process for searching is very similar to the process used when doing library searches.

In many cases, the first searches will result in a large list of irrelevant hits. One of the reasons for this is that many search engines automatically assume OR is intended between any of the words in the query. Thus, if one is looking for things about the University of Virginia, on many search sites, the hit will include "university" and "Virginia." Only some of these will contain both terms and relate to the desired subject. The Power Searches, Search Tips, or Help included with the search engine can assist in narrowing the search. Boolean search strategies will also help focus the search. Many search engines use a + (plus) in front of the term for AND and a − (minus) in front of the term for NOT. A blank space between terms can be considered as either an AND or an OR, depending on the search site.

► 11.3 EVALUATION OF INFORMATION

Although finding information that is specific for a topic can be a challenge, finding quality information can be even more of a challenge. One must always be sure to use high-quality information. The attributes of quality information provide a basis for developing criteria to evaluate information.

Information Attributes

Information attributes apply to all information, including health-related information. These attributes of information are used to develop criteria for evaluating the quality of information.

1. **Timely:** Information that is timely is true at this point in time. In other words, it is current. For example, in 1992, the Agency for Health Care Policy and Research released clinical practice guidelines on urinary incontinence. At that time there were close to 20 clinical practice guidelines published by this division of the US Government. There may be a copy of them in your school library. In 1996, the clinical practice guidelines on urinary incontinence were updated to reflect new findings. As of August 2004, only four of these clinical guidelines are still posted. They are located at http://www.ncbi.nlm.nih.gov/books/ bv.fcgi?call=bv.View..ShowSection&rid=hstat2.part.4408. The last updated guideline was posted in 2000, and the agency is now renamed Agency for Healthcare Research and Quality.

   When accessing information on the Internet or in a library, always check the date of the information at the site where the information is found. A word of caution applies when checking the date from an Internet site; the date may reflect the web page published date and not the article published date.

2. **Accurate:** Information is accurate when it does not contain errors or misleading information that could lead the reader to an incorrect conclusion. For example, using the search phrase "hiv does not cause aids" will result in several hits for sites that dispute a relationship between AIDS and the HIV virus. These sites contain inaccurate information.

3. **Verifiable:** Verifiable information can be checked at more than one source. There is consensus among experts and consistency on how the data are reported. Verifiable information is usually supported by quantifiable data. An example of verifiable information is the current nursing shortage. In this case, one might check government statistics, predictions from professional organizations, and health foundations such as the Pew Foundation. Although there may be slightly different numbers or predictions, each of these sites will confirm the existence of a nursing shortage.

4. **Accessible:** Accessible refers to how easy it is to obtain the information. For a number of years, MEDLINE was not generally available to the public. In the first 6 months that access to MEDLINE was offered free on the Internet, one third of all searches were conducted by the general public as opposed to professional health care providers. With the addition of MedlinePlus, this resource had become accessible to a widely diversified audience.

Information is accessible if one enters a search term for information and that information is in the search results. Four factors have a major influence. First are the terms or language used to store the information. If this is a bibliographic database, what words are in the title or in the abstract? How was the document indexed? If the information is located on the Internet, access depends on what words are used on the web page and the approach used by the Internet search engine to indexing. For example, does the Internet search engine search the entire document or only the first paragraph?

A second factor that determines access is the number of references that refers to the original document. In a bibliographic database, references are in the footnotes. Sometimes it is possible to click the footnote and be linked directly to the article. On the Internet, access is also determined by links. If there are several web pages that link to a document, one is more likely to find them either by browsing or by using a search engine.

The third factor that will determine accessibility is the ability to focus a search. Initial searches often find too much or too little information. One of the most effective approaches is to find one document that includes useful information and then use information from this document to find additional material.

A fourth factor that will determine accessibility is the functions added to the search engine software. For example, Elton B. Stephens Company has added reference linking. Reference linking offers three ways to link a particular article to other related resources. First, if a reference that is cited in the reference list of the original article is in the EBSCO database, a direct link from the cited reference to the actual reference will be provided. Second, clicking on a reference link at the top of the screen will create a list of references that have been cited in the original article. Finally, clicking the name of an author will create a list of other materials published by this author.

5. **Freedom from bias:** Biased information has been altered or modified in order to influence the reader. Sometimes the bias is blatant and easy to identify. Do an Internet search using the term "abortion" or "gun control." These are topics in which strong opposing opinions exist. Look at several sites to determine whether information is accurate and free from bias. Bias is easier to identify when one disagrees with the opinion being expressed or when the information is clearly inaccurate.

Sometimes the information is accurate, and the bias is subtle. For example, drug information provided by a drug company most likely includes information about side effects. The information, however, may be in small print near the end of the document. The indications for using the drug may be in larger print at the beginning of the document and reinforced with a graphic. Each time the drug is referred to in the document, the trade name is used as opposed to the generic name. These approaches influence the reader to consider the indications for the drug before its side effects and to think of the trade name before remembering the generic name.

6. **Comprehensive:** Comprehensive information is complete. Because there is always more that can be said about any topic, it can be difficult to determine whether the information is comprehensive. Information is not comprehensive if missing details mislead the reader. For example, there may be two hospitals in a local community where coronary artery bypass surgery is done. One hospital may have a higher postoperative death rate than the other. This information could lead to the conclusion that one hospital provides better care than the other. However, if the first hospital was a community hospital that took only low-risk patients and the second hospital was a major medical center for high-risk patients, the death rates data may not give a comprehensive picture of the quality of care at either hospital.

7. **Precise:** Information is comprehensive if all of the details are provided. However, the information lacks precision if the details are not specific. For example, a map on the Internet may include the specific street where a clinic is located. However, the map may fail to provide the street number for the clinic. Precision occurs when the details provided meet the specific information needs of the reader.

8. **Appropriate:** Appropriate refers to how well the information answers the user's questions. Is the information on target? For example, one may be looking for information on preparing clinic nurses for a new information system. There may be a great deal of information about the new system but nothing that helps to prepare the new users. The information that is found is precise, timely, accurate, and meets all of the other criteria of quality information. It just does not focus on the specific information needed.

9. **Clarity:** Information lacks clarity if one or more meanings can be applied to the same information. For example, "There are several sites on the Internet that provide health information. Some sites provide quality information while others do not. This is one of these sites." The reader is left to decide whether this is a site that provides good or poor quality information.

Criteria for Evaluating the Quality of Online Information

Knowing information attributes can help in the evaluation of online information. Those attributes include the source of the information, its accuracy and currency, and how easy it is to access and use the information online.

1. **Source:** When accessing and using information, try to start with a reliable source. Reliable sources are usually verifiable and accurate. The source of the information on the Internet refers to both author information and where the information is located on the Internet. Many times these two sources overlap. One may find information about the role of weight in diabetes on an Internet site maintained by the American Diabetic Association or find the information on the personal site of individuals well known for their research on diabetes and weight. Many times personal sites use a ˜ in the URL to direct you to a personal directory. When evaluating the author as a source, it is helpful to identify the author's name, title or position, degrees or education, and professional affiliation. Remember that this information may be included as part of the information on the web pages and may not be accurate. The author could state that he or she is the chairperson of the department of a major university but may in reality be a 10-year-old child learning to design a web page. It is up to the user of the information to validate the source.

   The URL is a major clue for the location of the information. Look at the following URL: http://www2.widener.edu/Wolfgram-Memorial-Library/webevaluation/webeval.htm.

   Widener is the name of the institution where the server is located.
   Edu indicates that this is an educational site.
   Wolfgram-Memorial-Library is the folder on the server where the document is located.
   Webevaluation is a subdirectory or subfolder where the document is located.

Webeval.htm is the actual document. The name of the document indicates that it deals with evaluation of web-based materials.

Reliable websites often provide information on both the author and the Internet location. For example, the University of Texas System Digital Library has created an excellent online tutorial at http://tilt. lib.utsystem.edu/ for learning to evaluate online information. Box 11.1 is an example of the type of information that one can expect to see on a reliable website.

Resources for Librarians and Educators

Copyright © 1998-2004. The University of Texas System Digital Library. This material may be reproduced, distributed, or incorporated only subject to the terms and conditions set forth in the TILT Open Publication License.

(The latest version is available at
http://tilt.lib.utsystem.edu/yourtilt/agreement.html.)

Box 11.1 Example of Reliable Web Site

2. **Current:** Current information is information that has been updated as new information has evolved. There are three dates that can be important to consider. The original date the information was generated. For example, if the site is quoting clinical guidelines, when were the guidelines produced? Second, what is the last date the content or information was updated? This is not the same as the last time the page was modified, which is the third date. Design features on the page may be modified and a new date put on the page; however, the information may not have been updated on that date.

Another clue that the information is current is the reliability of the links. There are two ways to evaluate the links. First, do they function? Links on the Internet change constantly. If a site is not well maintained, the links will become outdated and no longer function. Second, does this site link to current information? On a well-maintained site, links that no longer connect to current information are removed.

If historical data are maintained, it should be identified as such. Note the following example posted at http://www.health.gov/scipich/:

> On April 28, 1999, the Science Panel on Interactive Communication and Health (SciPICH), an independent body convened by the US Department of Health and Human Services (HHS), released its final report, Wired for Health and Well-Being: The Emergence of Interactive Health Communication.
>
> The panel is no longer active, and this site is maintained for historical purposes only.

3. **Easy to navigate:** Quality information is usually organized in a logical format. Logical technical approaches are then used to guide the user through the information. This may be as simple as a table of contents that provides an overview of the information in the document or as complex as the use of multiple frames. Sometimes a site map is used to provide an overview of the information at the site. The use of color and graphics can help or hinder the navigation of a site. A site may be comprehensive, but if the site is not well organized and the navigational aids do not function well, the user may never find the quality information located on the site. Because a search site may start the user anywhere in the site, effective navigational aids are important. They provide a clear overall picture of the website as a whole, as well as an at-the-moment location. A menu, a site map, arrows, and buttons should all flow together to provide direction. The use of standard terms such as Home or About is easier to understand than unique terms on a website.

4. **Objective information:** Objective information is free of bias. However, the Internet is also an excellent place for the expression of opinions as well as advertisement of ideas, products, and positions. Biases on the Internet are acceptable if they are clearly stated; http://democrats.org/ is the URL for the Democratic Party, and http://www.rnc.org/ is the URL for the Republican Party. One expects to find very different opinions on these sites.

5. **Error free:** Several of the criteria already listed will help to determine whether an online resource is error free. Additional clues are also helpful. First, watch for errors in spelling and grammar. If a site is sloppy with these kinds of details, it may also be sloppy with the accuracy of the information provided. Second, be cautious if the information is found on only one site and no other information verifying it exists at other sites. For example, an Internet site may describe a malaria epi-

demic in Alaska. Malaria is caused by a parasite that is transmitted from person to person by the bite of an infected Anopheles mosquito. These mosquitoes are present in almost all countries in the tropics and subtropics. Given these facts about the cause of malaria, would it be likely that there could be an epidemic in Alaska?

Health Care Information on the Internet

The problem:

> "Not all health information is created equal, and not everything out there is correct. When knowledgeable people have "surfed" the Web, they have found dangerously misleading or incomplete health information that looks quite legitimate on the surface. The medium itself contributes to the problem." (www.health.gov/scipich.IHC/problems.htm)

A good designer can make any web page look professional. Although poor design can indicate poor information, a good design does not guarantee good information.

Additional criteria for health information

The criteria that were already discussed deal with any information on the **Internet**. They apply to health care information but are not specific to health care information. There are, however, additional criteria that apply when the information is health related.

1. **Intended audience is clear:** Does the site clearly state who the intended audience is, including the skills and knowledge needed to interpret the information provided by the site? This information is often included in an area titled "mission" or "about us." Many sites will identify information as appropriate for the general public or health care professionals.
2. **Confidentiality of personal information:** Many health care sites collect personal health care data. For example, many sites have self-assessment areas. A quality site will clearly state what data are collected and how the data are used. Remember that anyone can publish anything on the web, including a statement of privacy that is incomplete or inaccurate. Be sure the site and the sponsors of that site are known before providing personal information to an Internet site.
3. **Source of the content references:** An Internet site that provides health information needs to be able to document the source of that information and the relationship of that source to the information. The

name of the organization or institution responsible for the content should be clear. The author's name, credentials, and personal or financial connections that could be a source of real or potential bias should be clearly indicated on the page. There should be an easily located resource for contacting the author on the page. Users of the information need to evaluate the source of the information and whether the sources listed are in fact real. The reference list itself can include references that do not exist.

4. **Sensitive to the health literacy of the intended audience:** Health literacy is "the degree to which individuals have the capacity to obtain, process, and understand basic health information and services needed to make appropriate health decisions" (Seldon, 2000). Basic to health literacy is the ability to read and comprehend information. Several tools can be used to evaluate the reading level of materials posted on the Internet. The word processing package presented in this book includes one such tool. Comprehension is a more difficult question. Comprehension deals with the health care background of readers and their ability to understand the information being presented. Because the Internet can be accessed by anyone, it is important for the site to help the reader with this question. It is helpful if the intended audience is well identified.

5. **Recognized by other authorities:** An excellent site with quality information will be recognized by others. If there are no links to the site and no references to this site, one needs to be concerned. For example, the Consumer and Patient Health Information Section of the Medical Library Association maintains a list of top 100 sites. This list is located at http://caphis.mlanet.org/consumer/index.html.

Sites with health care information criteria

The quality of health care information on the Internet is of concern to many health care providers. A number of sites located on the Internet provide guides for evaluating health care information.

Rollins School of Public Health at Emory University has developed a form that can be used to evaluate health-related sites on the Internet. The form is designed for health educators and clinicians to evaluate the appropriateness of websites for health education for their clientele. This form is located at http://www.sph.emory.edu/WELLNESS/instrument.html.

There are also organizations that accredit or recognize sites that meet specific criteria. One of the most recognized is Health On the Net Foundation. This is a not-for-profit organization that is located in Geneva, Switzerland. Among its many activities, the Health On the Net Foundation has developed a Code of Conduct for providers of health care information. The code is not intended to rate the quality or the information provided by a website. It defines a set of rules designed to make sure the reader always knows the source and the purpose of the data being read. This organization can be located at http://www.hon.ch/home.html. The Emory University form included a reference to this code on the evaluation form.

A second organization is the Utilization Review Accreditation Commission. The Utilization Review Accreditation Commission is an independent, nonprofit organization offering accreditation, certification, and other quality improvement activities for companies providing health services and information on the Internet. Their benchmarking activities cover health plans, preferred provider organizations, medical management systems, health technology services, health call centers, specialty care, workers' compensation, websites, and HIPAA privacy and security compliance, among other areas. Information about this organization is located at http://www.urac.org/.

► 11.4 USING INFORMATION

The final step in information literacy is the effective use of information. However, in this book, the discussion is limited to documenting information from the Internet.

Footnotes and Documentation

All information accessed on the Internet should be documented just as one would document information from any other source. Failure to document is plagiarism. Plagiarism is the act of stealing another person's ideas or work and presenting it as one's own. However, on the Internet, some additional issues exist. First, it is easy to forget that copyright laws also protect information posted on the Internet. This can even apply to e-mail messages posted to a listserv. The Office of Student Judicial Affairs, University of California, Davis, provides a number of suggestions for avoiding plagiarism. These suggestions are located at http://sja.ucdavis.edu/avoid.htm.

Second, just as it is easy to post information on the Internet, it is also easy to remove that information. Therefore, the citation for information obtained from the Internet should include some additional data, such as the date the information was developed. This information should be provided by the Internet site, and if it is not, the citation should indicate that the information source is not dated. Also, because data are frequently removed from the Internet the citation should indicate the date when the information was accessed. Several Internet sites give specific directions for formatting an Internet citation and how to include these dates.

Internet Sites for Citing Internet Information

The American Psychological Association (APA) is one of the most common formats used in health care. The APA maintains a website and includes information on how to use the APA format to cite Internet resources. It is located at http://www.apastyle.org/elecref.html. In addition to the APA, there are other accepted citation formats. Several of these are demonstrated on a site maintained by the General Library at the University of Texas at Austin, located at http://www.lib.utexas.edu/refsites/style_manuals.html.

Like the University of Texas at Austin, many libraries include this type of information on their websites. Often they will include a list of links to resources for citing Internet resources. Two sites that demonstrate this approach include http://www.nova.edu/library/eleclib/eref.html#cite and http://ww2.lafayette.edu/~library/guides/cite.html. The second site includes a list of components that should be included in any Internet citation.

SUMMARY

This chapter explored the concept of information literacy. It included strategies to identify an information need, find information, evaluate the quality of information, and cite information from the Internet. Quality health care requires good information. As a health care provider, it is important to search for the latest high-quality information and make appropriate use of that information in providing health care.

References

American Library Association. (2000). *Information literacy competency standards for higher education.* Retrieved on August 28, 2004, from http://www.ala.org/ala/acrl/acrlstandards/standards.pdf.

SciPICH (1998). Potential Problems with IHC Applications. Retrieved on December 29, 2004 from http://www.health.gov/scipich/IHC/problems. htm.

Seldon, CR, Zorn, M, & Ratzan, SC (2000). *Current Bibliographies in Medicine 2000–1: Health Literacy U.S. Department of Health and Human Services.* Public Health Service, National Institutes of Health Located at http://www.nlm.nih.gov/pubs/cbm/hliteracy.html#5.

Staggers, N., Gassert, C., Kwai, J. L., Milholland, K., Nelson, R., Senemeier, J., Stuck, D., & Welton, J. (2001). *Scope and standards of nursing informatics practice*. Washington, DC: American Nurses Publishing.

Exercise 1: Using a Search Site

Objectives

1. Use the help section of an Internet search site.
2. Conduct an Internet search using Boolean search strategies.
3. Identify a directory, search tool, meta-directory, and meta-search engine.

Activity

1. Access a search site.

   Type the following URL in a browser **Location** or **Address** text box: **http://www.yahoo.com**. *You are now on the home page of Yahoo.*

   On this page locate the following four areas: (1) Help, (2) Advance Search, (3) the area where the query is entered, and (4) the list of subjects within the directory.

2. Use a directory.

   Click the subject area that deals with **Health**. *The next page will be a subdirectory.*

   Click one of the Topics from the subdirectory. Look at the URL of this page to see whether there is a path statement that will tell you how deep you are in the directory. The path may look something like this: http://health.yahoo.com/health/centers/women/index.html.

3. Use a home navigational aid.

   Click the **Home** link to return to the Yahoo home page.

   Click the **Help** section. Does all of the help relate to searching Yahoo?

   Did you learn anything new on this page?

4. Use advanced search.

   Click the **Back** button on the browser to return to the Yahoo home page.

   Click **Advance Search**.

   Look around in this section, and note the various ways that one can focus a search.

   Click the **Back** button to return again to the Yahoo home page.

5. Find and orient to the new search site.

   Use Yahoo to find at least two other **Search** sites on the Internet.

   Use the same approach demonstrated with Yahoo to orient yourself to the search site.

6. Conduct a search.

   Go to the **Search site** that you prefer.

   Design a query to search for **Search Engine Tutorials**.

7. Compare online tutors.

   Select a **Tutorial** from the hits on your search and one of the following tutorials.

   Complete two tutorials.

   Which of the two did you find most informative? Why?

   http://academics.sru.edu/library/tutorials/internet/intro.htm

   http://www.mannlib.cornell.edu/reference/tutorials/search/index.html

   http://www.Webpro.co.za/services/search.htm

   http://www.notess.com/search/

   http://www.monash.com/spidap.html

   As you are looking for a site with tutorials for search engines, be sure to at least take a quick look at this site: http://www.lib.berkeley.edu/TeachingLib/Guides/Internet/FindInfo.html

8. Meta-search engine classifications.

   Meta-search engines can be classified in many ways. Some examples include classification by topic searched (medicine, law, art), by how sites are found and indexed (robots and people), and by how many search engines are being used to conduct the search at one time. There are sites on the web where lists of links to several search engines are presented. These sites classify the search engines in a variety of ways.

   Locate at least three sites that include 15 or more search sites.

   Locate sites where the search types are grouped under certain headings.

   Create a table that includes a column for (1) the site, (2) the classification, and (3) an example of a search site in that classification.

   Search sites may be classified in more than one way, and your groupings or classifications may overlap. Here are some sites to get you started. Do not include these sites in the five sites that you locate for this exercise.

   http://www.lib.berkeley.edu/TeachingLib/Guides/Internet/ToolsTables.html

   http://www.amdahl.com/internet/meta-index.html

   http://www.rcq.usherb.ca/ihea/ihea.htm

Exercise 2: Evaluating Information on the Internet

Objectives

1. Using the criteria mentioned in Chapter 11, develop a tool that can be used to evaluate the quality of information on the Internet.

2. Evaluate the effectiveness of the tool for a user who has limited health literacy.

Activity

1. Evaluate information sites.

   • Review three sites from the following:

http://www.virtualsalt.com/evalu8it.htm

http://library.albany.edu/internet/evaluate.html

http://www.ciolek.com/WWWVL-InfoQuality.html

http://www.ala.org/ala/alsc/greatwebsites/greatwebsitesforkids/greatwebsites. htm

http://www.library.ucla.edu/libraries/college/help/critical/index.htm

http://sosig.ac.uk/desire/internet-detective.html

2. Develop a tool that can be used to evaluate information on a website.

- Using information from the selected sites as well as from Chapter 11, design a tool for evaluating health information pages.
- Select two health-related Internet sites with information for the general public. One site should have high-quality information. The other site should have inaccurate information.

Ask a high school student or college freshman who would be expected to have a limited health care background to review the sites using your form.

3. Answer the following questions.

- Did the student collect information for all sections of your form?
- When information was missing, did he or she note this? For example, if the date the page was last updated was missing, did he or she note this?
- Did he or she validate the data or information that was collected? For example, if the author of the information at the Internet site indicated that he or she was a college professor, did the student check the directory of the college to see whether he or she was listed?
- Was the student able to differentiate the quality of the information at the two sites?
- If the student was correct, what factors influenced the student in making this decision? In other words, how was he or she able to recognize the quality of the information?
- If the student was incorrect, what factors misled the student? Remember that the student may be correct about one page and not the other.
- From this experience, how would you revise your form? What would you stress if you were teaching patients to evaluate information on the web?

Assignment 1: Evaluating Health Care Information on the Internet
Directions

1. Begin this assignment by designing two forms for evaluating health-related information at an Internet site. Design one form that can be used by a health care provider. The second form should be designed for use by the general public. The forms should be no longer than two pages and should include directions for use.

2. Pilot both forms with at least five users. Exercise 2 should be helpful to you in planning your pilot.

3. Write a paper about this project, including the following information. Explain the rationale for the design and content of each form. Describe how you selected your users and what happened when you piloted the forms with the users. Outline your findings or the results of your pilot. Redesign the forms based on your pilot and include the revised forms in your paper. Do not forget to cite references using the appropriate format.

4. After the paper is completed, design a poster presentation based on the paper. You may find PowerPoint helpful for this part of the assignment. Present the poster presentation to your classmates.

5. Turn in both the paper and the poster presentation.

Ensuring the Security and Integrity of Electronic Data

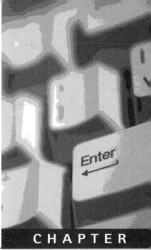

CHAPTER

12

OBJECTIVES

1. Discuss the concepts of privacy, confidentiality, and security as they apply to the management of electronic data.
2. Recognize common threats to privacy, confidentiality, and security of data stored in electronic systems.
3. Apply effective procedures for protecting data, software, and hardware.
4. Follow Health Insurance Portability and Accountability Act (HIPAA) regulations for protecting health care information.

The code of ethics for health care professionals consistently demonstrates that providing for the confidentiality and privacy of all patients, clients, and consumers is a major responsibility of health care providers. Meeting that responsibility is impossible if the health care provider does not understand how to follow current regulations and apply effective procedures with electronic data. In this chapter, the threats to privacy, confidentiality, and security are identified. Procedures for protecting data, software, and hardware are explained. Regulations for protecting health care information are clarified.

► 12.1 USING COMPUTER SYSTEMS FOR STORING DATA

Except for a few stand-alone clinics in rural areas, all health care organizations store some private data electronically. These data that are stored relate to the clients, the employees, and the institution. Although these computer systems are used for purposes other than the management of personal data, such as financial records and inventory management, the legal/ethical implications related to storing personal data are of primary concern.

Concerns with confidentiality and security are not limited to health care information systems. Many personal computers (PCs) now store a significant amount of confidential data. In addition, loss of any data from a computer can be a major source of problems. For example, if a student has spent several hours completing a term paper and if a computer virus wipes out the paper, it may be difficult to convince the instructor that the virus "ate the paper."

Four major concerns are related to electronically stored data, whether the data are stored on a health care information system or a PC:

1. Providing for privacy and confidentiality of data
2. Ensuring the integrity of the data
3. Protecting the hardware and software
4. Recognizing and prosecuting criminal abuse of computer data and equipment

► 12.2 PRIVACY AND CONFIDENTIALITY

To protect privacy and confidentiality, issues relevant to data storage and use must be addressed. Problems of ensuring privacy and confidentiality of data include data protection issues and data integrity issues.

Data protection issues	Access of data for unauthorized use
	Unnecessary storage of data
Data integrity issues	Incomplete or inaccurate storage of data
	Intentional or accidental manipulation of data

Personal Privacy and Confidentiality

With the advent of computers several companies, institutions and government agencies maintain databases of personal data. For example, personal information related to education is stored in university computers. This can include data related to learning disabilities. Information related to personal driving records is stored by the Department of Motor Vehicles. Social security benefits information is stored by the Social Security Administration, and mail-order companies store personal information such as phone numbers, addresses, and what items have been ordered. Health insurance companies have extensive information on personal health care. Knowing what data are stored is an important first step in protecting individual privacy.

Once warrantee or registration forms asking for name, address, and other information are completed, then that data may be sold to other companies. Simply using the Internet generates information about where individuals go on the Internet, who they interact with via chat rooms and listservs, and what products they buy. Several organizations have evolved in response to these issues and focus on educating the general public. One example is the Center for Democracy & Technology, which offers 11 specific approaches to protecting online privacy (*Center for Democracy & Technology's CDT'S Guide to Online Privacy*, n.d.).

Currently, many organizations now share personal data from their databases. By sharing information across these databases, it is possible to create a personal profile of an individual that is more extensive than the individual would have ever realized. An example of what data are being shared can be seen in the small print leaflets concerning privacy that are mailed with credit bills or bank statements. Another excellent example in health care is the MIB Group, Inc. MIB Group, Inc. is an association of over 500 United States and Canadian life insurance companies. By sharing information, these companies work together to assure the accuracy of health information supplied on the insurance application concerning the proposed insured (*MIB: About Us*, 2004). Because many people do not know these activities occur, few checks and balances exist to ensure the accuracy of this information.

Patient Privacy and Confidentiality

Because many people assume that information they share with their health care providers is held in confidence, they assume a level of protection that does not exist. Once that information is documented in a medical record, the confidentiality of that information is determined by who has access to that data. Besides physicians and other health care providers, health care information may be shared with insurance companies and government agencies such as Medicare or Medicaid. Legal access to these records is obtained when individuals agree to let others see these records. This usually occurs by signing consent forms or blanket waivers when receiving health care. With the increasing use of technology, medical information is stored in a variety of computer databases both in local institutions and in other places serving a number of health care institutions. With the passing of PL 104-191, the Health Insurance Portability and Accountability Act of 1996, Congress included provisions for a standard unique health identifier for each individual, employer, health plan, and health care provider in the health care system. To date, a process for issuing standard unique health identifiers for individuals has not been accepted and developed.

The Health Insurance Portability and Accountability Act (HIPAA) "applies to medical records maintained by health care providers, health plans, and health clearinghouses—and only if the facility maintains and transmits records in *electronic* form. A great deal of health-related information exists *outside* of health care facilities and the files of health plans and is therefore beyond the reach of HIPAA." (Private Rights Clearinghouse, 2004). Although the law also includes penalties for infringement of the integrity and confidentiality of the data, privacy advocates continue to be concerned about secondary uses of medical information, employer access, and unauthorized access.

Under both the HIPAA and the Patriot Act, some circumstances permit police access to medical records without a warrant (Burke & Weill, 2005). Furthermore, although HIPAA requires that people be informed about *how* their records may be used without consent, the act does not require that people be informed *when* their records are actually shared. In addition, the Patriot Act includes provisions that do not allow people to be told if their medical records are shared under the provisions of this act.

► 12.3 SAFETY AND SECURITY

Protecting the safety and security of patient data involves identifying the threats to computer systems and initiating procedures to protect the integrity of the data and system. There are two primary types of threats: threats to the integrity of data and threats to the confidentiality of the data. These threats can result from accidental or intentional human actions or natural disasters. Destruction of data, hardware, and software by natural disasters includes damage by water, fire, or chemicals; electrical power outages; disk failures; and exposure to magnetic fields.

The types of human actions that result in these threats can be divided into five areas (For the Record: Protecting Electronic Health Information, 1997):

1. Innocent mistakes: These are errors made by people who have legal access to the system and in the process of using the system, accidentally disclose data, or damage the integrity of data. This can be as simple as a physician recording data in the wrong medical record or a lab sending a fax to a wrong phone number. "Ontario's privacy commissioner issued a warning to all companies after a woman's confidential medical records ended up on the back of Toronto real estate flyers. The flyers, with pictures of houses for sale on one side and the woman's mammogram and pelvic exam results on the other, were among a batch of 10,000 from a Markham printer which were put in Toronto mailboxes earlier this week" (The Privacy Manager, 2003).

2. Inappropriate access by insiders for curiosity reasons: This is an intentional decision by a person with legal access to the system to abuse their access privileges. Browsing is a problem with many electronic record systems, and health records are not immune to this problem. The person is looking at medical records only to satisfy their own curiosity. Their access to the medical record provides no benefit to the patient.

3. Inappropriate access by insiders for spite or for profit: In 2002, Al Roker, the weatherman on NBC, had gastric bypass surgery to treat obesity. He told neither his mother nor his colleagues at the television station. He was admitted using a different name. Al describes his experience with privacy of medical data on a website he maintains. "The National Enquirer had a hospital employee violate my privacy and break several laws in providing them with my surgical and hospital information. Good for them. I'm sure they're proud" (Roker, 2004). The story in the National Enquirer included his preoperative weight, the time of surgery, and several other personal data items. This is an example of inappropriate access by insiders for profit.

4. An unauthorized intruder who gains access to patient data: Many hospitals rely on physical security, software, and user education to protect information stored inside a computer. The computers are located so that it is difficult for others to access and use the computers. Passwords and firewalls are used to control access. Within a few minutes of inactivity, the computer automatically logs off all users. Although these precautions help in securing access to patient data, they are not fool proof. People are one of the biggest threats to securing patient data.

5. Vengeful employees and outsiders, such as vindictive patients or intruders, who mount attacks to access unauthorized information, damage systems, and disrupt operations: Thus, most hospitals will

terminate computer access before informing an employee that they are being terminated.

▶ 12.4 COMPUTER CRIME

Since the advent of the Internet, new laws have been enacted to define computer crime. With its global connectivity, the Internet allows increased access to computers from external sites. However, it is still difficult to detect and prosecute many computer crimes. Many times the person initiating the criminal acts is not located in this country and may not be subject to US laws. A key resource for understanding computer crime and related issues is maintained by the US Justice Department. This includes a section especially designed for children located at http://www.cybercrime.gov/. Although the terms listed here are more readily identified with computer crime in areas other than health care, all types of crime could occur within a health care computer system.

Related Terms

Cybercrime	This refers to the use of the Internet to steal personal and other important information.
Cracker	This is a hacker who illegally breaks into computer systems and creates mischief.
Denial of Service	Denial of Service (DOS) is any action or series of actions that prevents any part of an information system from functioning. For example, using several computers attached to the Internet to access a website can cause the site to be overwhelmed and unavailable.
Data Diddling	This involves modifying valid data in a computer file.
Encryption	This is a method of coding sensitive data to protect it when sent over the networks.
Firewall	These are hardware and/or software systems used to protect computers or intranets from unauthorized access from outside the system or from the Internet.

Hacker	Originally, hacker referred to a compulsive computer programmer; it now has a more negative meaning and is often confused with "cracker."
Identity Theft	This occurs when someone uses another person's private information to assume his or her identity.
Logic Bomb	This is a piece of program code buried within another program, designed to perform some malicious act in response to a trigger. The trigger can involve entering a date or name, for example.
Phishing (pronounced "fishing")	This involves creating a replica of a legitimate web page to hook users and trick them into submitting personal or financial information or passwords (see Chapter 10).
Sabotage	This is the purposeful destruction of hardware, software, and data.
Software Piracy	This is unauthorized copying of copyrighted software.
Spamming	This is the act of sending unsolicited electronic messages in bulk. The most common form of spam is that delivered in e-mail as a form of commercial advertising; however, this is not the only use of spamming (see Chapter 10).
Theft of Services	This includes the unauthorized use of services such as a computer system.
Trapdoors	These are methods installed by programmers that allow unauthorized access into programs.
Trojan Horse	This involves placing instructions in a program that add additional, illegitimate functions; for example, the program prints information every time information on a certain patient is entered.
Time Bomb	This involves instructions in a program that perform certain functions on a specific date or time, such as printing a message or destroying data.
Virus	This involves a program that once introduced into a system replicates itself and causes a variety

of mischievous outcomes. Viruses are usually introduced from infected diskettes, e-mail attachments, and downloaded files.

Worm   This is a destructive program that can fill various memory locations of a computer system with information, clogging the system so that other operations are compromised.

Prosecution of Computer Crime

Prosecution of computer crime is difficult for several reasons. Some crimes are detected but not reported. When data are stolen, they are not always seen as valuable; thus, those responsible may not be prosecuted. Sometimes an institution is so concerned with the poor publicity that can result from reporting of this event that the event is not reported. Other crimes are not detected, although methods for tracking entry into computer systems are becoming increasingly sophisticated. Prosecution cannot occur if there is no detection.

Selected Laws Related to Computer Crimes

Freedom of Information Act of 1970   This law allows citizens to have access to data gathered by federal agencies. It deals with federal agencies only.

Federal Privacy Act of 1974   This law stipulates that there can be no secret personal files; individuals must be allowed to know what is stored in files about them and how it is used. This applies to government agencies and contractors dealing with government agencies, but not to the private sector.

US Copyright Law, 1976   This law stipulates that it is a federal offense to reproduce copyrighted materials, including computer software, without authorization.

Electronic Communication Privacy Act of 1986   This law specifies that it is a crime to own any electronic, mechanical, or other device primarily for the purpose of the surreptitious interception of wire, oral, or electronic communication. This law does not apply to an organization's internal communication such as e-mail between employees.

Computer Fraud and Abuse Act of 1984, amended in 1986	This law specifies that it is a crime to access a federal computer without authorization and to alter, destroy, or damage information or prevent authorized access . . . if such conduct causes the loss of $1,000 or more during any 1-year period.
Computer Security Act of 1987	This law mandated that the National Institute of Standards and Technology and Office of Personnel Management create guidance on computer security awareness and training based on functional organizational roles. In response, the National Institute of Standards and Technology created the Computer Security Resource Center located at http://csrc.nist.gov/index.html.
U.S. Copyright Law, 1995	This amendment protects the transmission of digital performance over the Internet, making it a crime to transmit something for which you do not have proper authorization.
National Information Infrastructure Protection Act of 1996	This law established penalties for interstate theft of information.
U.S. Copyright Law, No Electronic Theft Act, 1997	This addition to the copyright act creates criminal penalties for copyright infringement even if the offender does not benefit financially.
Digital Millennium Copyright Act of 1998	This legislation places the United States in conformance with international treaties that prevail in other countries around the world. The new act provides changes in three areas: protection of copyrighted digital works, extensions of copyright protection by 20 years, and addition of

criminal penalties and fines for attempting to circumvent the copyright. It provides for copyright protection for the creative organization and structure of a database, but not the underlying general facts, requires that "Webcasters" pay licensing fees to record companies, and limits Internet Service Provider's copyright infringement liability for simply transmitting information over the Internet.

Children's Online Protection Act of 2000

This law requires websites targeting children under the age of 14 years to obtain parental consent before gathering information on children.

The Patriot Act of 2001

This act gives federal officials greater authority to track and intercept communications that are deemed necessary for intelligence gathering and homeland security. With this act, law enforcement agencies require fewer checks to collect electronic data for the purpose of law enforcement and foreign intelligence gathering.

The Homeland Security Act of 2002

This act established a Department of Homeland Security as an executive department of the United States. It expanded and centralized the data gathering allowed under the Patriot Act.

Protection of Computer Data and Systems

The privacy and confidentiality of data as well as the safety and security of the entire system can be protected by procedures initiated by the health care agency. Steps taken by individual health care providers are also important to maintaining data security. Agency responsibilities include protecting data from unauthorized use, destruction or disclosure, and controlling data input and output. Individuals are also accountable for managing data responsibly.

To protect data from unauthorized use, destruction, disclosure, or inaccuracies agencies should

1. Develop ongoing educational programs to ensure users understand their responsibilities.
2. Restrict access to data by requiring passwords, personal identification numbers, and/or call-back procedures.
3. Develop encoding procedures for sensitive data.
4. Use transaction records to document access and routinely audit these records.
5. Develop biometric methods such as electronic signatures, fingerprints, iris scans, or retina prints to identify users.
6. Protect systems from natural disasters; locate them in areas safe from water and other potential physical damage.
7. Develop backup procedures and redundant systems so that data are not lost accidentally.
8. Develop and enforce policies for breaches of security.
9. Store only needed data.
10. Dispose of unneeded printouts by shredding.
11. Develop alerts that identify potentially inaccurate data such as a weight of 1,200 lbs. or a blood pressure of 80/130.

To manage data responsibly, individuals should

1. Avoid distractions and other factors that may result in data entry errors.
2. Refuse to share a password or sign in with another person's password.
3. Attend implementation classes and clearly understand institutional policies and procedures.
4. Keep the monitor screen and data out of view of others.
5. Develop passwords that include numbers and letters and that are not easy to identify.
6. Keep secure own password/means of access to data.
7. Report unusual computer activity and potential breaches of security.
8. Encourage patients to understand their rights to privacy and confidentiality.
9. Keep away materials that are damaging to computers, such as food, drink, and smoke.

Protecting Data on PCs

Most health care agencies store information on large computers and have policies for protecting these data. However, microcomputers are spread throughout the institution and are much more difficult to monitor. With the increased connectivity, many of these microcomputers are connected to a LAN that provides access to the Internet. The increased connectivity makes it easier to monitor the PCs but also increases the risk. These risks include inappropriate access as well as exposure to worms and viruses. Now that the Internet is used to access information, including health information, it is important to know how to safeguard information stored on the PC.

Although some of the same guidelines related to safety and security of larger computers are important for the PC, there are additional guidelines to protect the PC system and its data. Often individuals are concerned about the privacy of information on their computers and about what information may be accessed on their PC when using the Internet. The following is a summary of action steps to protect the data on a PC. Some apply to PCs in the work environment; others are related to PCs in the home environment. If the PC is in the work environment, check with the information technology (IT) department to see what their policies and procedures are regarding installation, firewalls, updates, configurations, and responsibilities.

Virus protection

- Install and routinely update a virus checker. The checker is only as good as the currency of the definitions it uses to scan for a virus. Most virus checkers can be configured to update its definition database automatically on a certain day and time. The computer must be connected to the Internet for this to occur. Make sure that users understand not to stop the program from checking for and updating its database. Most IT departments routinely configure their virus checker to do this.

- Configure the virus checker to scan all e-mail and downloaded files as they come in and to scan the computer hard drive(s) routinely. Do not open e-mail or attachments if the sender is unknown.

- Download data only from reputable systems that are regularly checked for viruses.

E-mail protection

- Do NOT set the mailer to open attachments automatically.

- If a filter is used to screen mail, remember to empty the junk mail box folder.

- Use whatever methods the e-mail system provides to protect mail from snooping, tampering, and forgery. Many of these are done at the mail server level on work PCs.

- Examine the implications related to where an e-mail address may be listed and the use of other information provided to the online service provider and other Internet resources that are used.

- Know the policies related to using e-mail. There is more protection if messages are transferred from the service provider to the user's computer than if they are left on the provider's server.

Software and data protection

- For those who access the Internet via a dial-up connection, do not stay connected to it when not actually using the Internet. This means to log off the ISP.

- For those using DSL or cable connections, install a personal firewall. If this is a work PC, check to see what precautions the IT department has in place.

- If others have access to the computer, install a password so that the password is required to sign on or set up user accounts. Users will only have access to their information and configurations and any shared data and programs.

- Be creative with passwords; avoid the obvious ones, such as initials or special dates, and do not tape them on the wall or under your keyboard! A combination of numbers and letters is often useful. Change passwords on a regular basis.

- Although IT departments have procedures for routinely backing up data on the network, this does not apply to local drives on a PC or laptop. Regularly perform system backups and rotate the tapes or disks used for the backup procedure. Because hard drives are large, many people backup only the data on the hard drive and not the application programs.

- If data are lost because of a virus, scan the backups before installing to be sure that the virus is not reinstalled.

- For personal PCs, store sensitive data on removable storage devices rather than on a hard drive. Place the removable storage device in a secure place. Remember this applies to personal data not to institutional data where the requirement may be to store ALL institutional data on a secure file server and to NOT remove any data via removable storage devices.

Hardware protection

- Use an approved surge protector and/or uninterrupted power supply to protect the hardware from damage during electrical problems.
- Do not eat or drink near the computer. Crumbs and spills can ruin the equipment.
- If the PC is in a work environment, physically secure it or keep the office locked. Place antitheft devices on laptops.

Personal identity protection

- Never give out personal information on a chat or a list server. If mail arrives asking for personal information, do not provide it. Although it might look like it is coming from a legitimate site, it may not be. ISPs and reputable businesses will NEVER ask for personal information such as passwords and credit card numbers over an e-mail system.
- Check NO. Many online companies give users the option to have their e-mail address used for sending future information. Checking NO should opt the user out of having their e-mail address passed on to others.
- Configure the browser to the appropriate security level. This can be done with Internet Explorer and Netscape Navigator.
- Use the secure server when given that option. Companies often provide the option to use a secure server. This provides additional protection when sending private information such as a credit card number via the Internet.
- Keep one credit card for Internet use only.
- Install software to scan and remove spyware from the computer.
- Look for the padlock icon. When using the Internet sites to send data, the padlock icon, usually in the lower part of the screen, signifies that data are encrypted and that a site is secure.
- Recognize that to make some websites work a "cookie" is placed on the computer. A cookie is a small file sent to the hard drive when the computer interacts with certain websites. It contains information about what was done on that website and, in some instances, communicates personal preferences when on the site. Cookies do not "scan the hard drive" and are read only by the site or site group that originally sent the file.

► **12.5 PROVIDING PATIENT CARE VIA THE COMPUTER**

Although most health care providers are aware of the computer as a tool for documenting care and managing the health care record, this is only the beginning of how computers are used to deliver care and communicate with patients, clients, and consumers. Telemedicine is used to deliver care in a variety of places across the country. Websites are fast becoming a major if not the major source of health information for the general public. The use of websites as a communication tool is discussed in Chapters 10 and 11. E-mail is becoming recognized as a valuable method of patient communication.

Telemedicine

Telemedicine is the delivery of health care and/or health-related data across telecommunication lines. The information may be exchanged using a videoconferencing approach and/or a web-based approach. The exchange may occur in real time or on an asynchronous schedule. Because these applications often cross state lines, they are subject to state privacy laws as well as HIPAA. In implementing HIPAA, the US Department of Health and Human Services proposes that Federal laws preempt state laws when they are in conflict with HIPAA regulatory requirements or when the state laws provide less stringent privacy protections. However, when states have *more* stringent privacy laws, the state law will preempt Federal law. With this interpretation of HIPAA, telemedicine practitioners are faced with a patchwork of state privacy standards. To comply with the provisions of HIPAA, the Federal Office for the Advancement of Telehealth has offered four recommendations:

- Train employees about security, and designate a privacy officer.
- Develop a Trading Partner Agreement that extends privacy protections to third-party business associates.
- Obtain patient consent for most disclosures of protected health information.
- Provide the minimum amount of information necessary (Office for the Advancement of Telehealth, 2001).

E-mail and Security Issues

Although physicians and other health care providers have been hesitant to use e-mail communication with patients, increasing numbers of patients are requesting this form of communication. Patients are especially interested in scheduling appointments, renewing prescriptions, and getting answers to questions. Health care providers are hesitant because of concerns related to security issues as well as the possibility that they would not be able to manage the increased workload. However, increasing numbers of health care providers are using this resource in their communication with patients. Two factors have encouraged this change. HIPAA requires that e-mail be encrypted and Danny Sands, a primary care physician and others, have become champions for patient–physician e-mail communication. As a result of their work, the American Medical Association and the American Medical Informatics Association have developed e-mail guidelines. These and other guidelines can be accessed at http://134.174.100.34/. However, safe use of e-mail communication requires educating both the health care provider and the health care receiver.

SUMMARY

Storing data and exchanging data via the computer raise several privacy, security, and confidentiality concerns. This chapter focused on issues related to confidentiality and privacy of data, as well as ensuring the integrity of the data, the software, and the hardware. Securing computers and the data they store is a challenge for large health care information systems and for individuals using PCs. The development of the Internet has created an entire new level of opportunity and concern. Protecting the privacy of patients and the integrity of their health-related data depends on carefully drafted laws and on educating both the provider and the consumer of healthcare. This chapter was an introduction to these issues.

References

Burke, L., & Weill, B. (2005). *Information technology for the health professions.* Upper Saddle River, NJ: Prentice Hall.

Center for Democracy & Technology, CDT's guide to online privacy: Getting started: Top ten ways to protect privacy. (n.d.). Retrieved September 18, 2004, from http://www.cdt.org/privacy/guide/basic/topten.html

For the Record: Protecting Electronic Health Information. (1997). Retrieved September 24, 2004, from http://www.nap.edu/openbook/0309056977/html/54.html

MIB: About us. (2004). Retrieved September 20, 2004, from http://www. mib.com/html/about_us.html

Office for the Advancement of Telehealth. (2001). *How might HIPAA affect telemedicine providers?* Retrieved September 23, 2004, from http://tele-health.hrsa.gov/pubs/hipaa.htm#telemed

Private Rights Clearinghouse. (2004). *Fact sheet 8: Medical records privacy.* Retrieved September 23, 2004, from http://www.privacyrights.org/FS/fs8-med.htm

Roker, A. (2004). *Al's journal.* Retrieved September 3, 2004, from http://www.alroker.com/journal.cfm

The Privacy Manager. (2003). Medical records put on flyer. Retrieved September 24, 2004, from http://www.theprivacymanager.com/archives/archives0302.htm

Exercise 1: Ensuring the Security and Integrity of Electronic Data

Objectives

1. Apply information about security and integrity of data to commonly encountered situations.

2. Clarify personal attitude about the legal/ethical use of computer hardware and software.

Activity

For each situation listed here, place a check by the term that best reflects your opinion of the behavior of the individual. Be prepared to discuss your responses.

1. Kevin gives his password to Beth, a friend of his who cannot seem to remember her password. The password allows Beth to access the school computer and printing facilities as well as Kevin's e-mail.

   Kevin:

   ETHICAL____ UNETHICAL____ COMPUTER CRIME____

   Beth:

   ETHICAL____ UNETHICAL____ COMPUTER CRIME____

2. A physical therapist gives his or her password to a friend who is a graduate student in physical therapy so that he or she may review a patient record and extract the data needed for a clinical paper.

Physical therapist:

ETHICAL___ UNETHICAL___ COMPUTER CRIME___

Graduate student:

ETHICAL___ UNETHICAL___ COMPUTER CRIME___

3. A copy of a commercial word processing package distributed as part of class materials is given to a friend who will be taking the course next term.

ETHICAL___ UNETHICAL___ COMPUTER CRIME___

4. Using a computer terminal, a health care worker breaks a security code and reviews confidential patient data. No use is made of the information. "I was just curious" is the response when caught.

ETHICAL___ UNETHICAL___ COMPUTER CRIME___

5. Brian is creating a web page and finds a terrific background on another page. He copies the background to use on his page.

ETHICAL___ UNETHICAL___ COMPUTER CRIME___

6. Several health care providers are collaborating on an important research study. The Hospital Board of Review has been slow to give permission for data collection via computerized patient records. The research team members, experienced with computer systems, decide to go ahead and begin data collection while waiting to hear from the review board.

ETHICAL___ UNETHICAL___ COMPUTER CRIME___

7. Terry lurks on a listserv that provides a thought-provoking discussion about AIDS. The student takes some of the ideas from the listserv and incorporates them into a paper that he or she is writing but does not credit the source of the ideas in order to ensure the privacy of people on the list.

ETHICAL___ UNETHICAL___ COMPUTER CRIME___

8. Judy downloads a file that is labeled shareware, useable for 45 days and if further use is desired, payment is requested. Judy really likes the program and continues to use it long after the trial period without sending any payment.

ETHICAL___ UNETHICAL___ COMPUTER CRIME___

9. Dr. Bob is teaching a computer course. The university purchased a site license for 25 copies of the software that he is distributing to students. However, 25 students are registered for the course. Dr. Bob makes a copy of the software for himself and distributes one copy to each student.

ETHICAL___ UNETHICAL___ COMPUTER CRIME___

10. James is completing his senior year as a nursing student in a BSN program. A patient he has cared for a few weeks ago obtained his e-mail address from the online university directory and has sent him an e-mail. In the e-mail, the patient discussed new and potentially serious symptoms. James forwards the e-mail to the

charge nurse on the unit where the patient was treated and to the senior resident involved in the patient's care.

ETHICAL___ UNETHICAL___ COMPUTER CRIME___

Exercise 2: The Use of Computers in Health Care
Objectives
1. Analyze common concerns related to the ethical use of computers in health care systems.
2. Articulate a position about the ethical use of computers.

Activity
1. You have been asked to be a part of a committee considering using computers to connect the main clinic and several satellite clinics, one of which is in the neighboring state. The committee has several tasks:
   a. Convince those who have recently joined the committee that computers will not be prone to unwanted access.
   b. Develop procedures for safeguarding the patient data that will be entered into the computer system.
   c. Ensure legal protection for the health professionals using the computers.
2. Using your word processing system, prepare a two- to three-page paper that summarizes the points that you would stress as the committee works on its tasks. Include your reference list. Submit your paper.

Exercise 3: Copyright and Privacy Issues
Objectives
1. Describe copyright and fair use.
2. Identify methods for adhering to copyright law when writing a research paper.
3. Identify some potential security problems when surfing the Internet.

Activity
Copyright. Access the following websites: http://www.lib.utsystem.edu/ copyright/ and http://www.sru.edu/pages/2629.asp. Complete the tutorial on the first site, and look over the articles on the second site.

Answer the following questions.
1. What is copyright?
2. What is fair use?
3. What is public domain?

4. What are the guidelines for including information in a research paper in order to be in compliance with the copyright law?

5. How do you cite a website in a reference list? How do you cite an e-mail message?

Submit your answers to these questions using your word processor.

Privacy. Use several different Internet search engines to search for your name and for the name of one of your faculty.

1. List each fact that you were able to learn about yourself from this search.

2. Write a description of your faculty using only the information that you were able to find on the Internet. If you were unable to find any information on your faculty member, do the exercise using one of the authors of this book.

Exercise 4: Preventing Computer Crime
Objectives

1. Apply information about computer crimes to prevent these crimes in commonly encountered situations.

2. Understand current laws as they apply to computer crimes.

Situation

During the school year you are living in a dorm and share a computer with your roommate. The rest of the time you live at home and share a computer with your family. In both cases you are concerned that you as well as the others involved are at risk of being the victim of a computer crime.

Activity

1. Review the materials that are available at http://www.cybercrime.gov/.

2. Write a set of guidelines that can be used in each situation described previously.

3. Describe how you would encourage others to use these guidelines.

Assignment 1: Using Internet Materials
Directions

1. You are a part of a student group that has been assigned the task of developing some guidelines for using materials on the Internet in such a way as to prevent copyright infringements.

2. Go to some of the following addresses or find your own sites to help develop your guidelines:

http://www.templetons.com/brad/copymyths.htm

http://www.bitlaw.com/copyright/fair_use.html

http://palimpsest.stanford.edu/bytopic/intprop/#faq

http://www.uwec.edu/library/tutorial/mod7/

3. Use your word processor and create a flyer that lists those guidelines using a variety of fonts, bold, italics, underlining, and other formatting features in an eye-catching format. Be creative.

4. Submit your flyer.

Assignment 2: Computer Use Guidelines
Directions

1. Identify the ethical/legal issues that you must consider in the situation.

2. Type these in outline format using your word processor.

3. Prepare a separate list of guidelines that you can give to the new users. Your guidelines should help to increase awareness of using the microcomputer in ways that will protect patient privacy/confidentiality and promote the safety and security of the computer data and equipment.

4. Submit your list of safety and security issues and your guidelines.

Situation. You are expecting an influx of personnel who will use the laptops now available in your health care agency. You want to encourage use but protect the misuse of this equipment. A variety of software is available on CD-ROMs as well as on the hard drives of the computers. You expect the personnel will use this equipment to prepare patient summaries, develop quality assurance reports, document supply inventories, and record patient visits.

Assignment 3: Issue Critique
Directions

1. Select one of the following statements to critique:

   a. "There is nothing wrong with breaking security if you accomplish something useful and leave things the way you find them."

   b. "The health care agency owns the data in its computer and is therefore free to do whatever it chooses with that data."

   c. "In the long run, when simple rules are followed, computer records are more secure than hard copy records."

   d. "There is nothing wrong with breaking security if the only records you are looking at are your own."

2. Using your word processor, prepare a one- to two-page paper identifying points that support or refute the statement you selected. End the paper by stating your position and your reasons for that position.

3. Submit your paper.

Assignment 4: Computer Ethics
Directions

1. Your health agency wants to post some rules on using computers ethically. Use the readings from this chapter and any other sources that you wish to create the "Ten Commandments of Computer Ethics."

2. Using your word processor, create an attractive flyer listing your Ten Commandments. Use color and graphics as you wish to make your flyer visually appealing and attractive.

3. Submit your flyer.

Assignment 5: E-Mail Guidelines
Directions

1. Use your word processor to create these guidelines. Be sure that the reading level is appropriate for the students.

2. Submit the guidelines.

Situation. In the school district where your children go to school, the school nurse has reported that both students and teachers are sending her e-mail using both the school intranet and the Internet. You have been asked to help her write a set of guidelines for the teachers and the students.

Health Care Informatics and Information Systems

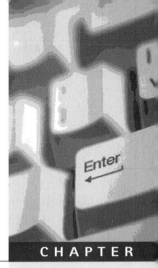

OBJECTIVES

1. Define health care informatics using the concepts of data, information, knowledge, and wisdom.
2. Describe automated health care delivery systems.
3. Discuss types of health care data and how the integration of these data influences the effectiveness of health care information systems.
4. Identify selected types and levels of computer-related personnel.
5. Differentiate between computer literacy, computer-assisted instruction, and health care informatics.

The revised *American Nurses Association's Scope and Standards of Nursing Informatics Practice* (Staggers et al. 2001) identified informatics compe-tencies that are required of all nurses, including beginning nurses, ex-perienced nurses, and informatics nurse specialists. "Informatics competencies for nurses may be organized into computer skills, information literacy skills, and overall informatics competencies" (Staggers et al., 2001, p. 24). In 2001, the

Institute of Medicine stated that "Education for the Health Professions is in need of a major overhaul" (Staggers et al., p. 1). This was followed by an Institute of Medicine summit focused on the reform of health professions education. A report based on the summit, *Health Professions Education: A Bridge to Quality* (Greiner & Knebel, 2003), identified five core competencies that are needed by all health professionals. These core competencies are patient-centered care, interdisciplinary teams, evidence-based practice, quality improvement, and informatics. Both of these publications establish the need for health care professionals to be computer, information, and informatics literate. This book is designed to provide an opportunity to learn the computer and information literacy skills needed by all health care professionals. In addition, it introduces the reader to informatics. This chapter introduces the health care provider to the discipline of health care informatics and to several types of automated systems commonly used in health care.

► 13.1 DEFINING HEALTH CARE INFORMATICS AND RELATED TERMS

Health care informatics is defined as "the study of how health care data, information, knowledge, and wisdom are collected, stored, processed, communicated, and used to support the process of health care delivery to clients, providers, administrators, and organizations involved in health care delivery" (Englebardt & Nelson, 2002, p. xx). It is concerned with the application of information and computer science concepts and theories to the delivery of health care. Health care informatics is an interdisciplinary science developed from the integration of information science, computer science, cognitive science, and the health care sciences.

Information science focuses on the study of information generation, transmission, and use. The study of information as a science is usually considered to have originated with Shannon and Weaver's theory of information (1949). Their work focused on the communication of information. Their communication model demonstrates the transmission of a message from a sender to a receiver and is the standard used in teaching communication concepts to health care providers. Since that time, the study of information theory has been approached from several different conceptual frameworks. The primary information model used to explain health care informatics was established by Blum (1986). Blum, in giving a historical overview of computers in health care, found the model useful in grouping medical applications according to the objects they processed. He identified three groups of applications: data processing, information processing, and knowledge processing.

Using Blum's model, Graves and Corcoran (1989) in their classic article, "The Study of Nursing Informatics," proposed that nursing informatics included nursing data, information, and knowledge. Later that year, Nelson and Joos (1989) proposed the addition of wisdom to this continuum. Understanding the definition of health care informatics requires an understanding of the terms: data, information, knowledge, and wisdom as well as an appreciation of the interrelationships between these concepts. The terms and their interrelationships are demonstrated in Figure 13.1.

Data

Data are raw facts. They exist without meaning or interpretation. Data are the attributes that health care professionals collect, organize, and name. The individual elements on a history and physical or a nursing assessment are data elements. For example, the observation that a patient's hair is red,

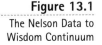

Figure 13.1

The Nelson Data to Wisdom Continuum

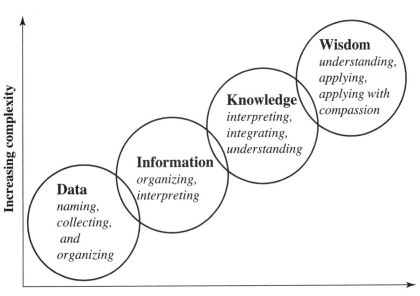

Increasing Interactions and Inter-relationships

that his weight is 150 pounds, or that his blood sugar is 200 are attributes or raw facts that can be interpreted in many different ways. In themselves, each of these data is meaningless. The red hair may be the result of illness, a hair color product, or just the natural color. The weight may be too high, too low, or the ideal weight for this individual. Depending on the circumstances, this blood sugar could be normal, indicate that the patient is improving, or indicate that the patient is becoming sicker. The process of populating the fields in a database, as described in Chapter 8, involves entering these types of data elements into the database.

Information

Information is a collection of data that has been processed to produce meaning. Some techniques that are used to process data include classifying, sorting, organizing, summarizing, graphing, and calculating. A number of tools are used to process data, including paper and pencil, short-term memory, and computers. Many of the exercises in this book demonstrate how computers can be used to present, classify, sort, organize, summarize, graph, and calculate data to produce meaningful information. These processes prepare data so that they can be interpreted. The actual interpretation of the data is a cognitive process whereby data are given meaning and become information. Several factors, including education, attitudes, emotions, and goals, influence how these data are interpreted. As a result, each individual gives a unique interpretation to the same collection of data. These interpretations can be similar, or they can be surprisingly different; however, they are never the same.

For example, a person with newly diagnosed type II diabetes has a blood sugar of 350. The client, the physician, and the nurse each place a different significance on this data element; each provides a different interpretation. In other words, this data element is meaningful, but the meaning is different for each individual involved. For example, a physician may interpret this data element as a need for more insulin. The nurse may interpret it as a need for additional patient education, and the client may assume that this blood sugar is the temporary result of the cake that was eaten the evening before the blood was drawn.

An **information system** is a system that processes data, organizing those data into meaningful units of information. This definition of an **information system** does not require that the system be automated.

However, in health care informatics, the focus is on automated **information systems** that are used in health care. Many different types of automated health care information systems exist. Several are described later in this chapter.

It is important to remember, however, that information from these systems may be interpreted and used differently by different health care providers. For example, a chart that tracks the increased independence of a client after a cerebral vascular accident presents vital nursing information. This same chart when interpreted by the physical therapist provides key rehabilitation information. Although members of both of these disciplines use this same information to make important decisions about the patient's plan of care, the chart has a different significance or meaning for the nurse and for the physical therapist. This is why the development of an effective interdisciplinary documentation system requires the involvement of each of the health care disciplines that will be using the system.

It is also important to realize that the same data can produce different types of information. A hospital information system processes order entry data to produce billing information. These same data may be processed by a clinical information system to develop a clinical pathway. Each of these information systems is using the same data, but in each case, the information produced is quite different.

Knowledge

Although information is built from data, knowledge is built from information. **Knowledge** is a collection of interrelated pieces of information. The interrelationships are as important as the individual items of information. An organized collection of interrelated information about a specific topic is usually referred to as a **knowledge base**. For example, the statement "this student has a good knowledge base in anatomy" would not sound correct if the word "base" was removed from the statement.

The information in a knowledge base is organized or structured so that interrelationships can be identified. The table of contents in any textbook provides an outline of a knowledge base. A well-presented lecture will explain how various facts or pieces of information interrelate. By understanding the information and the interrelationships, the learner can understand the concepts and theories that are inherent in the specific knowledge base being explained.

Once the learner develops a knowledge base, the learner uses this knowledge to interpret new data or even reinterpret old data producing new information. An individual's knowledge base plays a major role in determining how data and information are used in the process of decision making. For example, a diabetic client with an extensive knowledge base about diabetes could be expected to make different decisions than a person with a limited knowledge base.

A professional with an extensive knowledge base is usually referred to as a specialist or expert. In this discussion, a knowledge base is more than just a large collection of information. It is the interrelationships between the pieces of information that produce the knowledge base. An expert has built mental processes that provide quick access to a wide array of interrelationships. As a result, the expert has access to a new level of knowledge. An expert looks at a patient and sees the patient and his or her problems as a whole. The expert has a gestalt view. A novice looks at the same patient and sees only pieces of the information. A novice does not have the quick mental access to all of the interrelationships that the expert has and cannot always see the entire picture of what is happening with a patient. An expert can look at a client and understand immediately just how sick or anxious that client is. A novice on the other hand may see the same patient, collect the same data, and not reach the same conclusion. This is one of the reasons that the teaching learning process in a clinical setting can be such a challenge. The teacher with an expert background will process the same data and information differently than the student. The student will have no idea how the teacher was able to reach a diagnosis, and the teacher may not understand why the student could not see the "obvious."

A knowledge base can be stored and shared using a variety of media, including oral communication, textbooks, and online databases. As a person gains information, it is added to an internal knowledge base. It is this internal knowledge base that one first uses to interpret information and to make decisions. An individual will not go beyond this internal knowledge base unless that person determines that there is an information or knowledge gap. It is very difficult for even the expert to identify what is not known. This is a problem in health care where the amount of new knowledge and information is exploding. As a result, there is a keen interest in automated decision support systems that could identify information gaps and tap external knowledge bases.

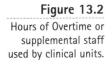

Figure 13.2

Hours of Overtime or supplemental staff used by clinical units.

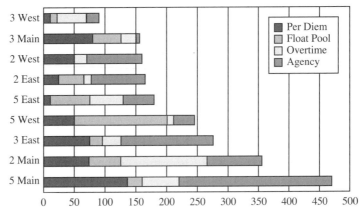

Automated decision support systems are systems that process information, identifying and demonstrating pertinent interrelationships. These systems may be as simple as the bar chart in Figure 13.2, which identifies overtime hours in a health care institution, or as complex as a fully automated staffing system. Complexity in this example refers to how much of the knowledge base is stored in the automated system and to the automated rules used to process the data. With a decision support system, the individual's knowledge base interprets the bar chart. Different nurse managers looking at this same bar chart can and do reach different conclusions about staffing on these units.

Although decision support systems can help in the decision-making process, they do not make decisions. For example, an automated scheduling system can be used to generate a work schedule for staff in a clinical setting. The automated system can contain an extensive online knowledge base. The system will "know" several facts about the staff as well as the institution's staffing rules. However, the scheduling system will not decide who will work when. The professional in charge is responsible for approving the schedule. Decision support systems are an aid to the decision maker. They provide the decision maker with a more complete picture of the interrelations between the information being considered. It is the decision maker who interprets the information and decides what action to take. This is the key difference between a decision support system and an expert system.

Wisdom

In health care, ethical decision making that ensures cost-effective quality care requires more than an empirical knowledge base. Knowing when and how to use this knowledge is referred to as wisdom. Knowledge makes it possible for a caregiver to explain the stages of death and dying. Wisdom makes it possible for the caregiver to use theories related to death and dying to help a terminal patient express anger and frustration. The development of wisdom requires not only empirical knowledge but also ethical, personal, and aesthetic knowledge. Currently, there is no way to automate wisdom but certain aspects of this concept are being built into automated systems. **Expert systems** are knowledge-based systems with built-in procedures for determining when and how to use that knowledge. In the future, the development of decision support systems for experts will require a better understanding of the concept of wisdom and how wisdom influences the decision-making process of expert practitioners.

▶ 13.2 AUTOMATED INFORMATION SYSTEMS IN HEALTH CARE

Computer technology has been infused into almost every aspect of health care delivery. This ranges from a stand-alone system used to make appointments in a private office to fully integrated computer-based patient records maintained by a large integrated health delivery system. This discussion of these systems is divided into three sections. First is an overview of the types of automated applications used in health care. This is followed by a discussion of the types of data that are processed in automated health care information systems—including a discussion of levels of integration. Finally, the systems are discussed in terms of nursing roles.

Automated Applications Used in Health Care Delivery

Automation in health care began in the late 1960s and early 1970s with systems designed to meet specific needs within health care. In most institutions financial applications developed first. These included, for example, payroll, billing, and general ledger. This was followed by the development of institution-wide applications to manage admission, discharge, and transfer (ADT) as well as applications to support the various clinical departments such as laboratory, radiology, or pharmacy. These departmental systems were usually stand-alone systems and were referred to as islands of information. The first attempts at communication between these applications were the development of order entry/results reporting systems. These systems, built on the ADT system, were located on the clinical units and communicated with the departmental systems. A unit clerk or nurse selected a patient from the ADT system and entered new orders. These orders were then communicated to the appropriate department. Once the orders were completed, the results were communicated back to the clinical units.

This section provides a review of the common types of applications used in health care. However, it is becoming increasingly difficult to classify the diverse applications into specific categories. As vendors have increased the scope of functions offered by their products, they increasingly overlap. In addition, several information systems companies have been purchased or merged. As a result, their products have been integrated or merged.

Clinical

Clinical information systems include a large group of automated systems that process patient data to support patient care. Examples of functions in clinical information systems include collecting patient assessment and health status data, developing care plans, managing the order entry process, keeping medication administration records, developing work lists, and producing reports such as patient problem lists. Two types that are of special importance are point-of-care documentation systems and departmental systems.

- *Documentation systems* are increasingly used as interdisciplinary tools. The primary uses for documentation systems include the development of plans of care, documentation of patient data, and access to clinical information. These systems can be interfaced to automated monitoring devices, thereby capturing vital signs and other data directly into the clinical record. Their primary benefits include decreasing the time used to document care while increasing the quality of the documentation and increasing access to client data.

- *Departmental systems* are systems that support the daily work or operations of a clinical department. The most common automated clinical departments include laboratory, radiology, cardiology, and pharmacy. Clinical departmental systems accept patient orders; schedule patients, equipment, and rooms; print labels and work lists; and maintain inventories. The primary benefit of these types of systems is the improved efficiency of the department.

Healthcare information systems

Healthcare information systems (HISs) were originally developed for hospitals. Today, however, they may be located in nursing homes, rehabilitation centers, or any other health care institution. There are four primary functions for health care information systems. First, they are often the backbone or primary system used to integrate or interface with the various applications throughout the organization. Second, they manage the ADT process. Third, they communicate information between the clinical units and the various hospital departments. This can include sending patient orders to hospital departments and reporting results back to the clinical units, as well as requesting supplies and equipment for the clinical units. These systems almost always interface with the financial systems that are used to track the charges and billing process for the institution. As part of the communication function, they may also support the institution's intranet. Finally, they are used to produce a number of reports that support the daily operations of the institution. For example, the HISs may be used to print a list of patients' diet orders. This list can then be used to distribute meal trays.

Financial systems

Financial systems include a combination of information systems that are used to manage and report the financial aspects of the institution. These include systems that track income such as billing and contract monitoring, systems used to develop and monitor capital and operating budgets, and systems that track costs to the institution such as payroll and cost accounting. These systems usually interface with the ADT and personnel systems. For example, the payroll system can interface with the time and attendance or scheduling system to track who has worked and the time that they worked.

Personnel systems

Personnel systems include a combination of systems that are used to track the characteristics of employees and/or the use of these employees within the institution.

- *Human resource management or personnel records systems* maintain individual employee records. For example, health care institutions must know the home address, salary scale, job title and description, professional license number and renewal date, along with a number of other details about each employee. Automated systems make it much easier to maintain accurate data and to search for information about individual employees as well as groups of employees.

- *Scheduling systems* are used to schedule the actual dates and times that an employee will be working or not working. These systems can keep a historical record of vacation, holiday, and sick time used.

Administrative systems

These systems automate the management of data used in the daily operations of the institution as well as data used for strategic and long range planning.

- *Classification systems* use patient data to classify patients by the amount and type of care required. For example, a patient with new second- and third-degree burns over 60% of the body may require 6 hours of professional nursing time every 8-hour shift. A second patient who is fifth-day postoperative from open-heart surgery may require 2 hours of professional nursing time. The data from classification systems can be used to decide the amount and type of staff assigned to a clinical unit. When classification data are used to make this determination, the classification system is also a staffing system.

- *Quality assurance systems* attempt to measure and report on cost-effective quality care resulting in a high level of patient satisfaction. Some examples of data that are processed in quality assurance systems include patient outcomes or variance reports, performance indicators for providers, infection reports, incident reports, patient satisfaction results, and costing data. These data can be reported for individuals or in aggregate format.

- *Material management systems* are used to manage the supplies and other inventory of an institution. These can include an online catalog that can be searched, an automatic interface to budget systems, automatic reordering of supplies, and alerts that can be issued when there is a significant increase or decrease in inventory orders.

Electronic health record

Electronic health record (EHR) systems grew out of the concept of a computer-based patient record. The EHR is a complete collection of an individual's health-related data. The data are collected and managed by an EHR system much as a database management system manages a database. Data from an individual's EHR can be stored in a clinical data repository. This can be conceptualized as a warehouse or large database when all data elements from all the different systems could be stored. This makes it possible to integrate the data and to obtain a different level of information. For example, by integrating the clinical data with the financial data, it would be possible to begin evaluating the cost of each problem on the patient problem list. For these systems to be truly effective, a data dictionary that defines each element is required. Although the development of the EHR has been evolving for several years, the development of these systems was stimulated in 2003 when the United States Department of Health and Human Services Secretary Tommy G. Thompson announced a government initiative to build a national electronic health care system that would allow patients and their doctors to access their complete medical records anytime and anywhere they are needed (US Department of Health and Human Services, 2003).

After this announcement, Level Seven (HL7), one of the world's leading healthcare standards developers, joined with both public and private organizations to develop an EHR Functional Model. Included in this effort are the Department of Health and Human Services, the Department of Veterans Affairs, the Health Information Management Systems Society, The Robert Wood Johnson Foundation, and the Institute of Medicine (HL7, 2004).

Setting specific systems

These systems include any of the functions already discussed; however, the functions are customized for the specific setting. This includes all functions related to clinical, financial, and personnel information management. Some examples of setting specific systems include home health systems, physician office systems, outpatient or ambulatory care clinics, nurse center clinics, and emergency room systems.

Types of Automated Data Used in Health Care Information Systems

To understand fully the impact of automated systems on health care, it is imperative that one considers the types of data that are processed. For the purposes of discussion, these data are classified into five major types. Four of these have previously been identified (Nelson, 2004). However, it is important to realize that any one datum by itself is without meaning and can in fact be used in any one of these five classifications but in a slightly different way.

Clinical or client data

These data include all data that are related to an individual client. A complete collection of the client data is stored in the EHR. An example of this type of data would be a patient's blood pressure or a list of the patient's problems.

Financial data

These types of data include all of the fiscal data related to the operation of the health care institution. Examples include the patient's bill or the budget for an individual unit.

Human resource data

These types of data include all data related to employees as well as individuals who have a contractual relationship with the institution such as physicians, nurses, students, or volunteers.

Material resources

These data refer to all of the tangible resources used in the operation of the health care institution. This includes everything from supplies that are purchased externally to supplies that are created internally.

Intellectual data

These data are all of the factual data that are stored in the various discipline or subject specific databases. Examples include a database with information about medications or a database with published articles and research results.

Levels of Data Sharing

The various types of data described previously are processed using health care applications. The effectiveness of these applications in supporting quality, cost-effective health care is influenced by the level of data sharing made possible by the overall logic and physical design of the total health care information system.

Stand-alone systems are systems that do not share data or information with any other computer system. A personal computer–based scheduling system located in one department would be a stand-alone system. If the schedule for an employee is changed on this system, that change will not occur in any other institutional system. The personnel and payroll systems would still show the original schedule. Stand-alone systems result in data redundancy in the system and database discrepancies.

Interfaced systems are systems that maintain their own database while sharing data across a network. For example, a laboratory system may be interfaced with a HIS. The patient orders from the HIS are passed directly to the laboratory system, and the laboratory results are passed directly back to the HIS. When several department systems are interfaced, the results have been referred to as spaghetti. Because most of these interfaced systems are from the different vendors and computer systems are constantly being updated, maintaining the interface code becomes a constant battle. Patient data can get lost in this complexity.

Integrated systems are systems that share a common database. The clinical data repository or warehouse system discussed earlier is such a system. All of the data related to a client, employee, or financial system are stored in one repository. Although this is a simple concept, the process of building a repository is very complex. Most health care institutions operate with a combination of stand-alone, interfaced, and integrated systems. Data are shared at four different levels.

Level 1 data sharing involves integration of a specific institution service or function. For example, an executive information system will pull census, personnel, and financial data to give an overall picture of the institution's operational status. A product line system will integrate patient data from several different systems to track how patients in that product line move through the organization.

Level 2 involves sharing data for an individual health care institution. Sometimes this refers to all patient data. Other times it refers to all institutional data including financial, personnel, and tangible resources.

Level 3 involves the sharing of data across all institutions owned by the organization. This type of system is referred to as an enterprise-wide system. This level of sharing has become increasingly important with the development of integrated health care delivery systems. One of the best examples of this level of integration in the Veterans Health Administration where there are plans for an individual patient's data to be accessible from any one of the 128 hospitals in the system. The integrated system of software applications that supports patient care at Veterans Health Administration healthcare facilities is called VistA. The keystone of this "system will be the Health Data Repository (HDR). The HDR will be a national databank for standardized, patient-specific clinical data. When the HDR begins operations in 2005, clinical data that are now dispersed over 128 individual VistA sites will be aggregated in a central repository." (VistA, 2004)

Level 4 involves sharing data outside of the institutions owned by the enterprise. This is a regional or community health information network. With this level of integration, a patient's record could be accessed from any health care institution. For example, if a person living in Pennsylvania was in a car accident in Florida, his or her health care record could be accessed from the emergency room in Florida.

In its early stages, health care computing was built on stand-alone systems. Today, the systems are becoming increasingly integrated. This sharing of data across disciplines within health care is one of the factors increasing the integration of services. As this trend continues, health care information systems are becoming more generic. For example, these systems are becoming patient-focused systems rather than medical or nursing systems. Although this trend is improving the comprehensiveness of the data, one approach to managing patient data will not meet the information needs for all disciplines. How to develop an integrated, patient-focused health care information system that meets the information needs of different disciplines is an important applied research question in health care computing.

Nursing Information Systems

The term nursing information system refers to a wide range of automated systems used by nurses in a variety of roles. The profession of nursing is traditionally discussed in terms of four domains of practice: clinical practice, administration, education, and research. Nursing information systems can also be discussed using these domains.

Clinical nursing information systems provide automated support to the nursing process. These systems are used to collect and record patient data for assessment or monitoring purposes, to develop plans of care, to print reminders and work lists, to document care, and to identify goal achievement. With the advent of health care reform and the development of clinical pathways, these systems are rapidly becoming multidisciplinary clinical information systems, as previously described under documentation systems.

Administrative nursing information systems support the administrative role and usually deal with the day-to-day operation of the clinical or nursing service department. These include systems such as classification systems, quality assurance systems, and staffing systems. With improved levels of data sharing, administrative systems are beginning to import their data from the clinical information systems. For example, a nurse documents a patient's postoperative status, and these data are used by the classification system to identify the amount of nursing care needed for this patient's care. Information from these types of administrative systems can be data for an executive information system (EIS). An executive information system is designed to assist senior managers by summarizing, integrating, and analyzing current information so that they can quickly and effectively monitor operations and trends across the organization. Executive information systems are then used to manage the institution and to serve as a basis for strategic and/or long-range planning.

Nursing educational information systems support nursing education and are used in teaching as well as in managing the educational process. Nursing education information systems were initially used in formal educational programs. Today, they are an integral part of staff development and are becoming common in patient education. The National League for Nursing has identified the importance of these systems with the establishment of the Educational Technology and Information Management Advisory Council (ETIMAC). The purpose of the Educational Technology and Information Management Advisory Council (ETIMAC) is "to promote the effective use of technology in nursing education, both as a teaching tool and an outcome for student and faculty learning, and to advance the integration of information management into educational practices and program outcomes" (National League for Nursing, 2004). The focus of these systems includes using technology in a traditional classroom as well as the use of technology to deliver distance education programs.

Nursing research information systems include a variety of different generic computing programs. Every software program in this book can be used in the research process. The development of automated health care information systems has had a major impact on what is possible within the field of nursing research. It is now possible to collect data from an automated database in seconds, whereas it would have required months of searching if the same data were stored in paper records. It is also important to note that although software programs can be helpful tools when doing nursing research, the use of such tools does not mean that one is doing informatics research. Health care informatics is a field of study in and of itself with a number of important research questions.

► 13.3 HEALTH CARE COMPUTING PERSONNEL

There are several levels and types of personnel who work in health care computing. Some personnel have their primary background in computer and information science, whereas others have their primary background in health care. A few are prepared in health care informatics. The educational preparation of people in health care computing varies from on-the-job training to postdoctoral preparation.

The Chief Information Officer or Director of Information Services

The chief information officer is administratively responsible for the operation of the information service department. Depending on the organization, this individual may be part of the executive team responsible for strategic and long-range institutional planning as well as the day-to-day operation of the department.

Systems Analysts

Systems analysts are personnel who work with users to define their information needs and design systems to meet those needs. Their education is usually in information or computer science with knowledge of health care acquired from on-the-job experience.

Programmers

Programmers are personnel who design, code, and test new software programs as well as maintain and enhance current applications. These individuals usually receive their educational preparation in computer science or as on-the-job training.

Systems or Network Administrators

Systems administrators are responsible for planning and maintaining multi-user computer systems maintained on a local area network. These individuals may have an associate or baccalaureate degree in computer or information science. They are often certified in the use of the software application used to manage the network.

Microcomputer Specialist

Microcomputer specialists are personnel who support personal computer users throughout the institution. They may install new software, troubleshoot or repair personal computers, answer user questions, and train users on new software.

Computer Operators

There are several types of computer operators. The title computer operator usually refers to an individual who actually runs a mainframe or minicomputer. These individuals usually have minimal interaction with health care providers. Microcomputer operators on the other hand work closely with users. They troubleshoot, upgrade, and repair computers as well as install software. Network managers provide this same type of service for local area networks.

Nursing Informatics Specialists

Nursing informatics specialists integrate "nursing science, computer science, and information science in managing and communicating data and information and knowledge in nursing practice" (Staggers et al., 2001, p. 32). These individuals have a degree in nursing and have become experts in the use of computers in health care.

SUMMARY

Literacy is the ability to read, write, and use numbers skillfully enough to meet the demands of society. Computer literacy is the ability to use a computer skillfully enough to meet the demands of society. Like literacy, the scope and depth of computer literacy needed by any one person can vary extensively. One person can be very literate with word processing, but unable to use any other program. Another person may have a general knowledge of several different programs. In today's automated world, all people need to have at least a basic understanding of computers. Health care professionals, like all other educated people, need a basic level of computer literacy.

Information literacy refers to the ability to access, evaluate, and use information. With the advent of computers, information literacy requires the ability to access databases, especially literature databases and the largest database of all—the Internet. Once information has been accessed, it requires the ability to evaluate the information. Inaccurate and incomplete information must be recognized. This is especially difficult if the reader has a limited knowledge base related to the information being accessed. Finally, information literacy requires the ability to use the information.

Health care informatics is specific to health care. Health care informatics uses tools from information science, computer science, cognitive science, and the health care sciences to help manage health care institutions and deliver quality health care.

References

Blum, B. I. (1986). *Clinical information systems.* New York: Springer-Verlag.

Englebardt, E., & Nelson, R. (2002). *Health care informatics: An interdisciplinary approach.* St. Louis: Mosby.

Graves, J., & Corcoran, S. (1989). The study of nursing informatics. *Image: Journal of Nursing Scholarship, 21*(4), 227–231.

Greiner, A., & Knebel, E. (Eds.). (2003). Institute of Medicine: Committee on the Health Professions Education Summit. *Health professions education: A bridge to quality.* Washington, DC: The National Academies Press. Available from http://www.nap.edu.

HL7. (2004). *EHR press releases.* Available from http://www.hl7.org/ehr//documents/press.asp#hhs

National League for Nursing. (2004). *Educational Technology and Information Management Advisory Council (ETIMAC).* Available from http://www.nln.org/aboutnln/AdvisoryCouncils_TaskGroups/etimac.htm

Nelson, R. (2004). Incorporating new technology: Nursing informatics. In L. Caputi & L. Engelmann (Eds.). *Teaching nursing: The art and the science* (pp. 555–588). Glen Ellyn, IL: College of Dupage Press.

Nelson, R., & Joos, I. (1989, Fall). On language in nursing: From data to wisdom. *PLN Visions,* 6.

Shannon, C. E., & Weaver, W. (1949). *The mathematical theory of communication.* Urbana, IL: University of Illinois Press.

Staggers, N., Gassert, C. Kwai, J. L., Milholland, K., Nelson, R., Senemeier, J., Stuck, D., & Welton, J. (2001). *Scope and standards of nursing informatics practice.* Washington, DC: American Nurses Publishing.

US Department of Health and Human Services. (2003). *News release: HHS launches new efforts to promote paperless health care system.* Available from http://www.hhs.gov/news/press/2003pres/20030701.html

Veterans Health Information Systems and Technology Architecture (VistA). (2004). Available from http://www.virec.research.med.va.gov/datasources-name/vista/vista.htm#history

Exercise 1: Literacy, Computer-Assisted Instruction, and Health Care Informatics

Objectives

1. Differentiate between computer literacy, information literacy, computer-assisted instruction, and health care informatics.

2. Identify available software programs, both generic and those related to health care.

3. Describe uses of each software group.

Activity

1. Make a list of all software programs that are available to you as a student in your current curriculum. Include the programs and databases in your library for accessing reference materials. This is the master list for this exercise.

2. Identify the programs on this list that are not specific to health care. For example, a word-processing program can be used in any field, not just health care. Classify the identified programs by their primary purpose. For example, Microsoft Word would be classified as a word-processing program. Write a brief statement explaining how each group of software would be useful for a health care student or employee.

3. Make a list of the databases in your library and briefly explain what literature is referenced in these databases. Give a brief description of the background or knowledge base the reader should have to evaluate the quality of information included in the references in each database.

4. Identify applications or computer programs that are used to teach health-related content. Select five of these programs, and describe the level of computer literacy necessary to use each program.

5. Identify one program that can be used to explain the concepts inherent in health care informatics. Explain how you would use this program to explain health care informatics concepts.

Exercise 2: Data, Information, Knowledge, and Wisdom
Objective

1. Develop a personal definition of health care data, information, knowledge, and wisdom.

Activity

Work in small groups (three to five people) to develop an answer for each of the following questions.

1. When patients complete a health assessment form, have they provided you with data or information? Explain your answer.

2. Does knowing a patient's diagnosis provide you with information or knowledge? Does your answer differ if you are referring to a medical or a nursing diagnosis?

3. What is your definition of health care knowledge? How does medical knowledge differ from nursing knowledge? How are they the same?

4. Can wisdom be taught? Explain your answer.

Assignment 1: Health Care Informatics: Job Descriptions

Directions

1. The health care setting where you are employed has decided to purchase and implement an EHR. Because computer and health care informatics content was included in your basic education program, you have been added to the implementation team with the title Informatics Specialist. Your first assignment is to write your job description. You have been referred to the following references.

   Staggers, N., Gassert, C., Kwai, J. L., Milholland, K., Nelson, R., Senemeier, J., Stuck, D., & Welton, J. (2001) *Scope and standards of nursing informatics practice.* Washington, DC: American Nurses Publishing.

   http://www.amia.org/working/ni/roles/roles.html

2. Type the job description using a word-processing program. Include a brief description of the job, a list of required and preferred qualifications, and a list of the job responsibilities.

Assignment 2: Health Care Informatics Education

Directions

1. Both the American Nurses Association and the Institute of Medicine discussed the need for health care professionals to be computer, information, and informatics literate. Develop an outline identifying the basic concepts that should be included in your education to become computer, information, and informatics literate.

2. Review your educational program, and identify what content from your outline is or is not included in your program.

3. When content is not included, identify where it should be added to your program.

4. Based on your analysis write a two-page position paper on health care informatics as part of health care education. Use your word-processing program to prepare your paper.

Assignment 3: Health Care Informatics

Directions

The table presented here includes several types of automated systems commonly used in health care today. Using references from your library and the Internet, identify common functions that would be associated with each type of system. The first one has been completed as an example of the level of detail needed with this assignment.

Type of System	Primary Functions
Laboratory	1. Data management for administrative functions. For example, create work lists of what laboratory work needs to be done, identify when and on whom the laboratory work must be done, an inventory of supplies used, and turnaround time. 2. Generate labels for automated or manual identification and tracking of a specimen from order generation to specimen collection to completion of a laboratory test. 3. Provide results reporting, either on paper or by computer. 4. Issue alerts on abnormal results, repeat orders, and so forth.
Home Health Care	
Medical Records	
Nursing	
Patient Classification	
Patient Monitoring	
Pharmacy	
Radiology	
Staff Scheduling	
Facilities Management	
Financial	
Human Resource Management	
Materials Management	
Managed Care System	
Quality Improvement	
Other	

Index

Page numbers followed by *f* denote figures; those followed by *t* denote tables